VMS

VISUAL MNEMONICS FOR PHYSIOLOGY AND RELATED ANATOMY

VMS

VISUAL MNEMONICS FOR PHYSIOLOGY AND RELATED ANATOMY

LAURIE L. MARBAS
Texas Tech University Health Sciences Center
Class of 2003
School of Medicine
Lubbock, Texas

ERIN CASE
Texas Tech University Health Sciences Center
Class of 2003
School of Medicine
Lubbock, Texas

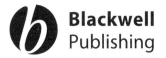
Blackwell Publishing

Blackwell Publishing, Inc.
350 Main Street, Malden, Massachusetts 02148-5018, USA
Blackwell Publishing Ltd
9600 Garsington Road, Oxford OX4 2DQ, UK
Blackwell Science Asia Pty Ltd
550 Swanston Street, Carlton South, Victoria 3053, Australia
Blackwell Verlag GmbH
Kurfürstendamm 57, 10707 Berlin, Germany

03 04 05 06 5 4 3 2 1
ISBN: 1-4051-0327-2

Library of Congress Cataloging-in-Publication Data

Marbas, Laurie L.
Visual mnemonics for physiology and related anatomy / Laurie L. Marbas, Erin Case.
p. ; cm. — (Visual mnemonics series)
Includes index.
ISBN 1-40510-327-2 (pbk.)
1. Human physiology—Study and teaching. 2. Human anatomy—Study and teaching. 3. Mnemonics.
[DNLM: 1. Physiology—Terminology—English. 2. Anatomy—Terminology—English. 3. Association Learning. QT 15 M312v 2003] I. Case, Erin. II. Title. III. Series.
QP39 .M374 2003
612'.0071—dc21 2002015313

A catalogue record for this title is available from the British Library

Acquisitions: Beverly Copland
Development: Julia Casson
Production: Jennifer Kowalewski
Cover design: Meral Dabcovich, Visual Perspectives
Interior design: Shawn Girsberger
Illustration remastering by Frank Habit
Typesetter: International Typesetting and Composition, in India
Printed and bound by Sheridan Books, in Michigan

For further information on Blackwell Publishing, visit our website: www.medirect.com

Notice: The indications and dosages of all drugs in this book have been recommended in the medical literature and conform to the practices of the general community. The medications described do not necessarily have specific approval by the Food and Drug Administration for use in the diseases and dosages for which they are recommended. The package insert for each drug should be consulted for use and dosage as approved by the FDA. Because standards for usage change, it is advisable to keep abreast of revised recommendations, particularly those concerning new drugs.

CONTENTS

PREFACE

Visual Mnemonics is a study tool that aids in quickly learning and memorizing material presented in anatomy and physiology. Two significant features of *Visual Mnemonics* are the long-term retention of material and the increased rate of learning. This allows the student more time to study the fraction of material not covered in the *Visual Mnemonics* book.

These illustrations were created to assist in my own studying, because I was always short on time to efficiently memorize facts, and then I was frustrated because I couldn't remember them longer than an hour after the test. As a mom of three small children, my time for studying is limited and must be high yield 100% of the time. These illustrations allowed me, and many classmates, to do that. Several classmates stated to me that their grades improved 10 points from one exam to the next. Also, we all agree that the long-term retention is incredible compared to traditional study methods of memorizing from lists or notecards.

I have attempted to combine as many pertinent facts and functions into the illustrations as possible. This book is not meant to be an end all to your studying but it certainly can provide an efficient and more stimulating method of studying the material that is contained in the illustrations.

Some tips on using the pictures: look at them after you have read your class notes or gone to class, etc. Then you will know what material is not covered in this book and what material is deemed important in your particular curriculum. Also, write on them, color them, redraw them, add your own drawings to them—the more the illustrations are manipulated, the more information will be retained in long-term memory. Some students rewrite notes to study, etc.—write this information in the book. It will be concise and everything will be in one place for you.

—Laurie Marbas

ACKNOWLEDGMENTS

Throughout my medical education I have been blessed with many opportunities which I thank the Lord for everyday. A special thank you must go to my grandmother, Maxine Turner, for helping me care for my three children while I attended school. Without her none of this would have been possible. My husband, Patrick Marbas, is also deserving of a tremendous debt of gratitude for making many sacrifices for me, including driving 100 miles one-way to work everyday for two years, so that I could attend medical school. In addition, much love to my three beautiful children, Emily, Jonathan, and Gabriel, for playing quietly while I study and giving me hugs of encouragement when I needed it the most.

Also, thank you to Dr. Dalley for helping me with this project and allowing us to use some of his mnemonics. I would also like to say thank you to my mother, Patricia Lockridge, for her creative support and encouragement.

Finally, I would like to thank Erin Case for her supportive friendship during this project.

—Laurie Marbas

A special thank you must go to Laurie for her support, encouragement, and great friendship. I truly thank her for this wonderful opportunity in allowing me to contribute to this series of books. I would also love to thank my husband, Jay, for all the late-night typing. A great thanks goes to my mom, Christine, and Jay for their help with my daughter, Violet. I would also like to thank Dr. Dalley, Dr. Pelley, all the great folks at Blackwell Publishing, and Nehal Shah.

—Erin Case

FACULTY ADVISOR

Bernell K. Dalley, Ph.D.
Assistant Dean for Admissions and Student Affairs
Texas Tech University Health Sciences Center
School of Medicine
Lubbock, Texas

REVIEWERS

Simon Adanin
Class of 2004
Chicago College of Osteopathic Medicine
Chicago, Illinois

Jonathan Hero Chung
Class of 2004
Washington University School of Medicine
St. Louis, Washington

Umesh Dave
Class of 2004
Nova Southeastern University College of Osteopathic Medicine
Ft. Lauderdale, Florida

Alicia-Maria Fernandez
Class of 2003
Chicago College of Osteopathic Medicine
Chicago, Illinois

Clair Palley
Class of 2004
University of Kentucky School of Medicine
Lexington, Kentucky

Sean I. Perkins
Class of 2002
University of Kansas School of Medicine
Wichita, Kansas

NOTES

DALLEY'S RULES OF EXCEPTIONS*

- All muscles with "Palato" in the name are innervated by CN X (with fibers that began with CN XI) except tensor veli palatini, which is V3, a branch of CN V.
- All muscles of pharynx (with pharyngo(eous) in their name) are innervated by CN X (with fibers that began with CN XI) except stylopharyngeus, which is innervated by CN IX.
- All muscles of tongue (with glossus(o) in name) are innervated by CN XII except palatoglossus, which is innervated by CN X.

All intrinsic muscles of larynx are innervated by recurrent laryngeal except cricothyroid, which is innervated by the external laryngeal nerve.

*Reprinted with permission from Dr. Bernell Dalley, Texas Tech University Health Sciences Center School of Medicine, Lubbock, TX.

See Tables 1.1 and 1.2 in Appendix.

Bones

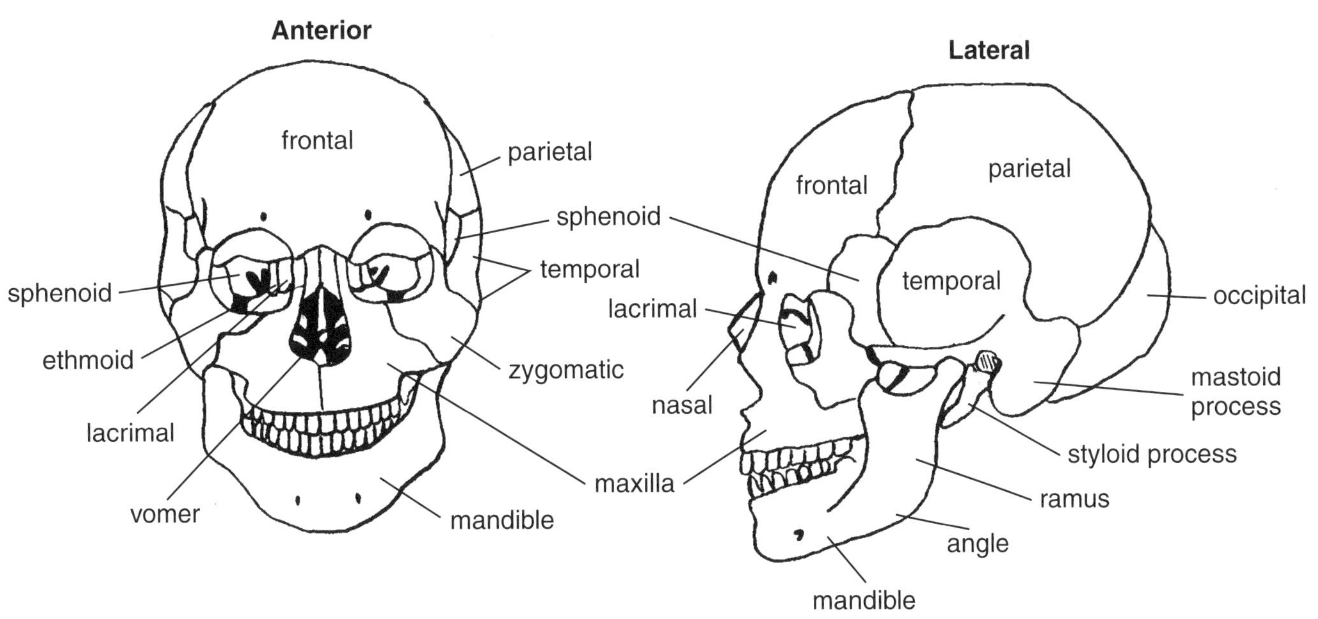
Anterior
frontal
parietal
sphenoid
temporal
sphenoid
ethmoid
zygomatic
lacrimal
vomer
maxilla
mandible
Lateral
frontal
parietal
sphenoid
temporal
occipital
lacrimal
nasal
mastoid
process
styloid process
maxilla
ramus
angle
mandible

Arteries

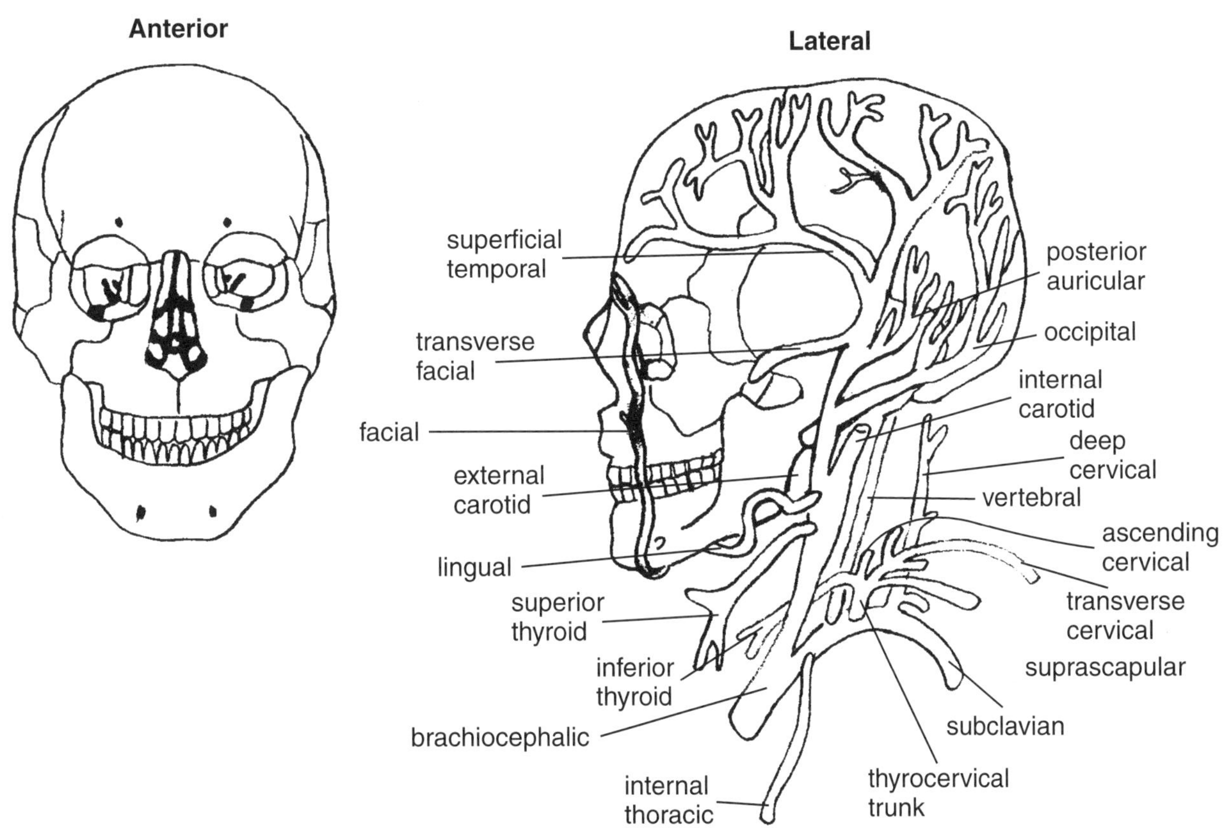
Anterior
Lateral
superficial
temporal
posterior
auricular
transverse
facial
occipital
internal
carotid
facial
deep
cervical
external
carotid
vertebral
ascending
cervical
lingual
transverse
cervical
superior
thyroid
suprascapular
inferior
thyroid
brachiocephalic
subclavian
internal
thoracic
thyrocervical
trunk

NOTES

See Tables 1.1 and 1.2 in Appendix.

Nerves

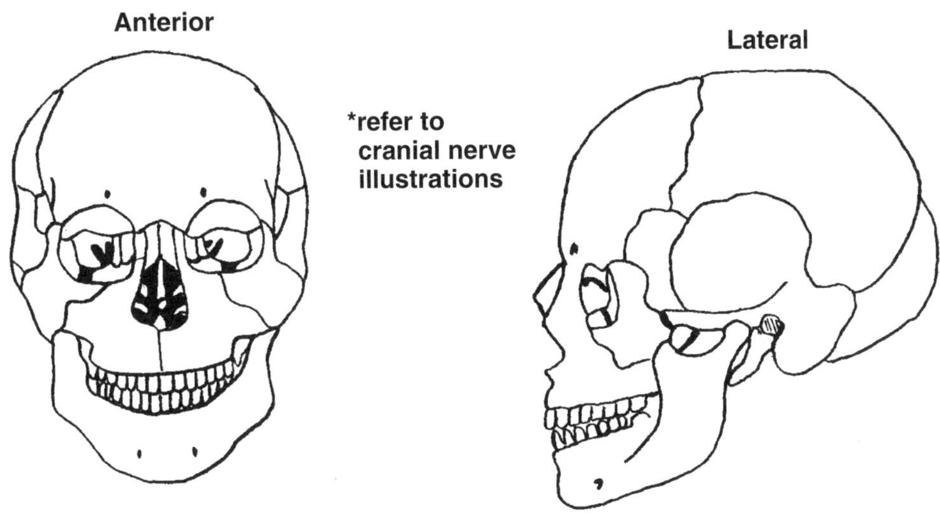

Muscles

Anterior

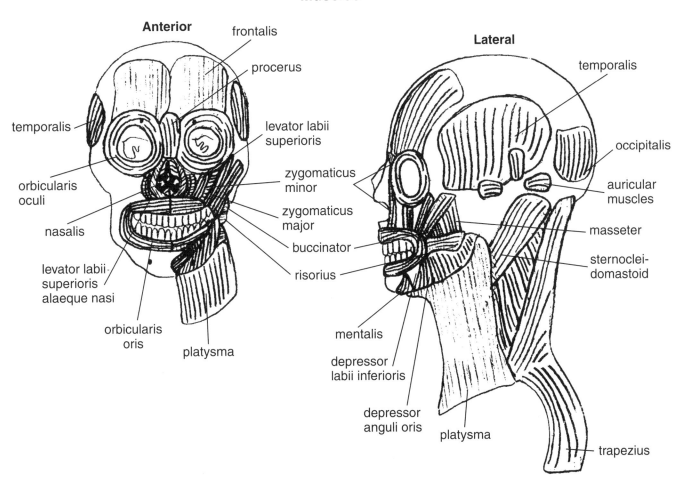

frontalis
procerus
temporalis
levator labii superioris
orbicularis oculi
zygomaticus minor
nasalis
zygomaticus major
buccinator
levator labii superioris alaeque nasi
risorius
orbicularis oris
platysma

Lateral

temporalis
occipitalis
auricular muscles
masseter
sternocleidomastoid
mentalis
depressor labii inferioris
depressor anguli oris
platysma
trapezius

NOTES

See Tables 1.1 and 1.2 in Appendix.

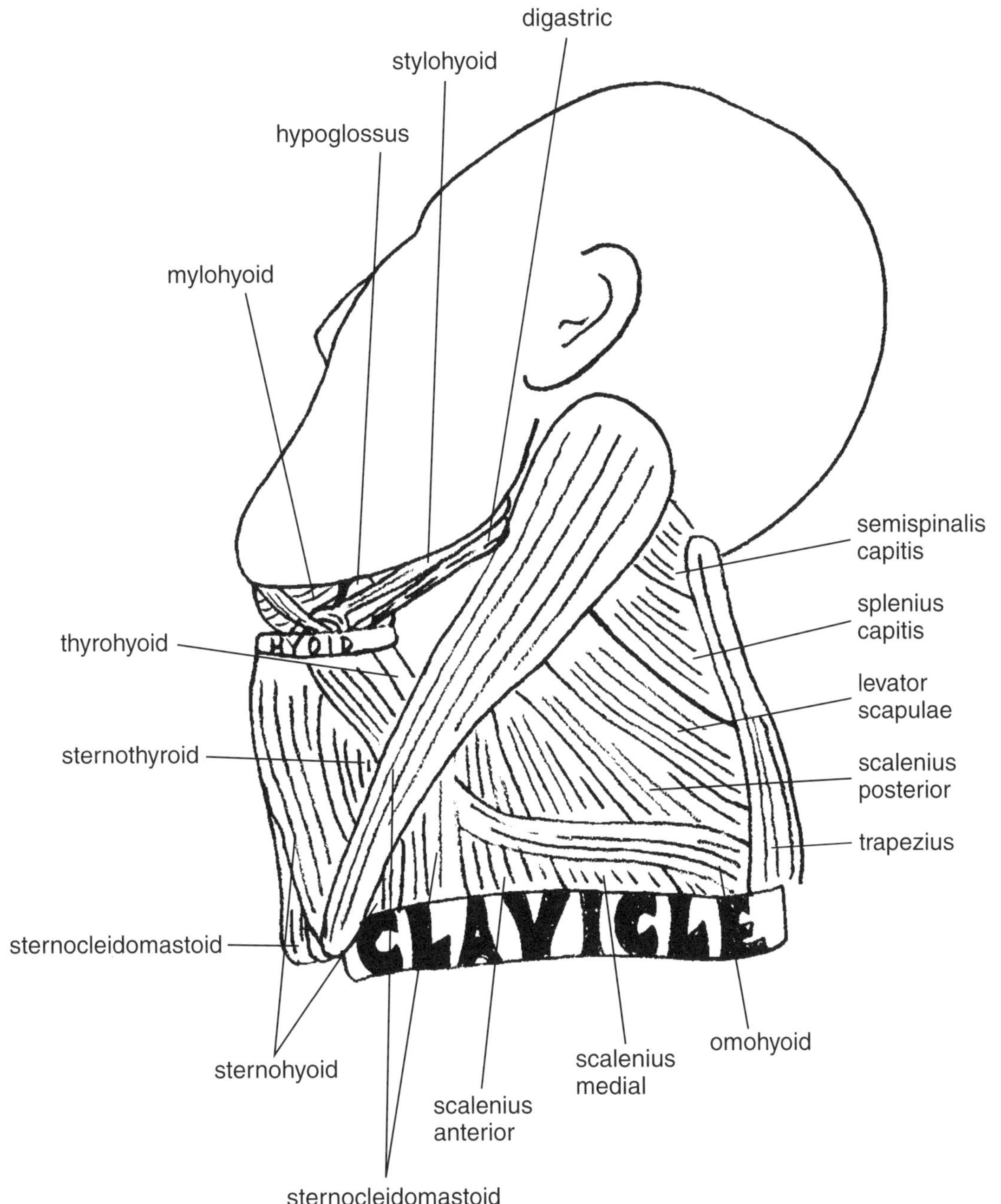
digastric
stylohyoid
hypoglossus
mylohyoid
HYOID
thyrohyoid
sternothyroid
sternocleidomastoid
semispinalis capitis
splenius capitis
levator scapulae
scalenius posterior
trapezius
CLAVICLE
sternohyoid
scalenius anterior
scalenius medial
omohyoid
sternocleidomastoid

NOTES

CLINICAL CORRELATIONS CN I

- Anosmia—loss of sense of smell
  - occurs with aging due to progressive reduction of olfactory cells
  - usually unilateral
  - may be a clue to fracture in cribriform plate with clinical symptom of CSF rhinorrhea
- Olfactory hallucinations and "uncinate fits"
  - olfactory hallucinations—false perceptions of smell that may be caused by temporal lobe lesions
  - an irritating lesion that affects the lateral olfactory area (deep to uncus); may induce temporal lobe epilepsy (uncinate fits), which result in imaginary unfavorable odors and involuntary lip and tongue movements

See Tables 1.1 and 1.2 in Appendix.

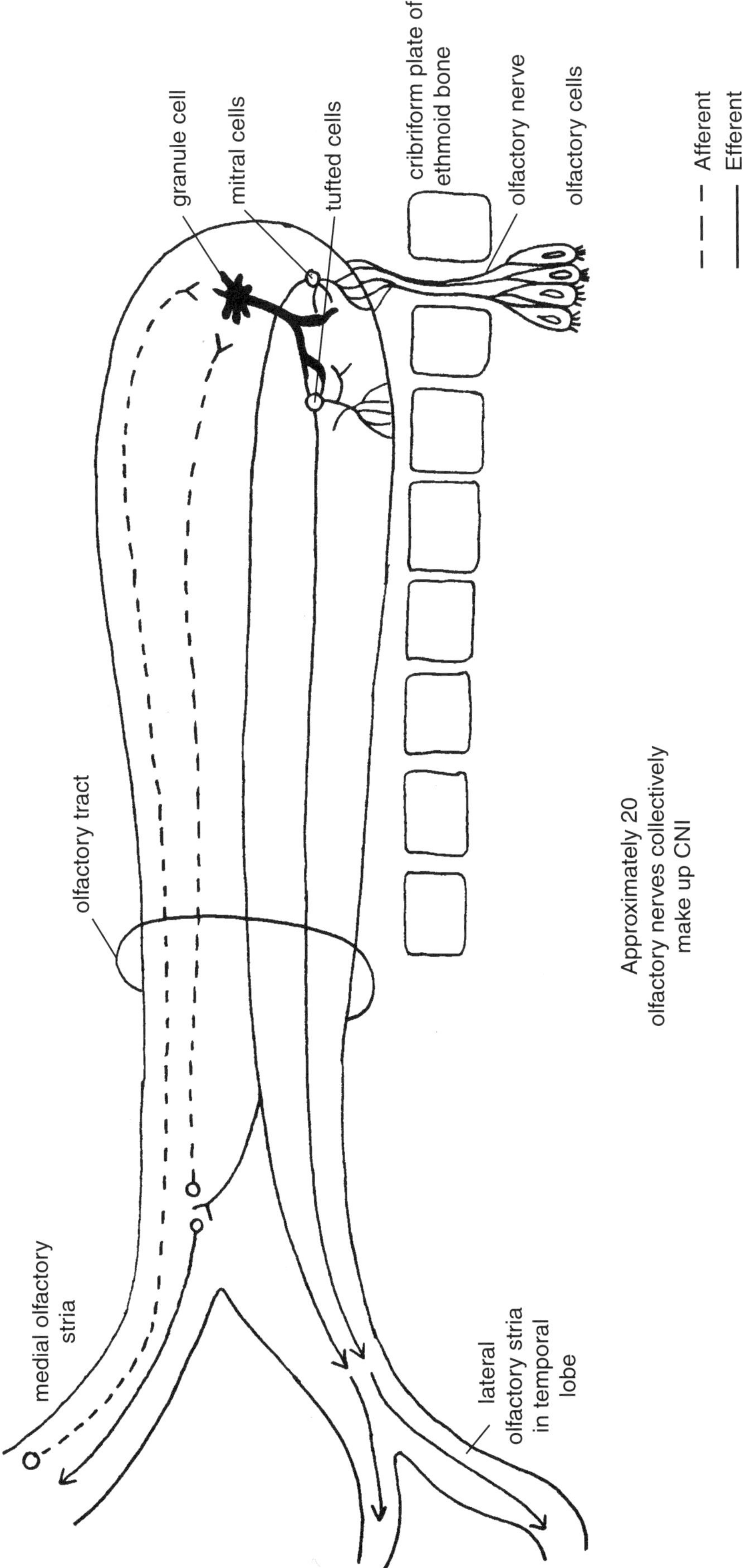
granule cell
mitral cells
tufted cells
cribriform plate of ethmoid bone
olfactory nerve
olfactory cells
Afferent
Efferent
olfactory tract
Approximately 20 olfactory nerves collectively make up CNI
medial olfactory stria
lateral olfactory stria in temporal lobe

NOTES

CLINICAL CORRELATIONS CN II

- Papilledema
  - caused by increased intracranial pressure (↑ CSF pressure in subarachnoid space that surrounds optic nerve → constricts central vein → resulting in decreased return of retinal venous blood)
- Optic neuritis
  - optic nerve lesions that cause decreased visual acuity secondary to inflammation or demyelination of nerve
- Bitemporal hemianopsia
  - results from lesion in optic chiasm → loss of both temporal visual fields resulting in "tunnel vision"

See Tables 1.1 and 1.2 in Appendix.

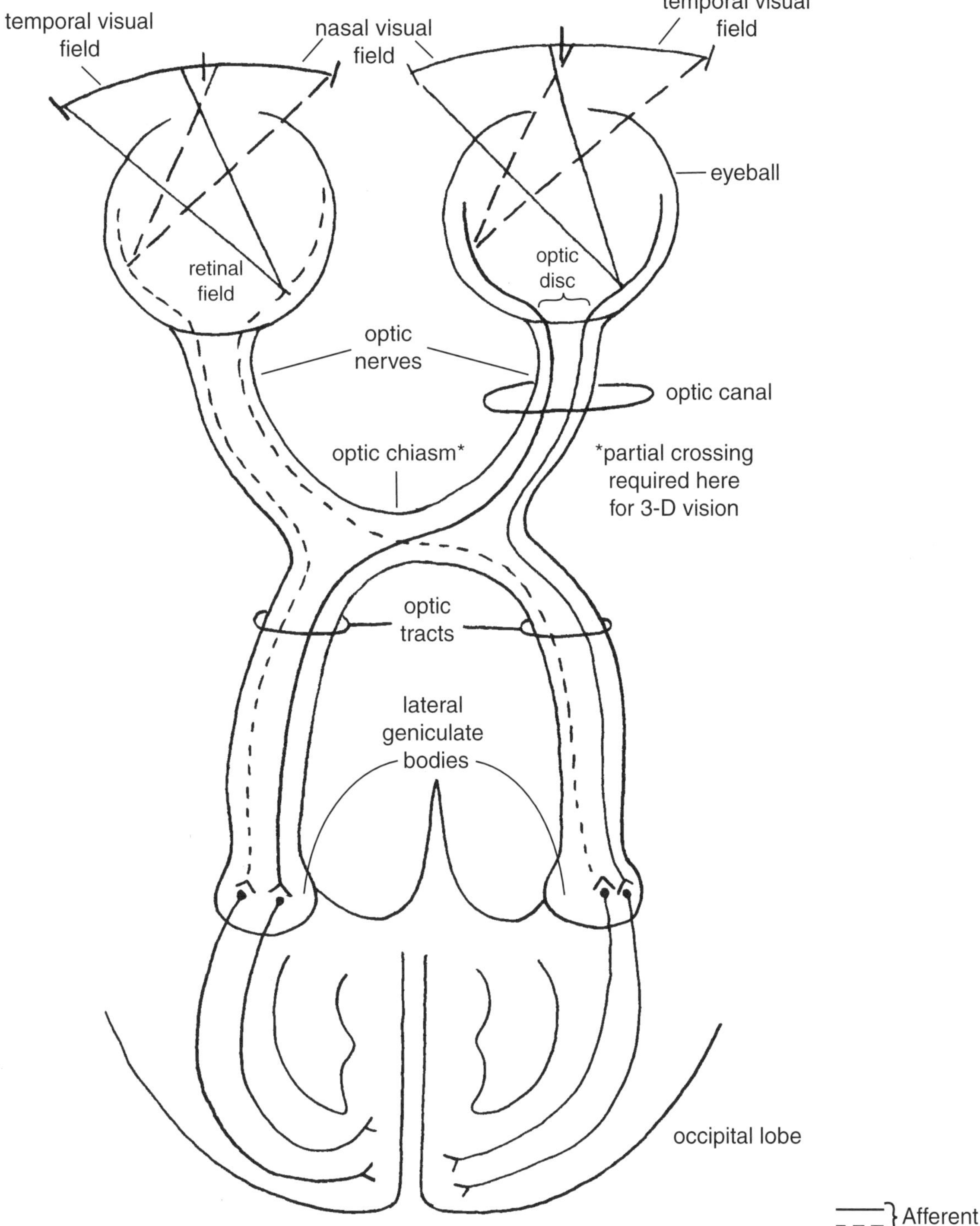
temporal visual field
nasal visual field
temporal visual field
eyeball
retinal field
optic disc
optic nerves
optic canal
optic chiasm*
*partial crossing required here for 3-D vision
optic tracts
lateral geniculate bodies
occipital lobe
Afferent

NOTES

CLINICAL CORRELATIONS CN III, CN IV, CN VI

CN III OCULOMOTOR

- Lesion would result in paralysis of all extraocular muscles except lateral rectus and superior oblique
- The sphincter pupillae in the iris and the ciliary muscle in the ciliary body would also be paralyzed
- Signs of lesion affecting CN III
    - ptosis—drooping of the upper eyelid
    - no pupillary (light) reflex
    - pupillary dilation
    - down and out abduction of eyeball
    - no accommodation of the lens
        - adjustment of ↑ convexity for near vision
- CN III compression
    - autonomic fibers are superficial; therefore rapid ↑ intracranial pressure will be apparent first by ipsilateral slowness of the pupillary response to light

CN IV TROCHLEAR

- Rarely paralyzed alone
- Lesion causes paralysis of superior oblique and inability to move eyeball inferomedially
- May be torn in head injuries over long course
- Characteristic feature of injury is diplopia (double vision) looking down as when going downstairs
    - person can compensate for nerve damage by inclining head anteriorly and to the side of the normal eye

CN VI ABDUCENS

- Can be stretched when intracranial pressure is increased
- Lesion causes paralysis of lateral rectus muscle resulting in medial deviation of affected eye
- Diplopia present in all ranges of eye movement except when gazing
- Paralysis probable when circle of Willis aneurysm present

See Tables 1.1 and 1.2 in Appendix.

Nerves of the Orbit from Lateral Side

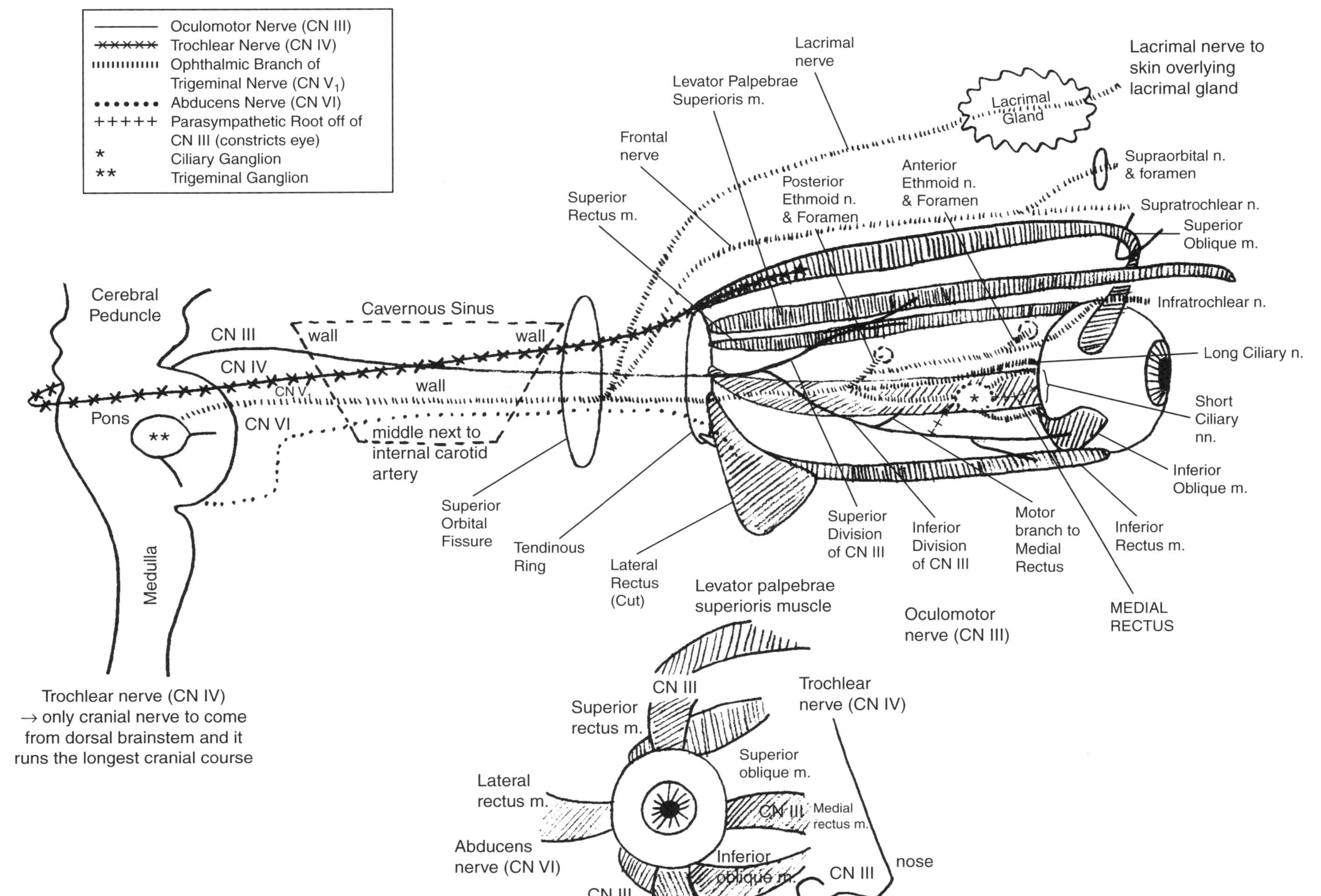
Oculomotor Nerve (CN III)
Trochlear Nerve (CN IV)
Ophthalmic Branch of Trigeminal Nerve (CN V1)
Abducens Nerve (CN VI)
Parasympathetic Root off of CN III (constricts eye)
Ciliary Ganglion
Trigeminal Ganglion
Lacrimal nerve
Levator Palpebrae Superioris m.
Lacrimal nerve to skin overlying lacrimal gland
Lacrimal Gland
Frontal nerve
Supraorbital n. & foramen
Posterior Ethmoid n. & Foramen
Anterior Ethmoid n. & Foramen
Superior Rectus m.
Supratrochlear n.
Superior Oblique m.
Infratrochlear n.
Cerebral Peduncle
Cavernous Sinus
wall
wall
CN III
CN IV
wall
CN V1
Long Ciliary n.
Pons
CN VI
middle next to internal carotid artery
Short Ciliary nn.
Inferior Oblique m.
Superior Orbital Fissure
Tendinous Ring
Lateral Rectus (Cut)
Superior Division of CN III
Inferior Division of CN III
Motor branch to Medial Rectus
Inferior Rectus m.
MEDIAL RECTUS
Medulla
Levator palpebrae superioris muscle
Oculomotor nerve (CN III)
CN III
Trochlear nerve (CN IV)
Superior rectus m.
Superior oblique m.
Lateral rectus m.
CN III
Medial rectus m.
Abducens nerve (CN VI)
Inferior oblique m.
CN III
nose
CN III
Trochlear nerve (CN IV) → only cranial nerve to come from dorsal brainstem and it runs the longest cranial course
* revised with permission from TTUHSC-SOM, Lubbock, TX

CLINICAL CORRELATIONS CN V

- Injuries occur via trauma, tumors, aneurysms, or meningeal infections
  - paralysis of mastication muscles resulting in deviation of jaw toward side of lesion
  - loss of facial sensation
  - loss of corneal and sneezing reflexes
- Trigeminal neuralgia
  - attacks of pain

See Tables 1.1 and 1.2 in Appendix.

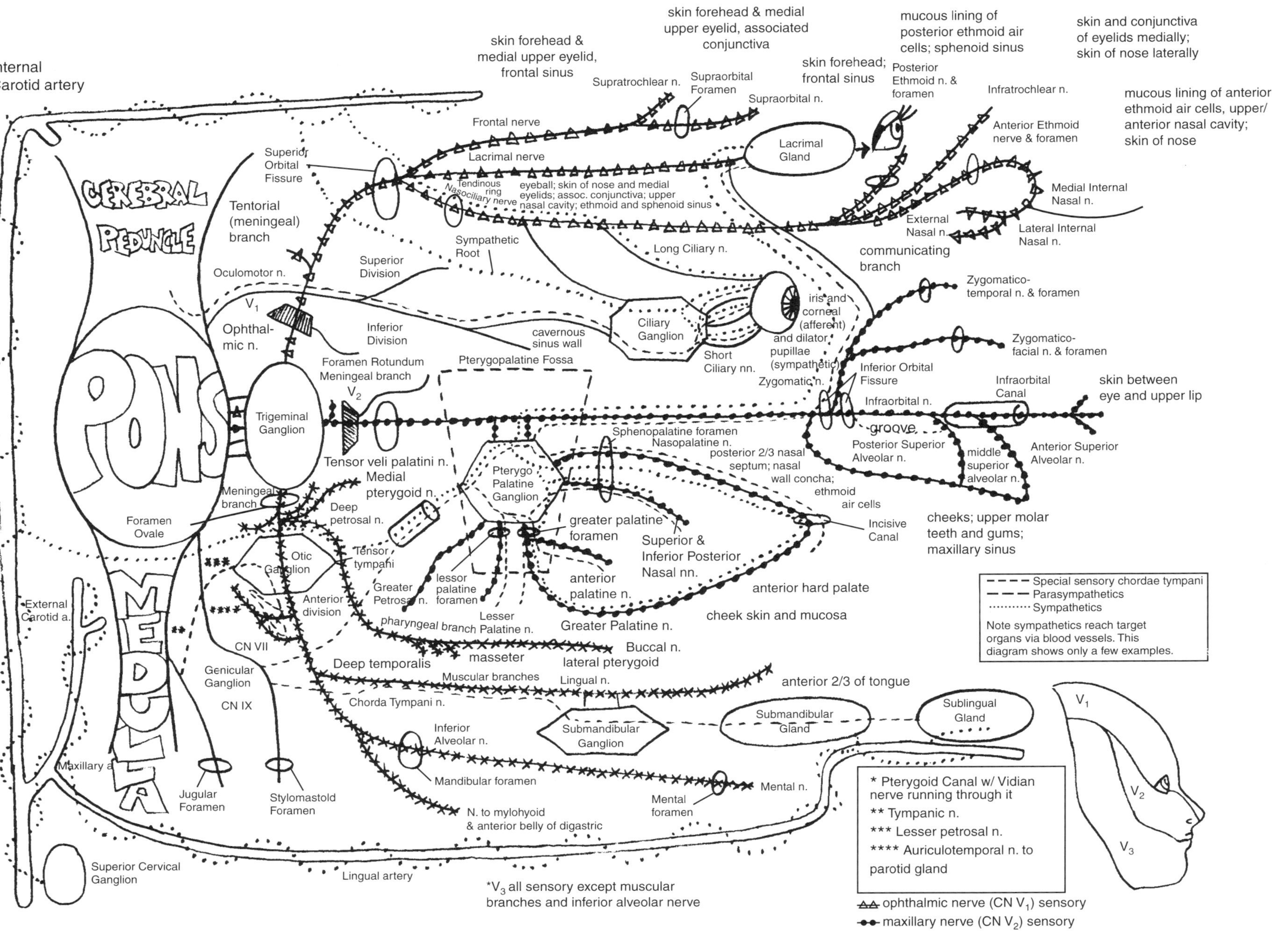
dura of the anterior cranial fossa
mucous lining of posterior ethmoid air cells; sphenoid sinus
skin and conjunctiva of eyelids medially; skin of nose laterally
mucous lining of anterior ethmoid air cells, upper/anterior nasal cavity; skin of nose
skin forehead & medial upper eyelid, associated conjunctiva
skin forehead; frontal sinus
skin forehead & medial upper eyelid, frontal sinus
Internal Carotid artery
Supratrochlear n.
Supraorbital Foramen
Supraorbital n.
Posterior Ethmoid n. & foramen
Infratrochlear n.
Anterior Ethmoid nerve & foramen
Frontal nerve
Lacrimal nerve
Lacrimal Gland
Superior Orbital Fissure
Tendinous ring
Nasociliary nerve
eyeball; skin of nose and medial eyelids; assoc. conjunctiva; upper nasal cavity; ethmoid and sphenoid sinus
Medial Internal Nasal n.
External Nasal n.
Lateral Internal Nasal n.
CEREBRAL PEDUNCLE
Tentorial (meningeal) branch
Sympathetic Root
Long Ciliary n.
communicating branch
Oculomotor n.
Superior Division
Zygomatico-temporal n. & foramen
V_1
Ophthalmic n.
Inferior Division
cavernous sinus wall
Ciliary Ganglion
iris and corneal (afferent) and dilator pupillae (sympathetic)
Short Ciliary nn.
Zygomatico-facial n. & foramen
Foramen Rotundum
Meningeal branch
Pterygopalatine Fossa
Zygomatic n.
Inferior Orbital Fissure
Infraorbital Canal
skin between eye and upper lip
PONS
V_2
Trigeminal Ganglion
Infraorbital n.
groove
Sphenopalatine foramen
Nasopalatine n.
posterior 2/3 nasal septum; nasal wall concha; ethmoid air cells
Posterior Superior Alveolar n.
middle superior alveolar n.
Anterior Superior Alveolar n.
Tensor veli palatini n.
Medial pterygoid n.
Pterygo Palatine Ganglion
Meningeal branch
Deep petrosal n.
Foramen Ovale
greater palatine foramen
Superior & Inferior Posterior Nasal nn.
Incisive Canal
cheeks; upper molar teeth and gums; maxillary sinus
Otic Ganglion
Tensor tympani
lessor palatine foramen
anterior palatine n.
anterior hard palate
External Carotid a.
Anterior division
Greater Petrosal n.
Lesser Palatine n.
pharyngeal branch
Greater Palatine n.
cheek skin and mucosa
Special sensory chordae tympani
Parasympathetics
Sympathetics
Note sympathetics reach target organs via blood vessels. This diagram shows only a few examples.
MEDULLA
CN VII
Buccal n.
masseter
lateral pterygoid
Deep temporalis
Genicular Ganglion
Muscular branches
Lingual n.
anterior 2/3 of tongue
CN IX
Chorda Tympani n.
Submandibular Gland
Sublingual Gland
Submandibular Ganglion
Inferior Alveolar n.
V_1
Maxillary a.
Mandibular foramen
Mental n.
Jugular Foramen
Stylomastoid Foramen
N. to mylohyoid & anterior belly of digastric
Mental foramen
V_2
V_3
* Pterygoid Canal w/ Vidian nerve running through it
** Tympanic n.
*** Lesser petrosal n.
**** Auriculotemporal n. to parotid gland
Superior Cervical Ganglion
Lingual artery
*V_3 all sensory except muscular branches and inferior alveolar nerve
ophthalmic nerve (CN V_1) sensory
maxillary nerve (CN V_2) sensory
mandibular nerve (CN V_3) sensory/motor

NOTES

CLINICAL CORRELATIONS OF FACIAL NERVE: CN VII

- Most frequently paralyzed of all cranial nerves
- Lesion near origin or near geniculate ganglion
  - loss of motor, gustatory (taste), and autonomic functions
  - motor paralysis of facial muscles on ipsilateral (same) side
- Central lesion
  - paralysis of lower face muscles on contralateral (opposite) side
  - forehead wrinkling unimpaired
- Bell's palsy
  - common disorder resulting from CN VII damage
  - sudden loss of muscle control of entire left or right side of face

See Tables 1.1 and 1.2 in Appendix.

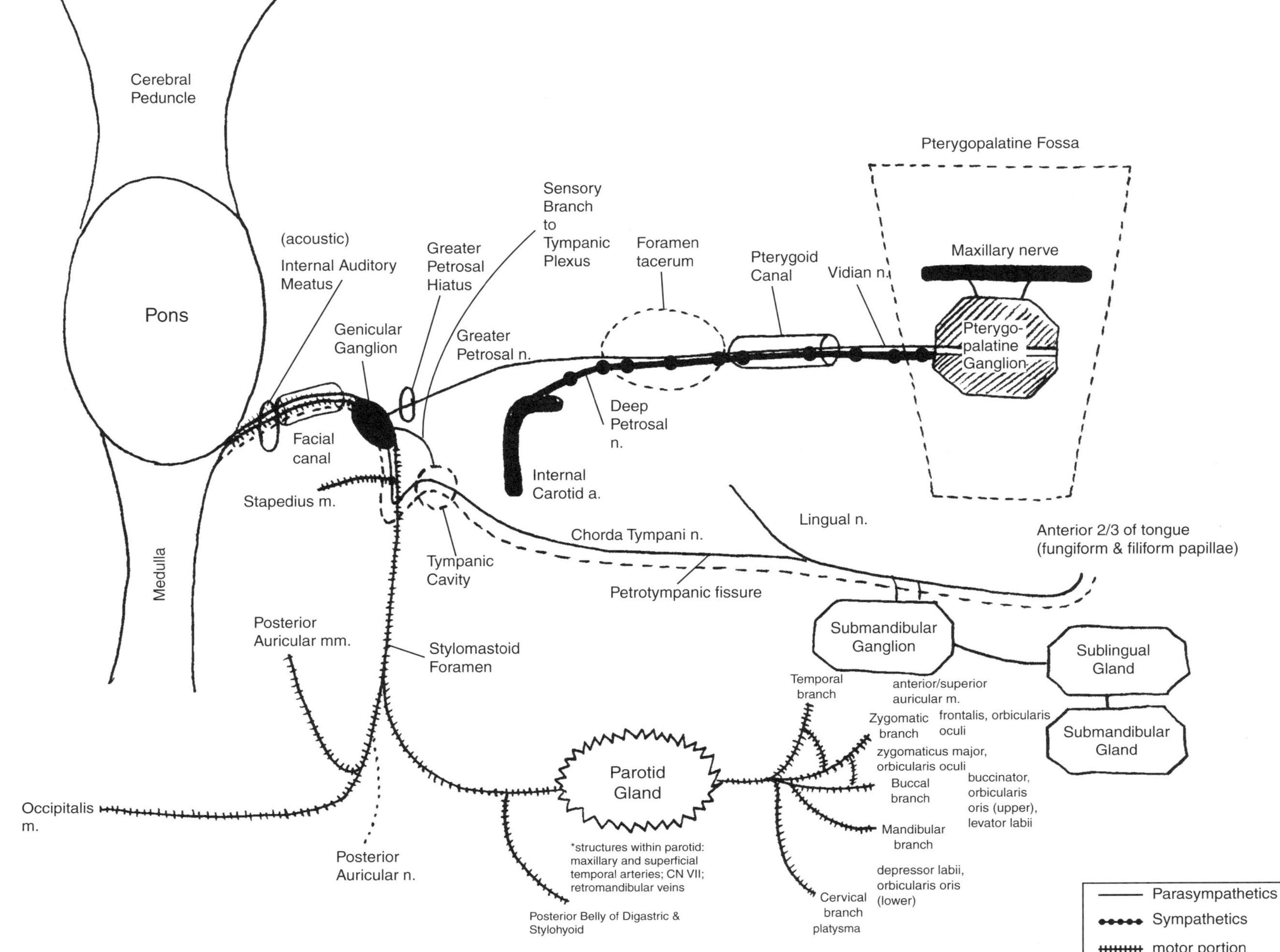
Cerebral Peduncle
Pons
Medulla
(acoustic)
Internal Auditory Meatus
Genicular Ganglion
Facial canal
Stapedius m.
Greater Petrosal Hiatus
Greater Petrosal n.
Sensory Branch to Tympanic Plexus
Foramen tacerum
Pterygoid Canal
Vidian n.
Pterygopalatine Fossa
Maxillary nerve
Pterygo-palatine Ganglion
Deep Petrosal n.
Internal Carotid a.
Lingual n.
Chorda Tympani n.
Tympanic Cavity
Petrotympanic fissure
Anterior 2/3 of tongue (fungiform & filiform papillae)
Submandibular Ganglion
Sublingual Gland
Submandibular Gland
Posterior Auricular mm.
Stylomastoid Foramen
Occipitalis m.
Posterior Auricular n.
Parotid Gland
*structures within parotid: maxillary and superficial temporal arteries; CN VII; retromandibular veins
Posterior Belly of Digastric & Stylohyoid
Temporal branch
anterior/superior auricular m.
Zygomatic branch
frontalis, orbicularis oculi
zygomaticus major, orbicularis oculi
Buccal branch
buccinator, orbicularis oris (upper), levator labii
Mandibular branch
depressor labii, orbicularis oris (lower)
Cervical branch
platysma
Parasympathetics
Sympathetics
motor portion
special sensory

* revised with permission from TTUHSC-SOM, Lubbock, TX

CLINICAL CORRELATIONS CN VIII

- Conducts two special senses
  - hearing (audition)
  - balance (vestibular)
- Receptor cells located in membranous labyrinth embedded in temporal lobe
- Sound transmission
  - sound waves → TM → bony ossicles → fluid movement in cochlea → stimulates hair cells → activation of auditory area of CN VIII
- Vestibular apparatus responds to changes in head position

See Tables 1.1 and 1.2 in Appendix.

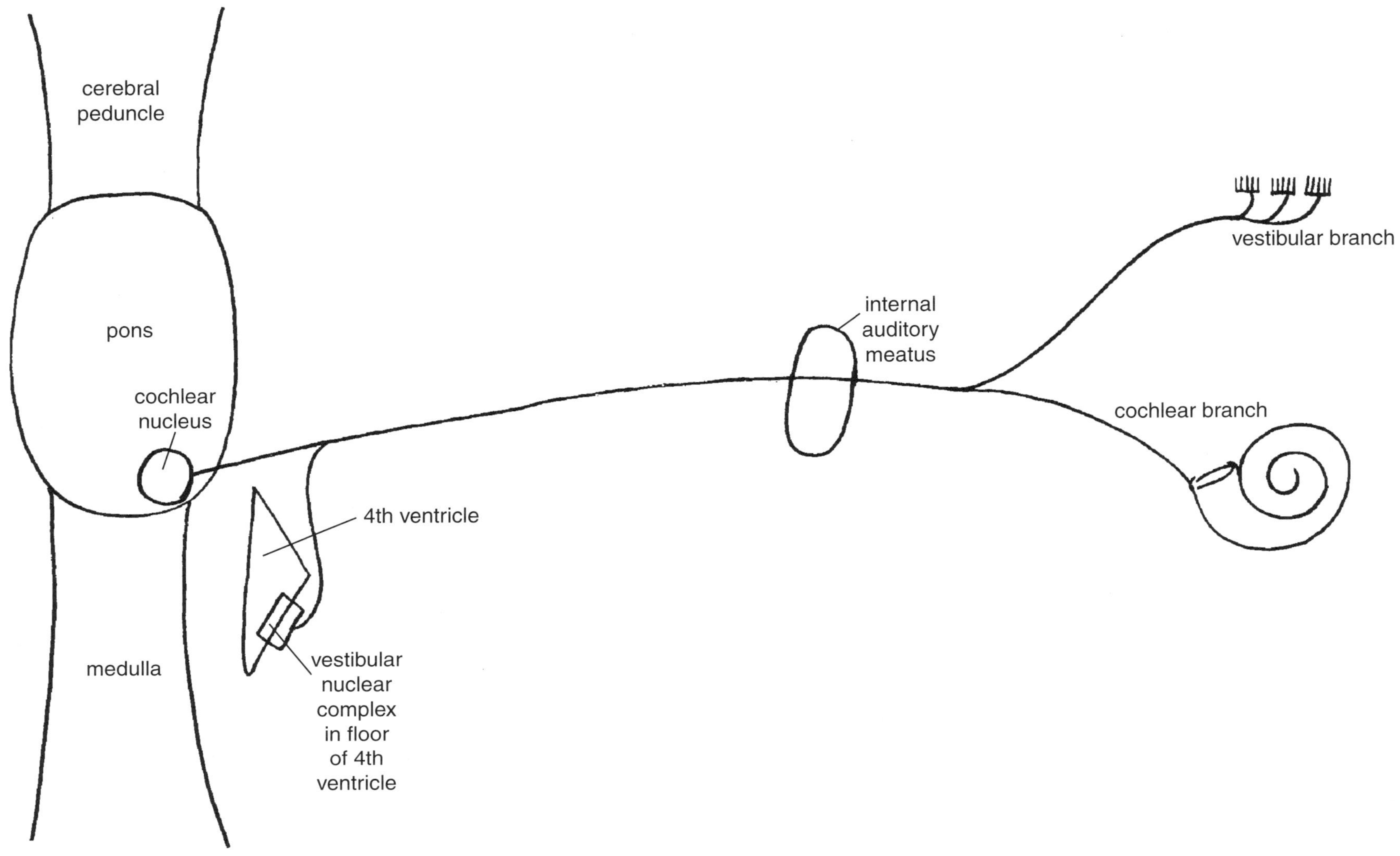
cerebral peduncle
pons
cochlear nucleus
medulla
4th ventricle
vestibular nuclear complex in floor of 4th ventricle
internal auditory meatus
vestibular branch
cochlear branch

NOTES

CLINICAL CORRELATION CN IX

- Taste lost in posterior one-third of tongue; gag reflex absent on the side of lesion

See Tables 1.1 and 1.2 in Appendix.

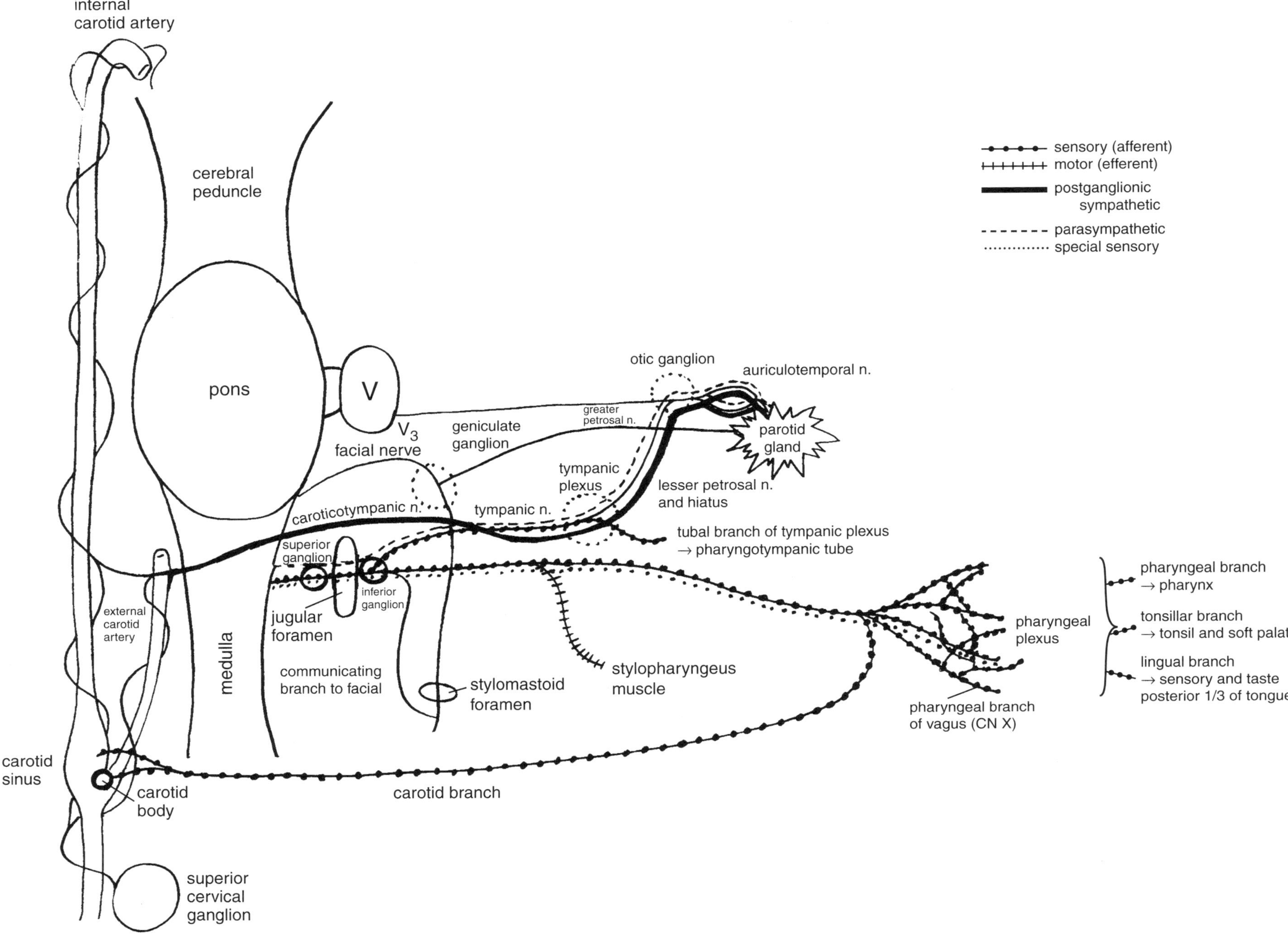
internal carotid artery
cerebral peduncle
pons
V
V_3
facial nerve
geniculate ganglion
greater petrosal n.
otic ganglion
auriculotemporal n.
parotid gland
tympanic plexus
lesser petrosal n. and hiatus
caroticotympanic n.
tympanic n.
tubal branch of tympanic plexus → pharyngotympanic tube
superior ganglion
inferior ganglion
jugular foramen
external carotid artery
medulla
communicating branch to facial
stylomastoid foramen
stylopharyngeus muscle
pharyngeal plexus
pharyngeal branch of vagus (CN X)
pharyngeal branch → pharynx
tonsillar branch → tonsil and soft palate
lingual branch → sensory and taste posterior 1/3 of tongue
carotid sinus
carotid body
carotid branch
superior cervical ganglion
sensory (afferent)
motor (efferent)
postganglionic sympathetic
parasympathetic
special sensory

NOTES

CLINICAL CORRELATIONS CN X

- Vagus innervation:
  - all palate except tensor veli palatini
  - all pharyngeous except stylopharyngeous
  - all laryngeal
    - recurrent laryngeal except cricothyroid
  - external branch of superior laryngeal
- Injury to pharyngeal branches resulting in swallowing difficulty
- Injury to superior laryngeal nerve resulting in loss of superior larynx sensation and cricothyroid muscle paralysis (the voice is weak and tires easily)
- Injury to recurrent laryngeal nerve resulting in hoarseness; dysphonia (difficulty in speaking) → paralysis of vocal cords
  - both: aphonia → complete loss of voice
  - inspiratory stridor → high-pitched respiratory sound
    - caused by cancer of larynx and thyroid gland

See Tables 1.1 and 1.2 in Appendix.

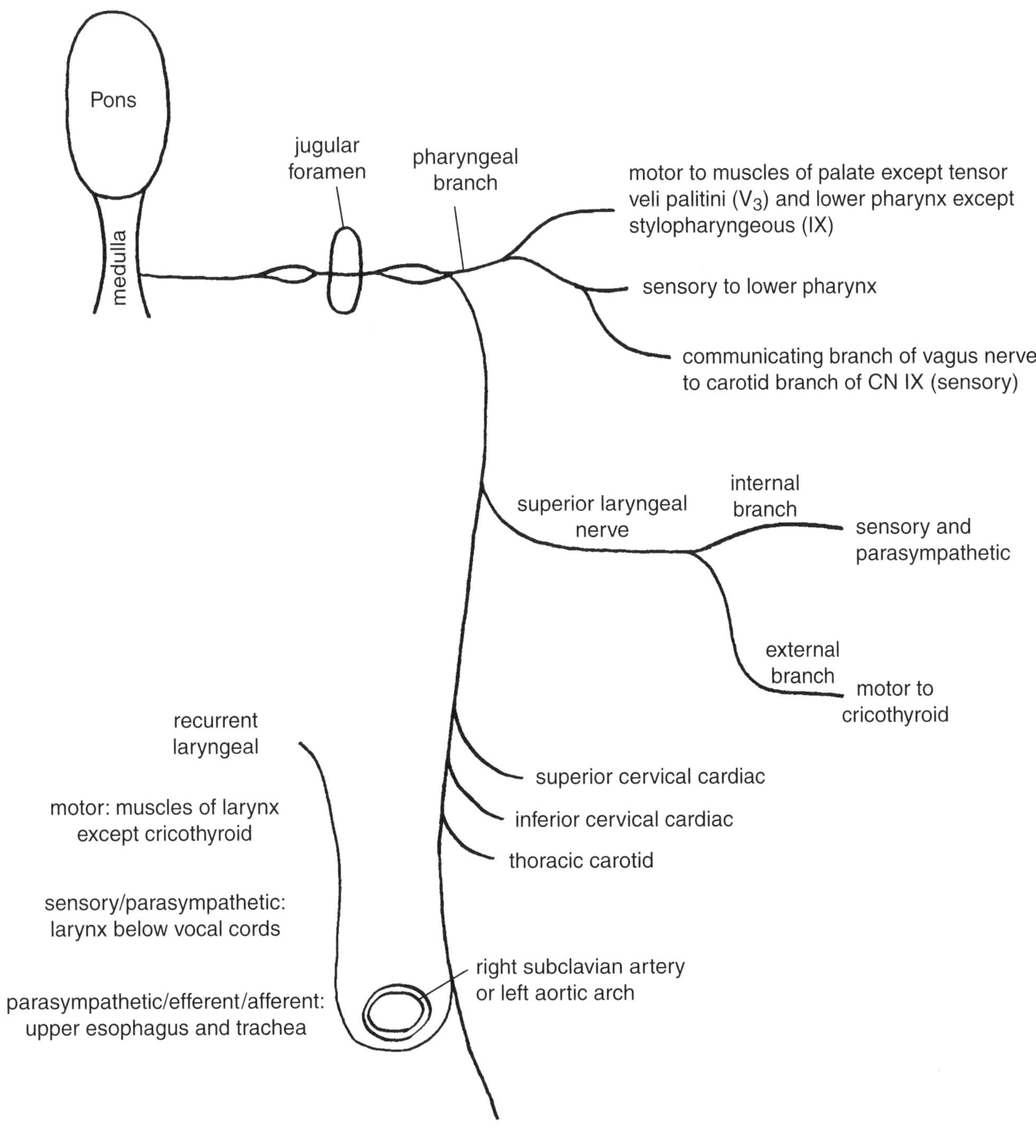
Pons
medulla
jugular
foramen
pharyngeal
branch
motor to muscles of palate except tensor
veli palitini (V_3) and lower pharynx except
stylopharyngeous (IX)
sensory to lower pharynx
communicating branch of vagus nerve
to carotid branch of CN IX (sensory)
superior laryngeal
nerve
internal
branch
sensory and
parasympathetic
external
branch
motor to
cricothyroid
recurrent
laryngeal
motor: muscles of larynx
except cricothyroid
sensory/parasympathetic:
larynx below vocal cords
parasympathetic/efferent/afferent:
upper esophagus and trachea
superior cervical cardiac
inferior cervical cardiac
thoracic carotid
right subclavian artery
or left aortic arch

See Tables 1.1 and 1.2 in Appendix.

CLINICAL CORRELATIONS CN XI

- Injury to spinal root: because nerve passes through posterior cervical triangle, it is susceptible to injury during surgical procedures in cervical region
- Lesions produce weakness and atrophy of trapezius and sternocleidomastoid → impairment of rotary movement of neck and chin to opposite side
- Trapezius weakness results in difficulty shrugging shoulders and winging of the scapula (worsens on shoulder abduction)

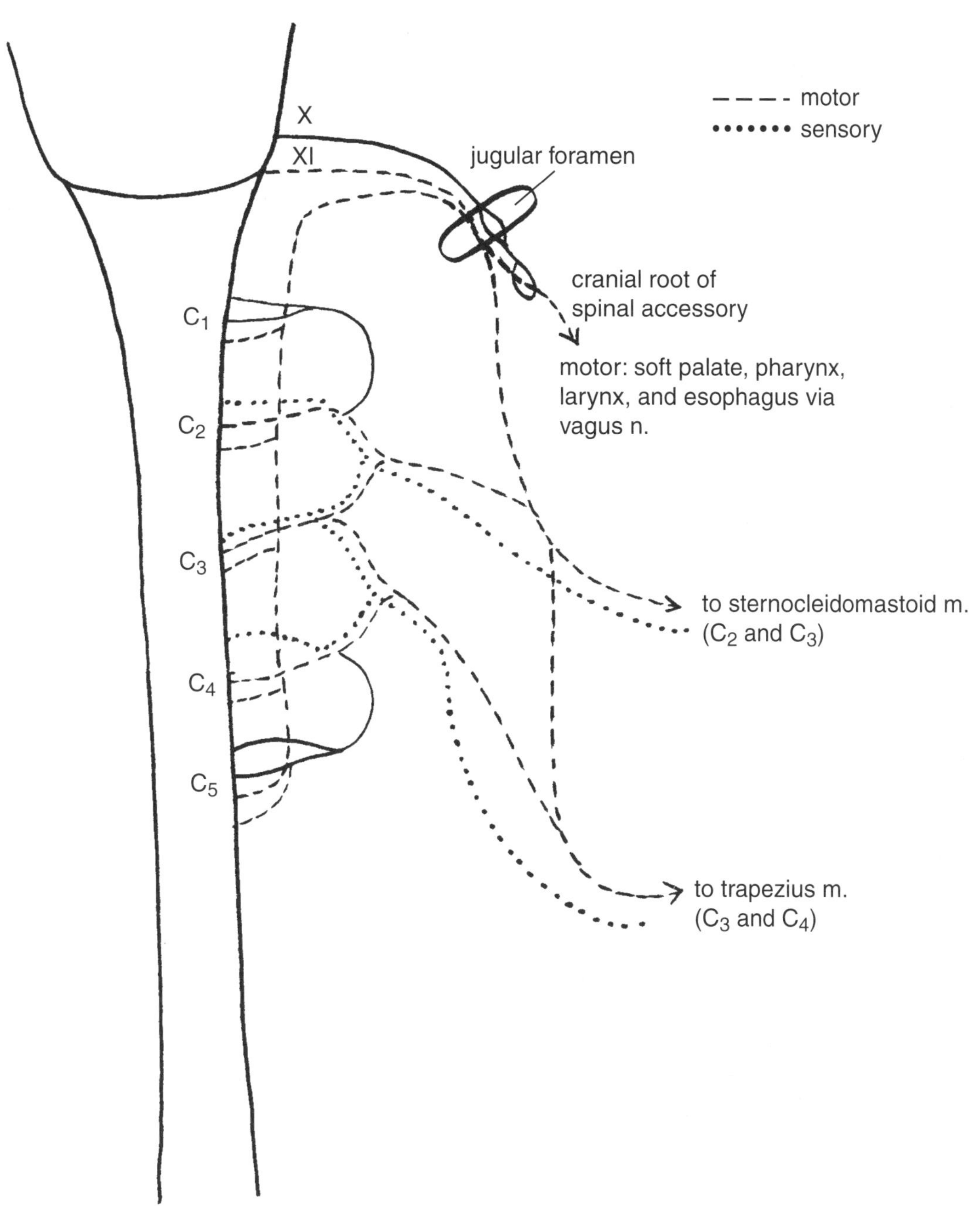
– – – - motor
••••••• sensory
X
XI
jugular foramen
cranial root of
spinal accessory
motor: soft palate, pharynx,
larynx, and esophagus via
vagus n.
C_1
C_2
C_3
C_4
C_5
to sternocleidomastoid m.
(C_2 and C_3)
to trapezius m.
(C_3 and C_4)

NOTES

CLINICAL CORRELATIONS CN XII

- Innervates all tongue muscles except palatoglossus
  - hyo-
  - stylo-
  - genio-
- Injury paralyzes the tongue's ipsilateral side
- Tongue atrophies
- When tongue is protruded, tip deviates toward the paralyzed side (lower motor neuron injury)

See Tables 1.1 and 1.2 in Appendix.

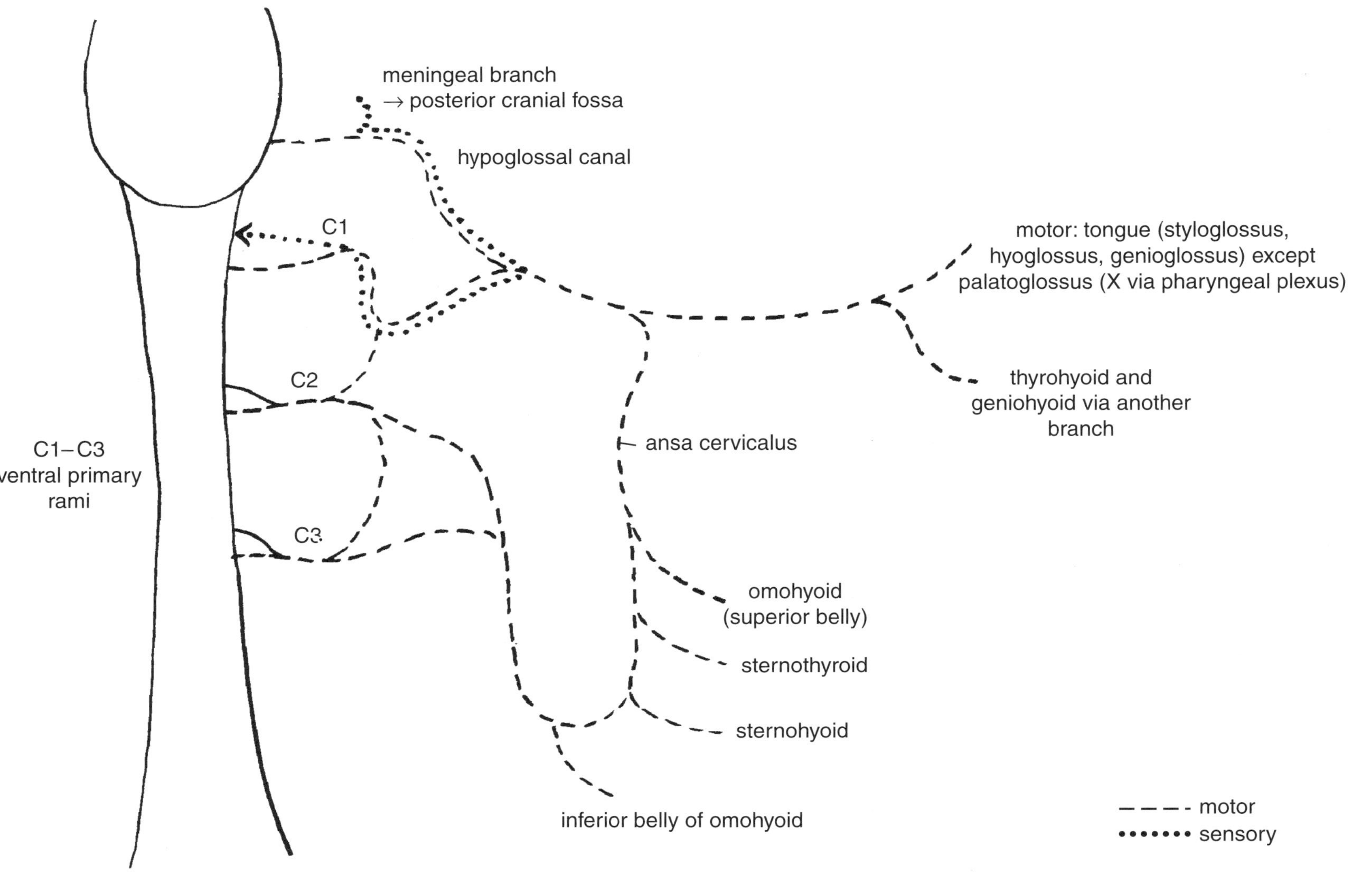
meningeal branch
→ posterior cranial fossa
hypoglossal canal
C1
motor: tongue (styloglossus, hyoglossus, genioglossus) except palatoglossus (X via pharyngeal plexus)
C2
thyrohyoid and geniohyoid via another branch
C1–C3 ventral primary rami
ansa cervicalus
C3
omohyoid (superior belly)
sternothyroid
sternohyoid
inferior belly of omohyoid
– – – - motor
••••••• sensory

NOTES

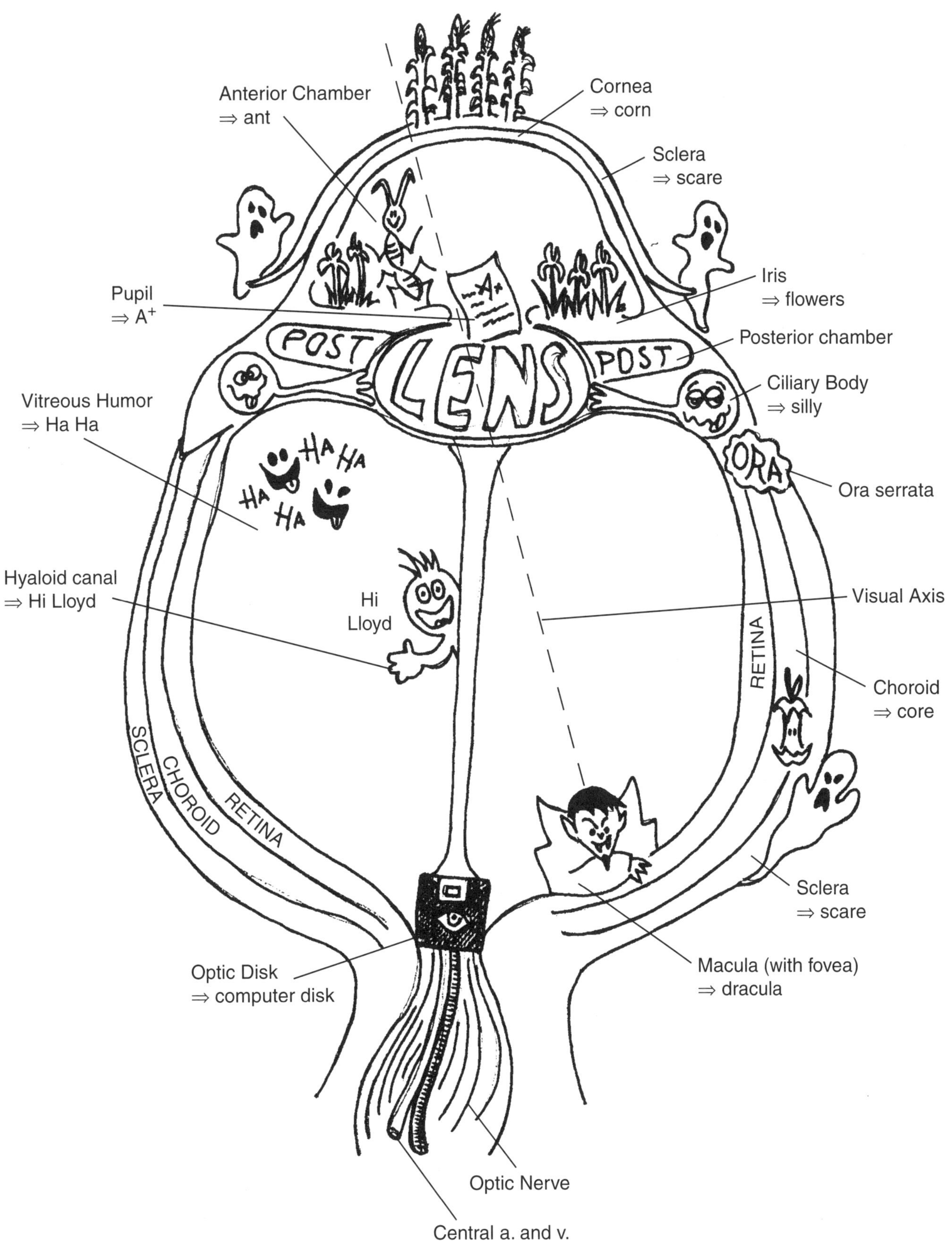
Anterior Chamber
⇒ ant
Cornea
⇒ corn
Sclera
⇒ scare
Iris
⇒ flowers
Pupil
⇒ A+
POST
LENS
POST
Posterior chamber
Ciliary Body
⇒ silly
Vitreous Humor
⇒ Ha Ha
HA HA
HA
HA
ORA
Ora serrata
Hyaloid canal
⇒ Hi Lloyd
Hi
Lloyd
Visual Axis
RETINA
Choroid
⇒ core
SCLERA
CHOROID
RETINA
Sclera
⇒ scare
Optic Disk
⇒ computer disk
Macula (with fovea)
⇒ dracula
Optic Nerve
Central a. and v.

NOTES

COMPARISON OF RODS AND CONES

RODS

⇒ fishing rod
- Long outer segment
  ⇒ long fishing rod
- Night vision
  ⇒ moon
- High sensitivity
- Sensitive to scattered light
- Lower visual acuity
- Not present in the fovea
  ⇒ running away from fovea
- No color vision
- Slow response
  ⇒ rod standing still
- One type of rod

CONES

⇒ ice cream cone
- Short outer segment
- Larger synaptic terminal
- Day vision
  ⇒ sun
- Low sensitivity
- Sensitive to direct light
  ⇒ direct rays
- Higher visual acuity
- Present in the fovea
- Color vision
  ⇒ rainbow
- Fast response
  ⇒ cone running
- Three types of cones: **S** (blue), **M** (green), **L** (red)
  ⇒ cone holding up three fingers

Comparison of Rods and Cones

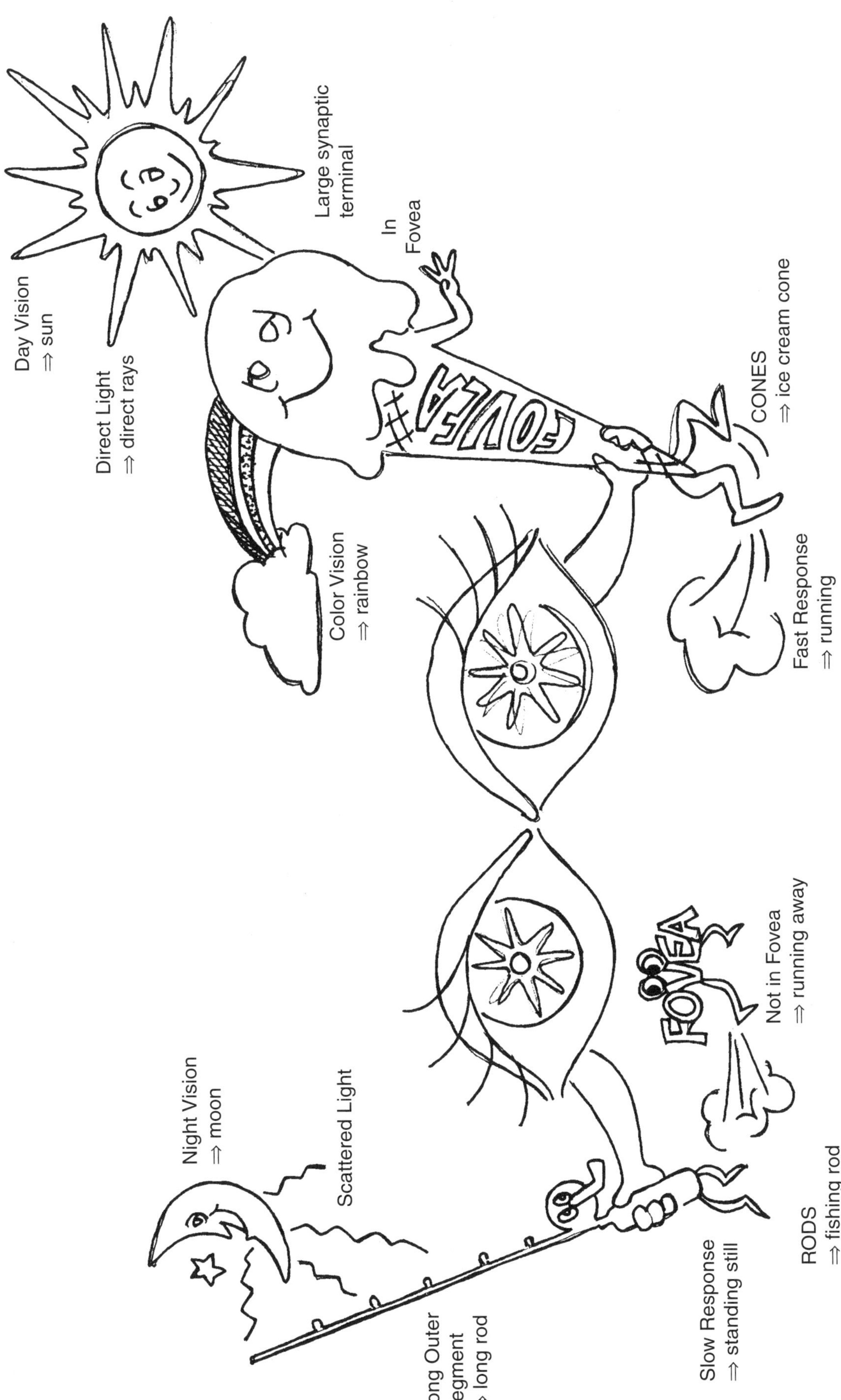
Day Vision
⇒ sun
Direct Light
⇒ direct rays
Large synaptic
terminal
In
Fovea
FOVEA
CONES
⇒ ice cream cone
Color Vision
⇒ rainbow
Fast Response
⇒ running
Night Vision
⇒ moon
Scattered Light
Not in Fovea
⇒ running away
FOVEA
Long Outer
Segment
⇒ long rod
Slow Response
⇒ standing still
RODS
⇒ fishing rod

NOTES

LAYERS OF THE RETINA

- Retinal pigment epithelium absorbs stray light
  retinal pigment epithelium ⇒ pig
- Rods and cones comprise the photoreceptor layer
- Bipolar cells and photoreceptors synapse in the outer plexiform layer
  outer plexiform layer ⇒ O flexed form
- Bipolar cells and ganglion cells synapse in the inner plexiform layer
- Ganglion cell axons form the optic nerve
  Inner plexiform layer ⇒ I flexed form
  ganglion ⇒ gang
- Several rods synapse on a bipolar cell, whereas only a few cones synapse on a bipolar cell
- Interneurons include horizontal cells (outer plexiform layer) and amacrine cells (inner plexiform layer)
  horizontal ⇒ horizon
  amacrine ⇒ I'm cryin'
- Blind spot results from the lack of rods and cones on the optic disk

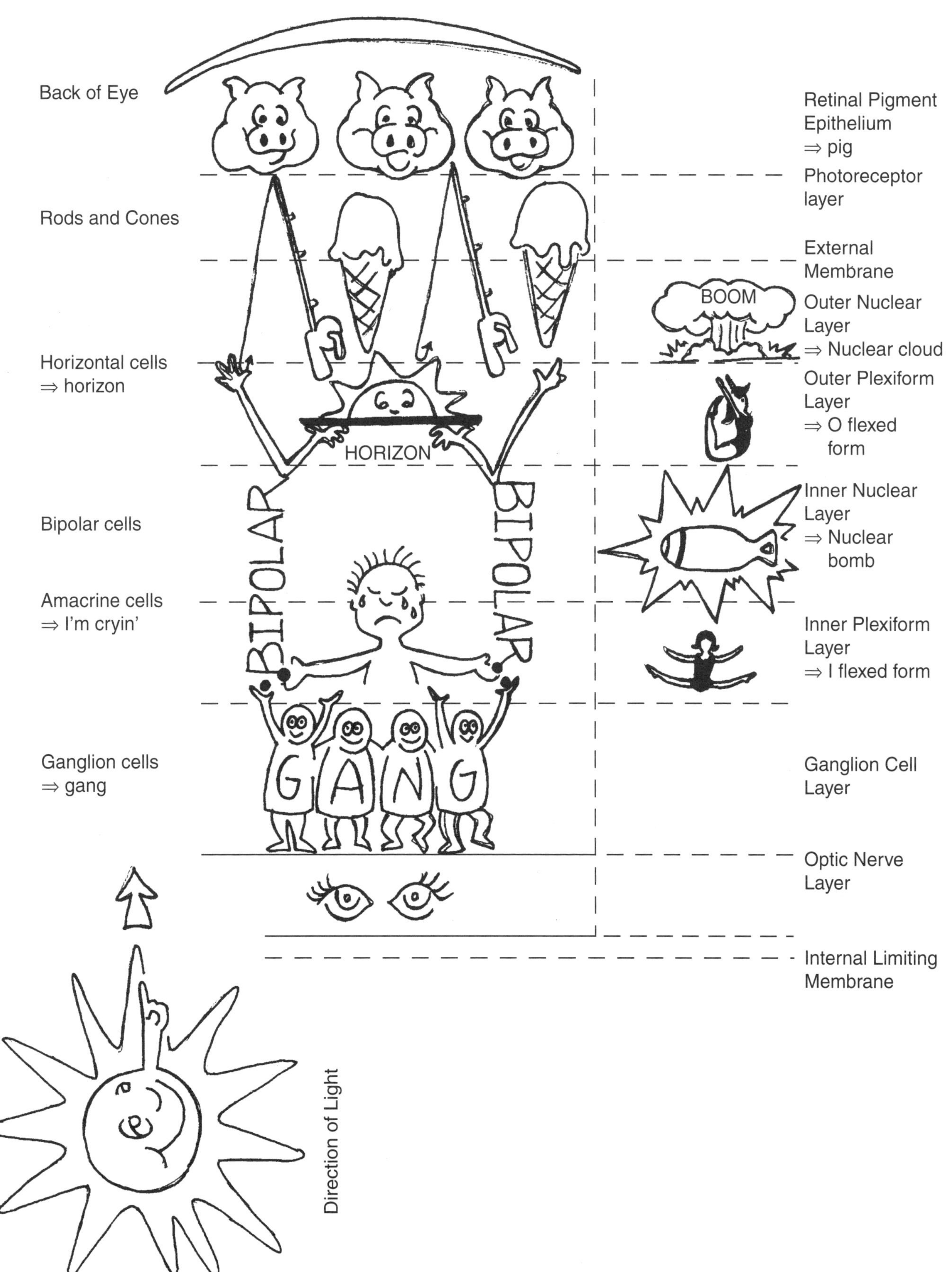
Back of Eye
Rods and Cones
Horizontal cells
⇒ horizon
Bipolar cells
Amacrine cells
⇒ I'm cryin'
Ganglion cells
⇒ gang
Retinal Pigment
Epithelium
⇒ pig
Photoreceptor
layer
External
Membrane
BOOM
Outer Nuclear
Layer
⇒ Nuclear cloud
Outer Plexiform
Layer
⇒ O flexed
form
HORIZON
BIPOLAR
BIPOLAR
Inner Nuclear
Layer
⇒ Nuclear
bomb
Inner Plexiform
Layer
⇒ I flexed form
GANG
Ganglion Cell
Layer
Optic Nerve
Layer
Internal Limiting
Membrane
Direction of Light

NOTES

EXTRAOCULAR MUSCLES AND NERVES

SO_4 LR_6 R_3 = Superior Oblique (CN IV), Lateral Rectus (CN VI), and the Rest are CN III

- Intorsion caused by superior muscles
- Extorsion caused by inferior muscles
- Superior oblique (SO) introverts, abducts, depresses
- Inferior oblique (IO) extorts, abducts, elevates

CN III Oculomotor palsy

- Eye deviates down and out; unopposed SO_4 LR_6
- Ptosis from levator palpebrae paralysis
- Dilated, fixed pupil from disruption of parasympathetics
- Paralysis of accommodation

CN IV Trochlear palsy

- Vertical diplopia
- Head tilting to compensate
- Extorsion of eye

CN VI Abducens palsy

- Horizontal diplopia
- Deviating eye turns inward
- Head turning to compensate

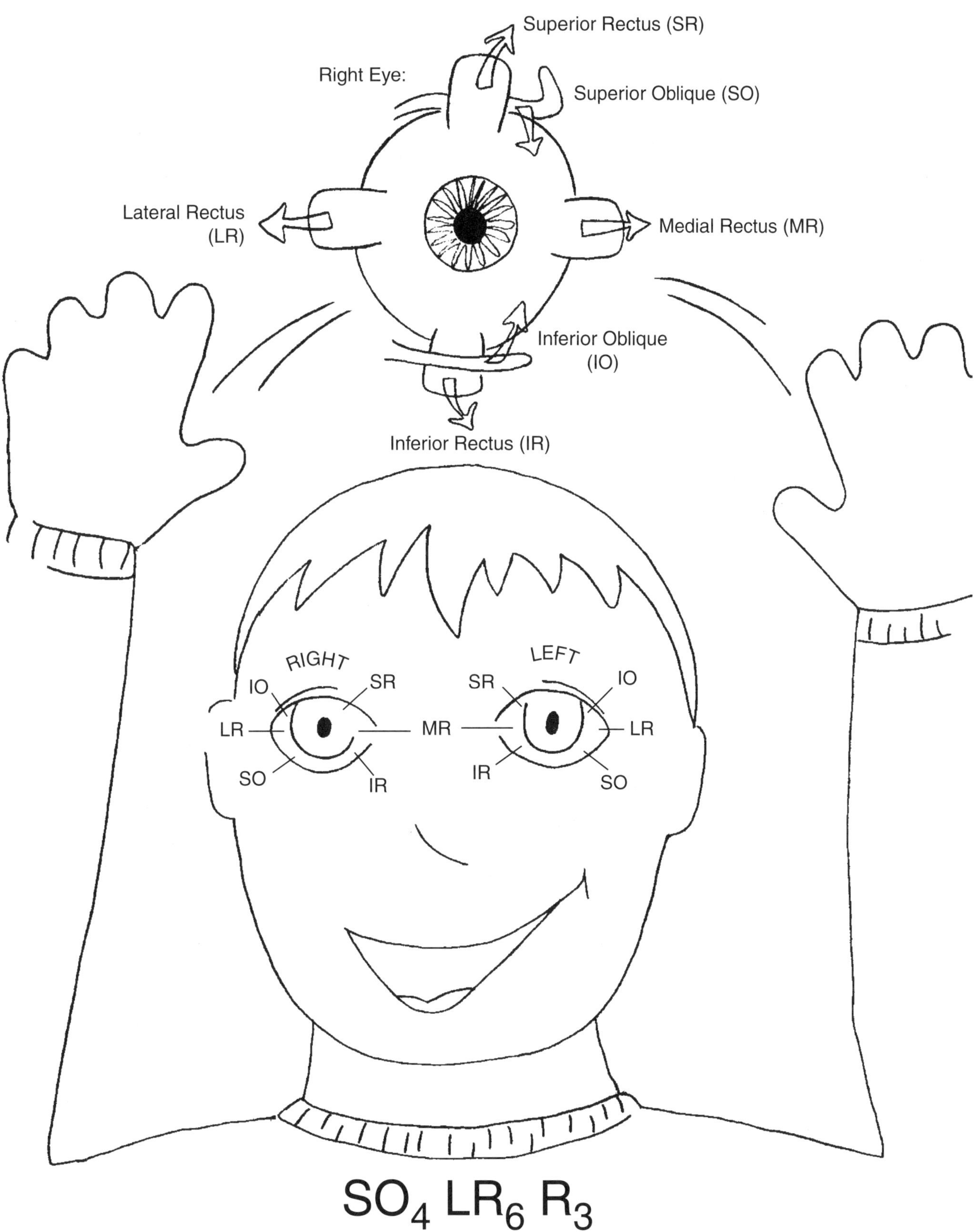
Superior Rectus (SR)
Right Eye:
Superior Oblique (SO)
Lateral Rectus (LR)
Medial Rectus (MR)
Inferior Oblique (IO)
Inferior Rectus (IR)
RIGHT
LEFT
IO
SR
LR
MR
SO
IR
SR
IO
LR
IR
SO

$SO_4\ LR_6\ R_3$

NOTES

VISUAL FIELD DEFECTS

- Fibers from each nasal portion of both retinas cross at the optic chiasm
- Fibers from each temporal portion of both retinas remain ipsilateral
- The right optic tract contains fibers from the left nasal hemiretina and the right temporal hemiretina
- The left optic tract contains fibers from the right nasal hemiretina and the left temporal hemiretina
- The lateral geniculate body of the thalamus receives the optic tract
  lateral geniculate body ⇒ genie is lateral
- The lateral geniculate body radiations form the geniculocalcarine tract, which projects to the occipital lobe of the cortex
  occipital ⇒ ox

	DEFICIT	LOCATION OF LESION
1	Anopsia of right eye	Optic nerve
2	Heteronymous hemianopsia	Optic chiasm
3	Homonymous hemianopsia	Optic tract
4	Upper quadrant anopsia	Meyer's loop
5	Lower quadrant anopsia with macular sparing	Upper bank of calcarine fissure
6	Upper quadrant anopsia with macular sparing	Lower bank of calcarine fissure
Meyer's Loop ⇒ my R Calcarine Fissure ⇒ Cal's car		

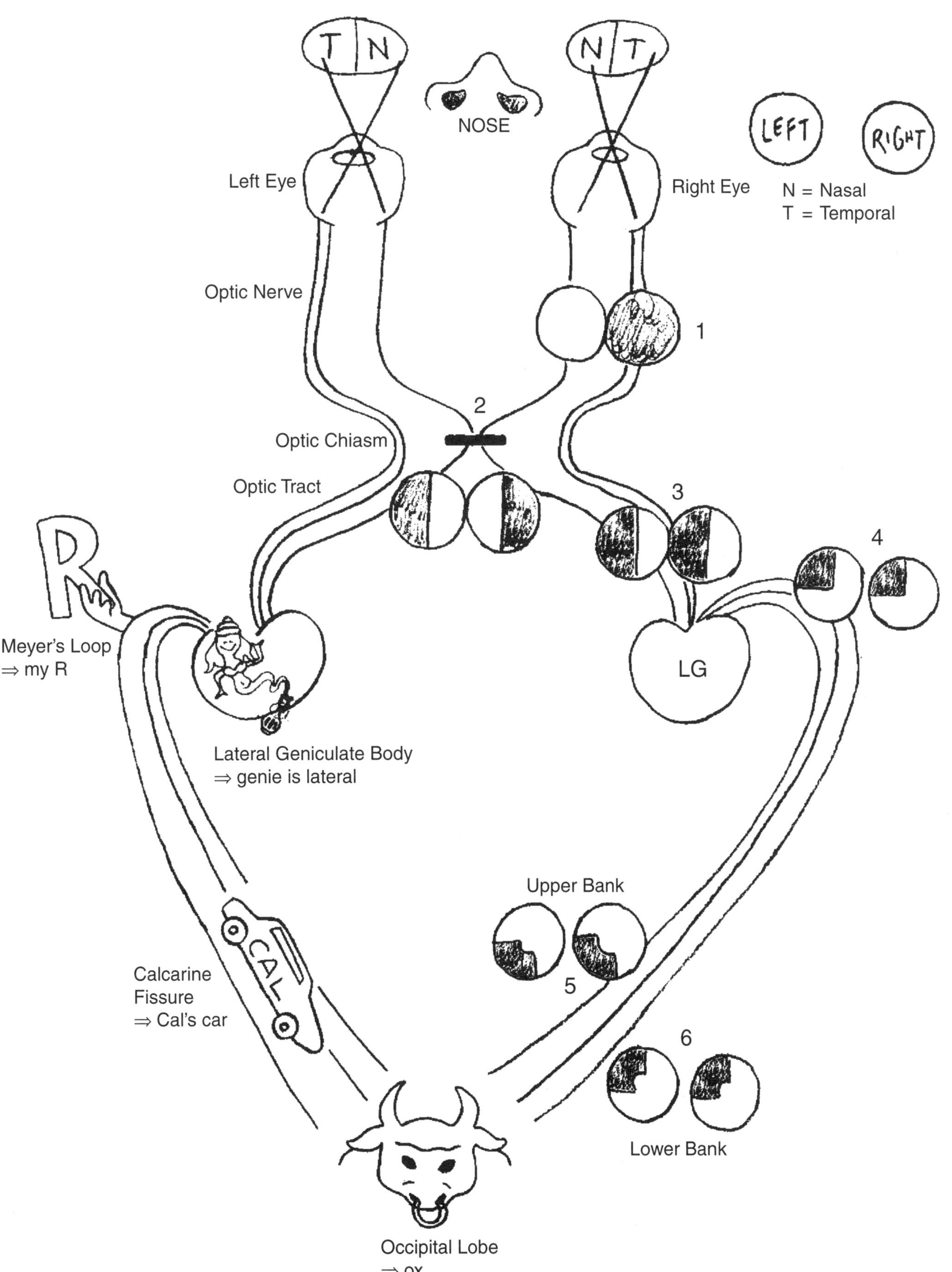
T N
N T
NOSE
LEFT
RIGHT
Left Eye
Right Eye
N = Nasal
T = Temporal
Optic Nerve
1
2
Optic Chiasm
Optic Tract
3
4
R
Meyer's Loop
⇒ my R
LG
Lateral Geniculate Body
⇒ genie is lateral
Upper Bank
5
CAL
Calcarine
Fissure
⇒ Cal's car
6
Lower Bank
Occipital Lobe
⇒ ox

NOTES

PHOTOTRANSDUCTION CASCADE

Dark state

- Rhodopsin is composed of 11-*cis*-retinal and opsin
  rhodopsin ⇒ road
  11-*cis*-retinal ⇒ sister

Photoisomerization

- Absorption of light by the retina converts 11-*cis*-retinal to all-*trans*-retinal
  absorption of light ⇒ sun
  all-*trans*-retinal ⇒ trans-am

Transduction

- Meta-rhodopsin II activates transducin, a G-protein
  transducin ⇒ deuce
- Transducin activates a phosphodiesterase, which converts cGMP to 5'-GMP decreasing cGMP levels
- As cGMP levels decrease, Na^+ channels close and the rod's cell membranes hyperpolarize
  sodium ⇒ salt shaker
- As the rod's cell membranes hyperpolarize, glutamate release decreases
  hyperpolarization ⇒ hyper polar bear
  glutamate ⇒ glue
- Degree of hyperpolarization increases as the light entering increases

Re-isomerization

- Isomerase converts all-*trans*-retinal back to 11-*cis*-retinal; 11-*cis*-retinal binds to opsin and becomes light-sensitive rhodopsin

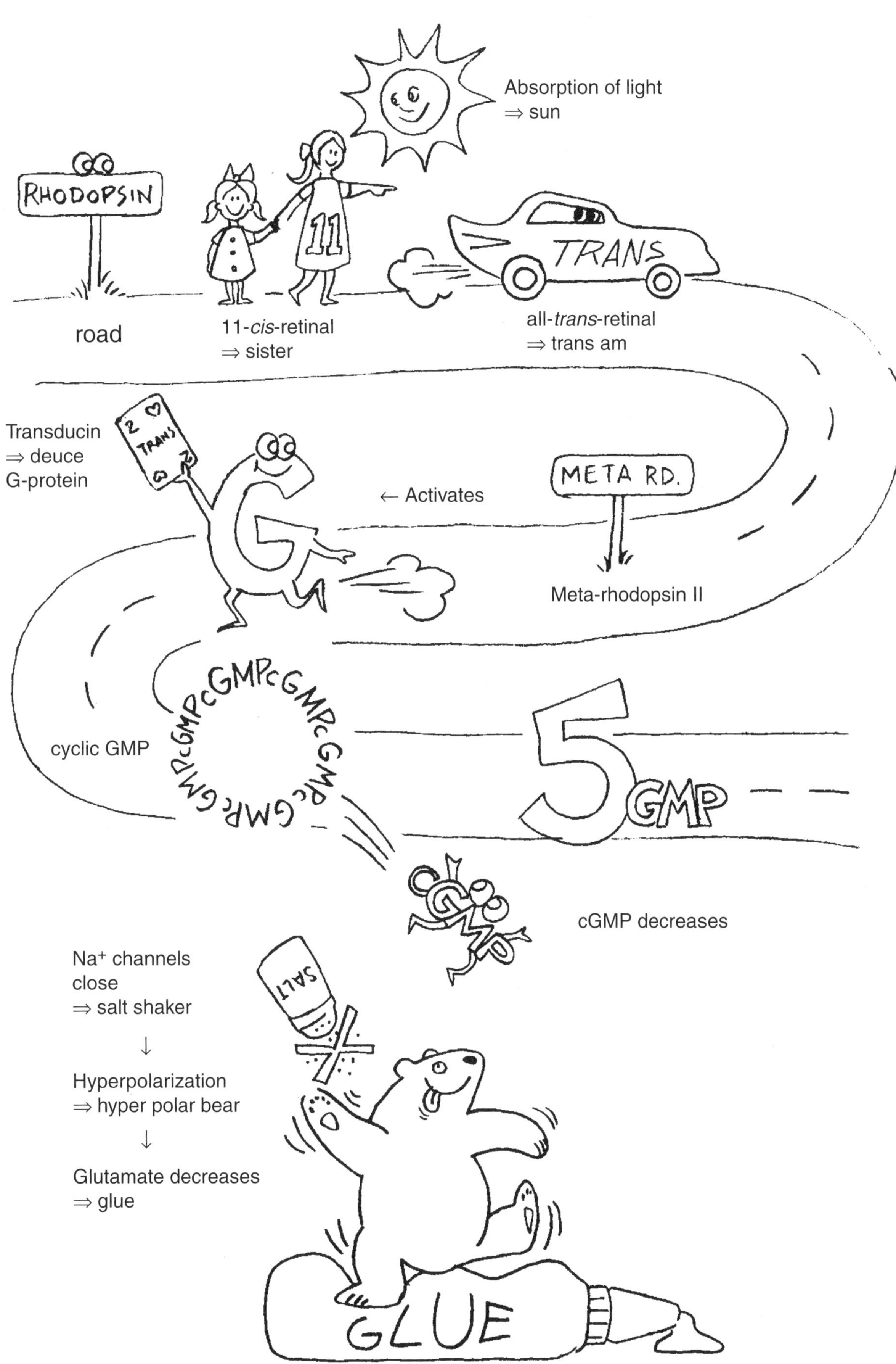
Absorption of light
⇒ sun
RHODOPSIN
11
TRANS
road
11-*cis*-retinal
⇒ sister
all-*trans*-retinal
⇒ trans am
Transducin
⇒ deuce
G-protein
2 ♡ TRANS
← Activates
META RD.
Meta-rhodopsin II
cGMPcGMPcGMPcGMPcGMPcGMP
cyclic GMP
5GMP
cGMP
cGMP decreases
Na⁺ channels
close
⇒ salt shaker
SALT
↓
Hyperpolarization
⇒ hyper polar bear
↓
Glutamate decreases
⇒ glue
GLUE

NOTES

EAR ANATOMY

- Three compartments of the ear
  - outer ear → sound enters the external auditory meatus on its way to the tympanic membrane
  - middle ear → contains three ossicles (malleus, incus, stapes) that transmit sound waves from the tympanic membrane to the oval window; air-filled cavity
  - inner ear → contains cochlea, vestibule, and semicircular canals; fluid-filled cavity

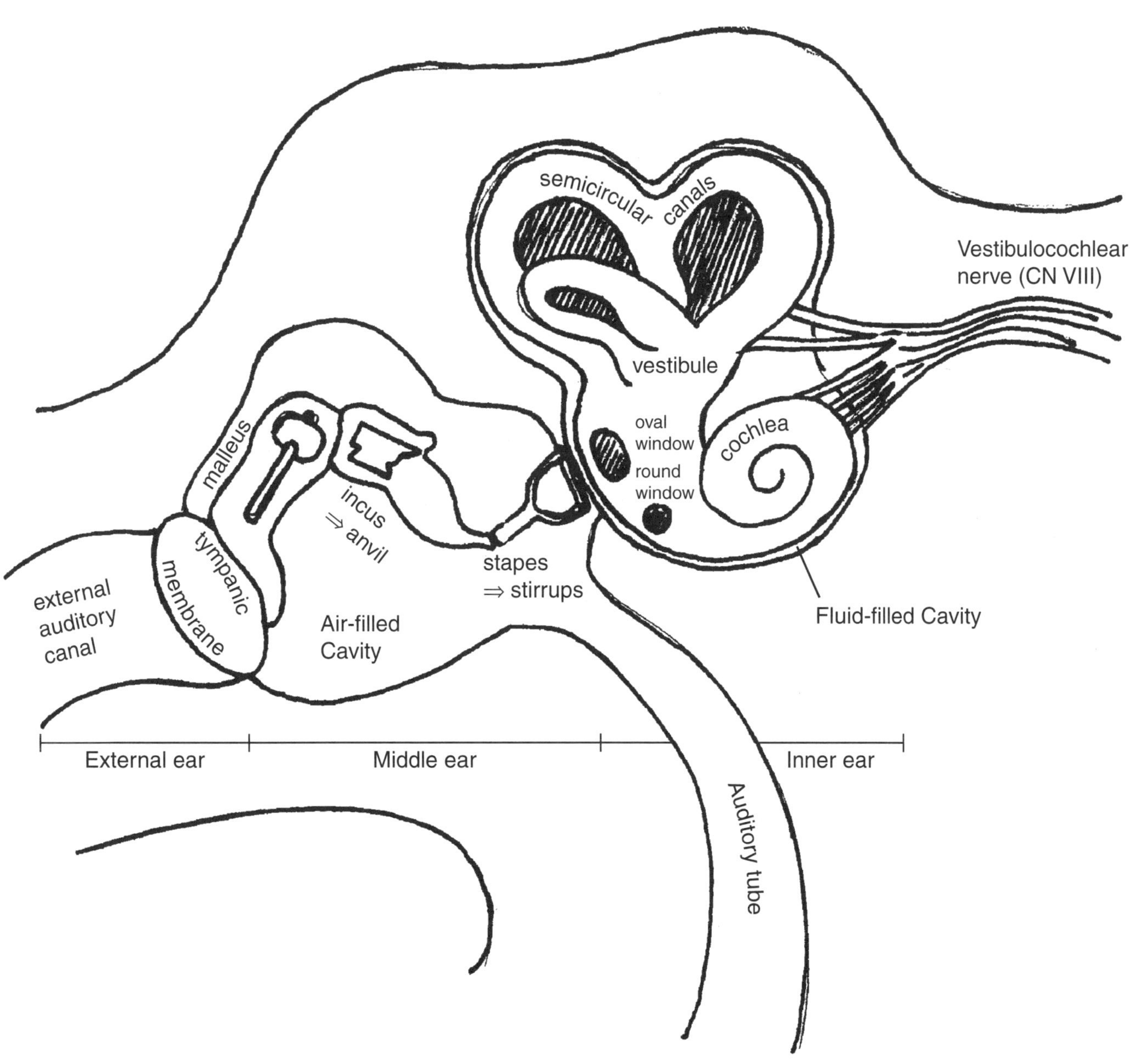
semicircular canals
Vestibulocochlear
nerve (CN VIII)
vestibule
malleus
oval
window
round
window
cochlea
incus
⇒ anvil
tympanic
membrane
stapes
⇒ stirrups
external
auditory
canal
Air-filled
Cavity
Fluid-filled Cavity
External ear
Middle ear
Inner ear
Auditory tube

NOTES

What do you see through an otoscope?

(Hopefully not too much ear wax)

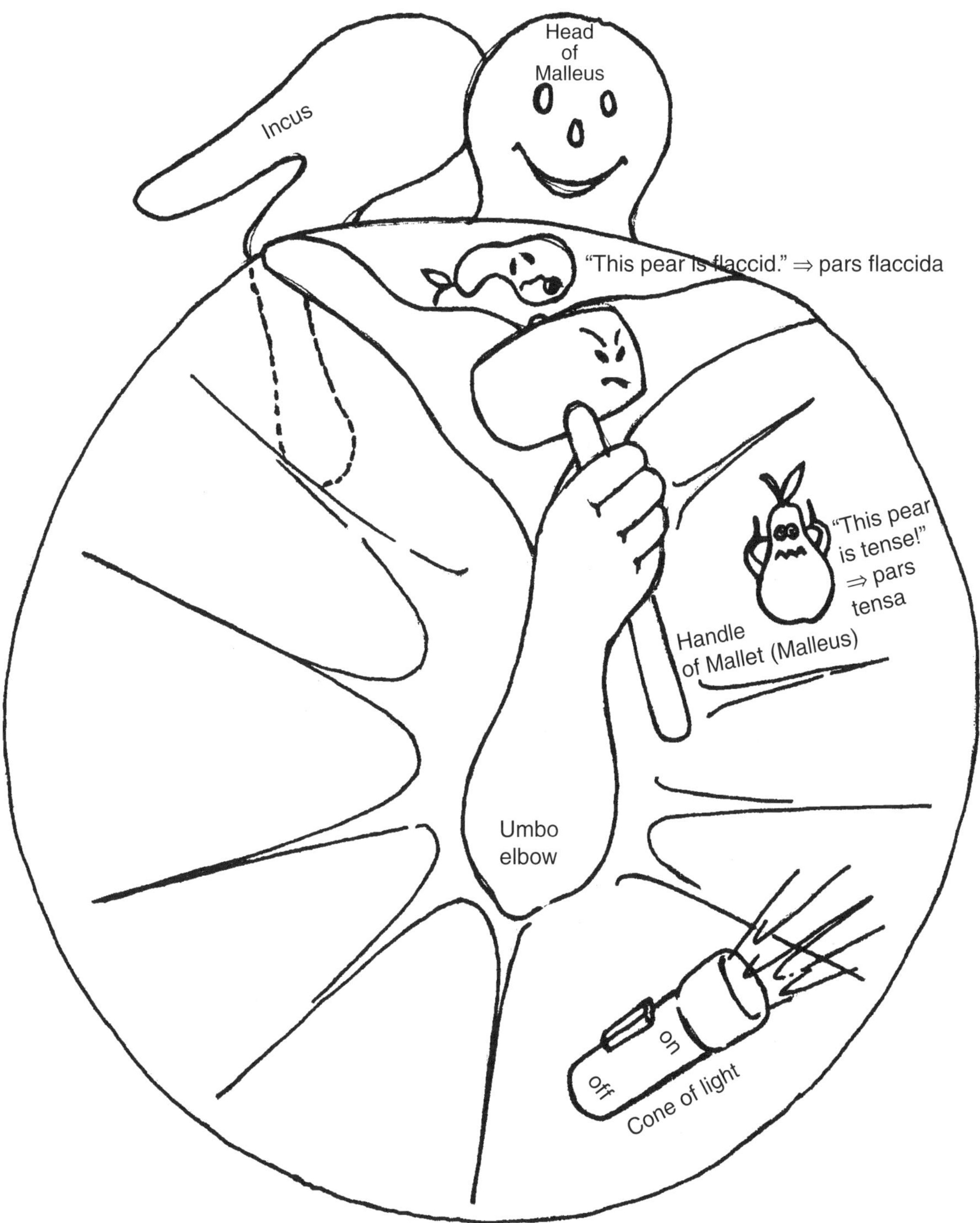

NOTES

MIDDLE EAR MUSCLES

Stapedius muscle

- Attaches to the neck of the stapes
- Pulls the stapes posteriorly, which prevents too much vibration of the oval window and protects the inner ear during a loud noise
- Innervated by cranial nerve 7 or the facial nerve

Tensor tympani muscle

- Attaches to the handle of the malleus
- Pulls the handle of the malleus medially, which causes the tympanic membrane to become tense
- Innervated by the mandibular branch (V3) of the trigeminal nerve (cranial nerve 5)

Stapedius Muscle

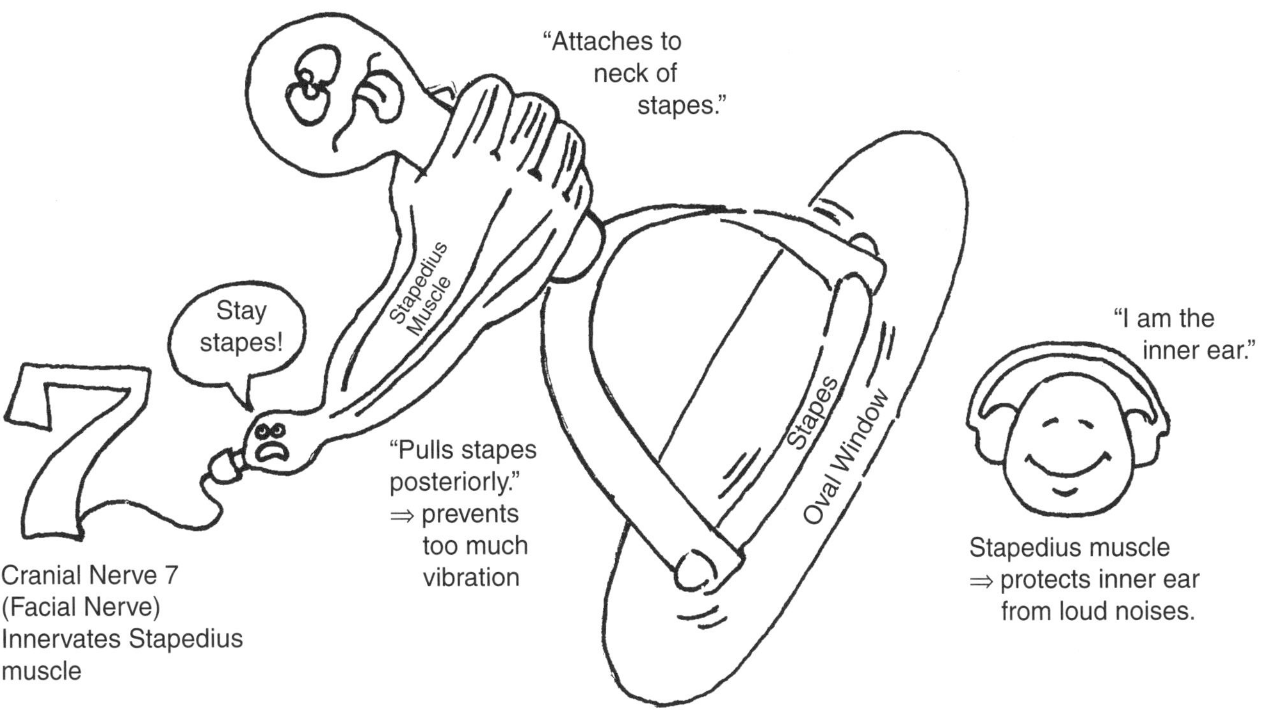

Tensor Tympani Muscle

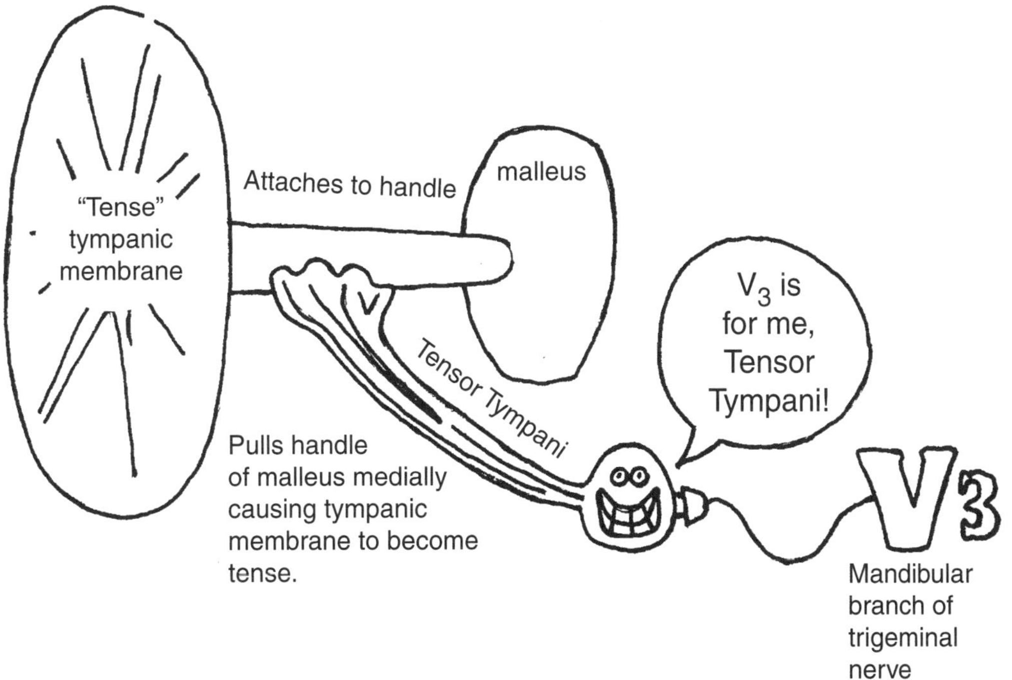

NOTES

VESTIBULE, COCHLEA, AND SEMICIRCULAR CANALS UP CLOSE

COCHLEA

- Three tubular compartments: scala vestibuli, scala tympani, and scala media
- Scala vestibuli and scala tympani communicate at the helicotrema containing perilymph, which has a high sodium content
- Scala media lies between the scala vestibuli and scala tympani containing endolymph, which has a high potassium content; the organ of Corti is attached to the basilar membrane at the base of the scala media
    - Organ of Corti: contains inner (few) and outer (many) hair cells that synapse with the spiral ganglion (cell bodies of CN VIII); cilia of hair cells are embedded in tectorial membrane
    - basilar membrane: low frequencies detected at the apex near the helicotrema; high frequencies detected at base near oval and round windows
    - sound transmission: refer to sound transmission illustration

VESTIBULE AND SEMICIRCULAR CANALS

- Semicircular canals: three perpendicular canals filled with endolymph detect angular acceleration; receptors (hair cells) located at end of canals and embedded in cupula detect rotation when fluid movement bends the stereocilia either toward or away from the kinocilium (longest cilium on each hair cell); toward kinocilium results in depolarization (activation), away results in hyperpolarization (inhibition)
- Saccule and utricle of vestibule detect linear acceleration

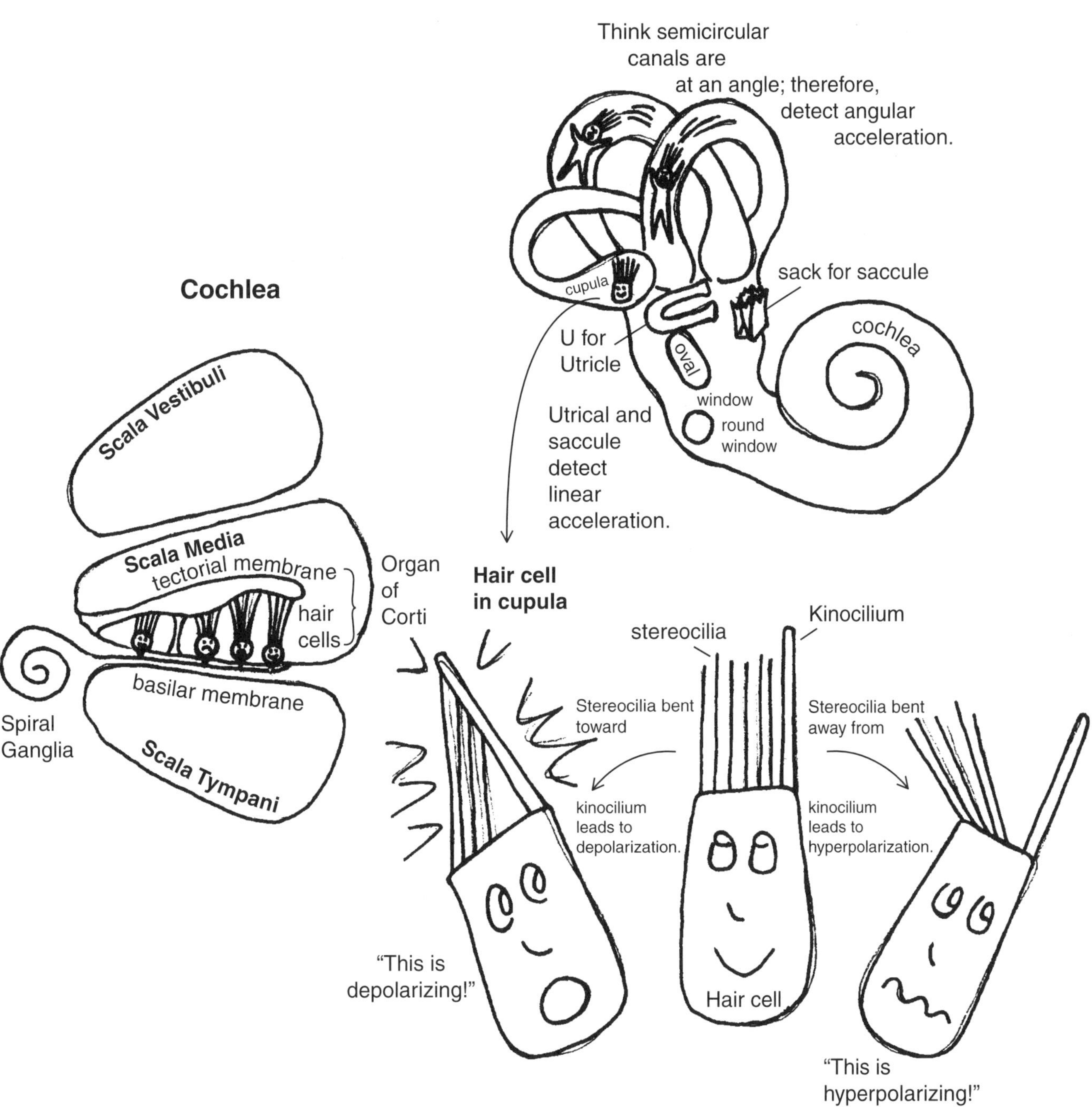
Vestibule and Semicircular Canals
Think semicircular canals are at an angle; therefore, detect angular acceleration.
cupula
U for Utricle
sack for saccule
oval
window
round window
cochlea
Utrical and saccule detect linear acceleration.
Cochlea
Scala Vestibuli
Scala Media
tectorial membrane
hair cells
Organ of Corti
basilar membrane
Spiral Ganglia
Scala Tympani
Hair cell in cupula
stereocilia
Kinocilium
Stereocilia bent toward
kinocilium leads to depolarization.
Stereocilia bent away from
kinocilium leads to hyperpolarization.
"This is depolarizing!"
Hair cell
"This is hyperpolarizing!"

NOTES

SOUND TRANSMISSION

(1) sound waves enter external auditory meatus → (2) vibrate tympanic membrane → (3) vibrates three ossicles in following order → Malleus (hammer) → Incus (anvil) → Stapes (stirrups) → stapes attached to oval window → (4) therefore, transmitting vibrations to the perilymph of scala vestibuli → (amplification of sound energy) → vibrations now transmitted through fluid instead of air → vibrations travel through scala vestibuli → (5) communicate with scala tympani at helicotrema → (6) as vibrations travel through scala tympani, basilar membrane vibrates (high frequency at base of basilar membrane near oval and round window; low frequency at apex of basilar membrane near helicotrema) → vibration of organ of Corti attached to basilar membrane → (7) hair cells bend because of attachment to tectorial membrane → change in K+ conductance → different directions cause depolarization or hyperpolarization → oscillating potential → (8) activation of cochlear nerves

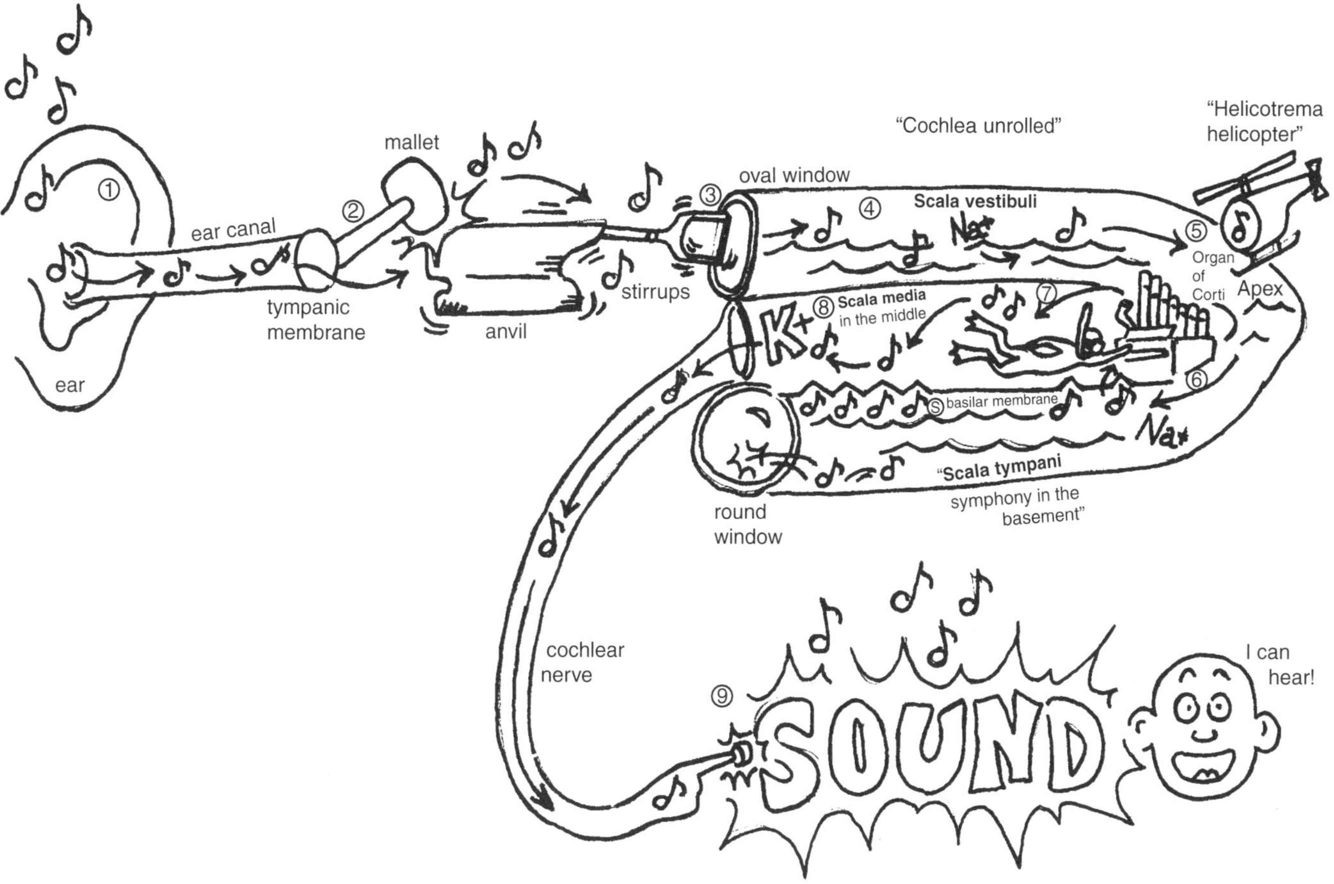
ear
①
ear canal
②
tympanic membrane
mallet
anvil
stirrups
③
oval window
"Cochlea unrolled"
④
Scala vestibuli
Na+
"Helicotrema helicopter"
⑤
Organ of Corti
Apex
⑦
⑧ Scala media in the middle
K+
⑤ basilar membrane
⑥
Na+
"Scala tympani symphony in the basement"
round window
cochlear nerve
⑨
SOUND
I can hear!

NOTES

HEART CIRCULATION

Deoxygenated blood from head and lower body enters right atrium through superior and inferior vena cava → through tricuspid valve to right ventricle → to pulmonary arteries → to lungs → pulmonary veins → left atrium → through mitral valve to left ventricle → to aorta then to body

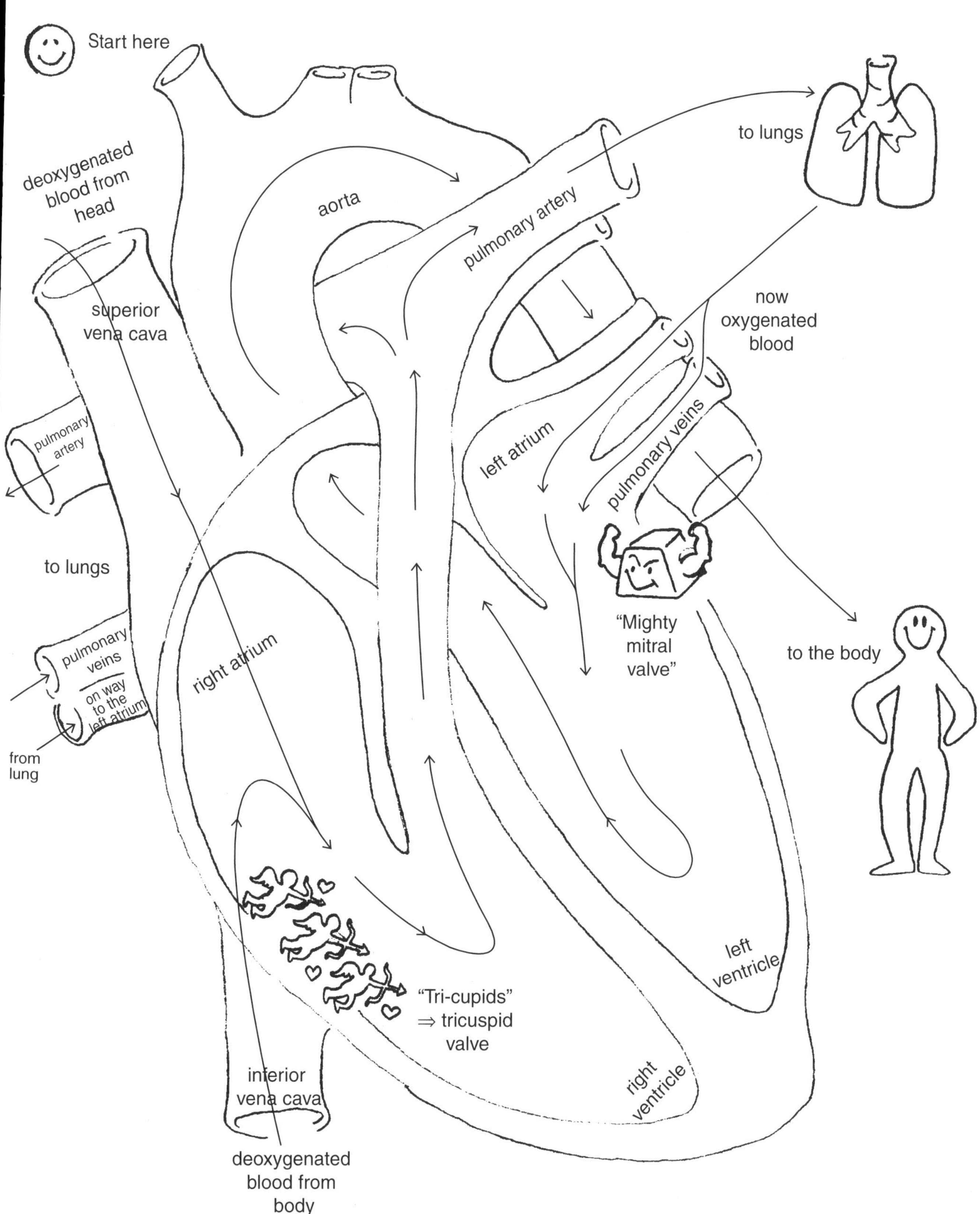
Start here
deoxygenated blood from head
aorta
pulmonary artery
to lungs
superior vena cava
now oxygenated blood
pulmonary artery
left atrium
pulmonary veins
to lungs
"Mighty mitral valve"
to the body
pulmonary veins
on way to the left atrium
right atrium
from lung
"Tri-cupids"
⇒ tricuspid valve
left ventricle
right ventricle
inferior vena cava
deoxygenated blood from body

NOTES

FETAL CIRCULATION

Placenta → umbilical vein (oxygenated blood) → ductus venosus → inferior vena cava → right atrium → foramen ovale → aorta → head and brain → superior vena cava → right atrium → right ventricle → pulmonary trunk → ductus arteriosus (connects pulmonary trunk to aorta moving blood to lower body) and pulmonary arteries to lungs → blood diverted to descending aorta eventually returns to placenta via two umbilical arteries

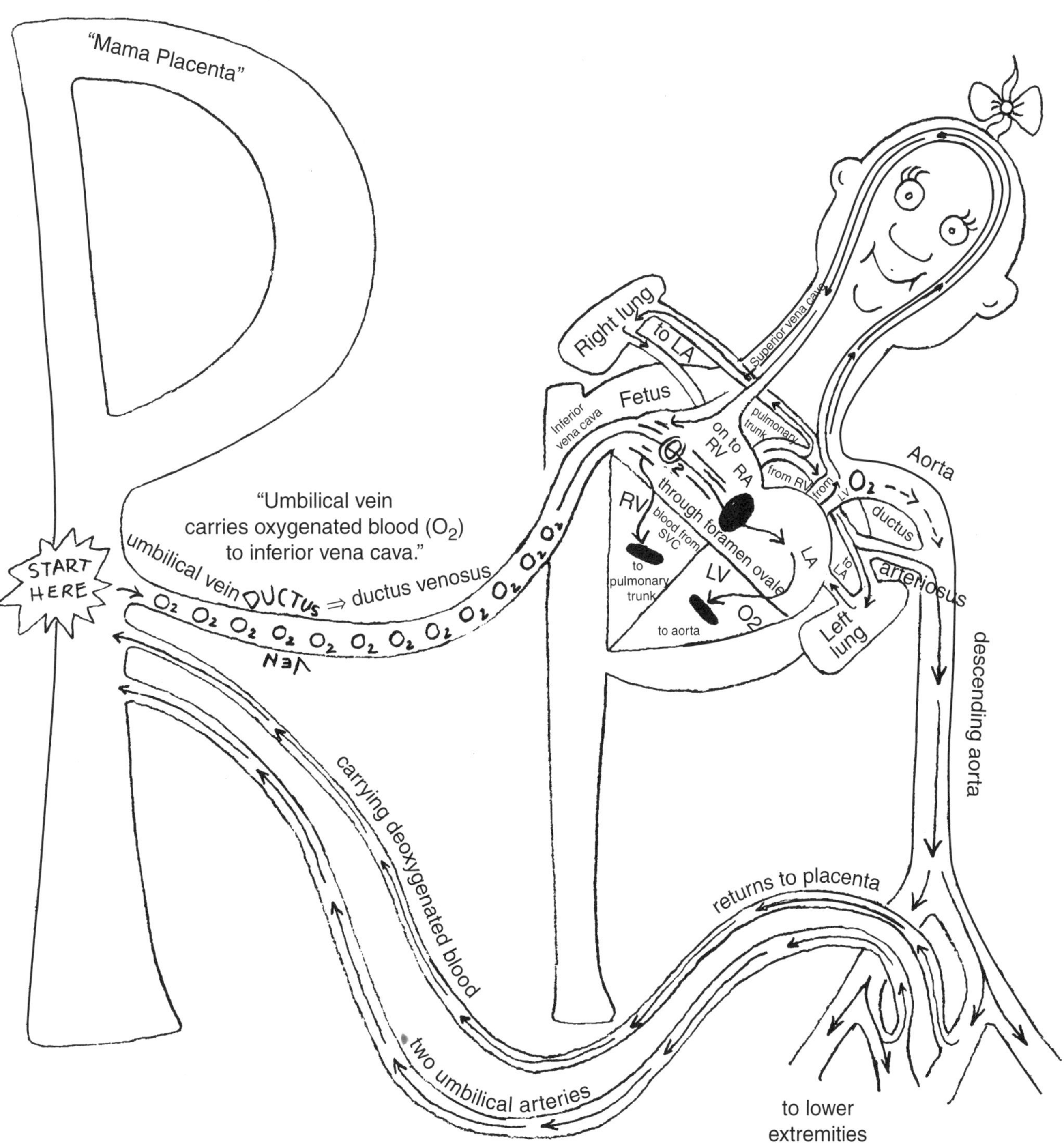
"Mama Placenta"
Right lung
to LA
Superior vena cava
Fetus
Inferior vena cava
pulmonary trunk
on to RV
RA
from RV
from LV
Aorta
"Umbilical vein carries oxygenated blood (O_2) to inferior vena cava."
RV
through foramen ovale
blood from SVC
ductus
LA
START HERE
umbilical vein DUCTUS ⇒ ductus venosus
to pulmonary trunk
LV
to LA
arteriosus
to aorta
Left lung
descending aorta
carrying deoxygenated blood
returns to placenta
two umbilical arteries
to lower extremities

NOTES

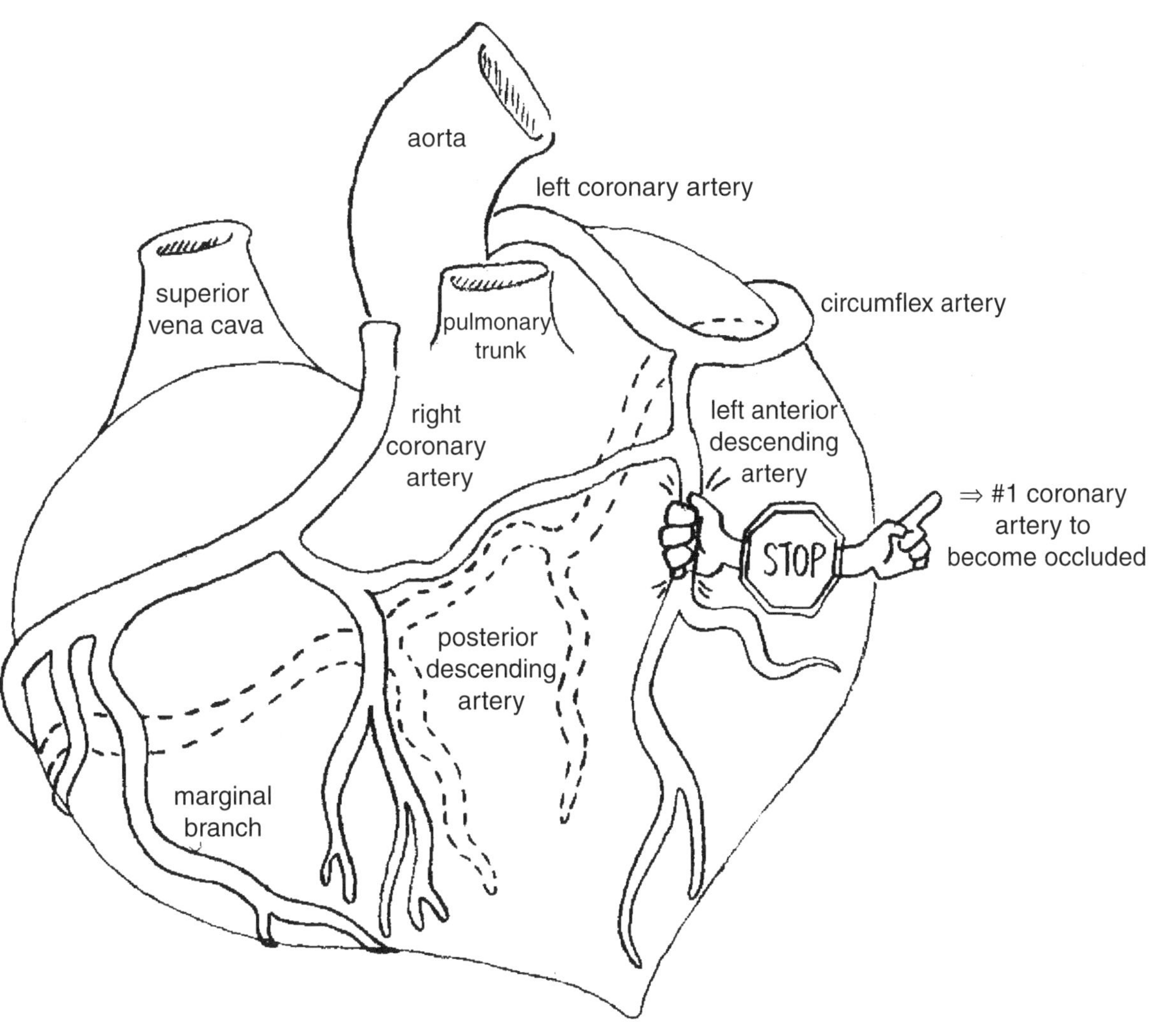
aorta
left coronary artery
superior vena cava
pulmonary trunk
circumflex artery
right coronary artery
left anterior descending artery
⇒ #1 coronary artery to become occluded
STOP
posterior descending artery
marginal branch

NOTES

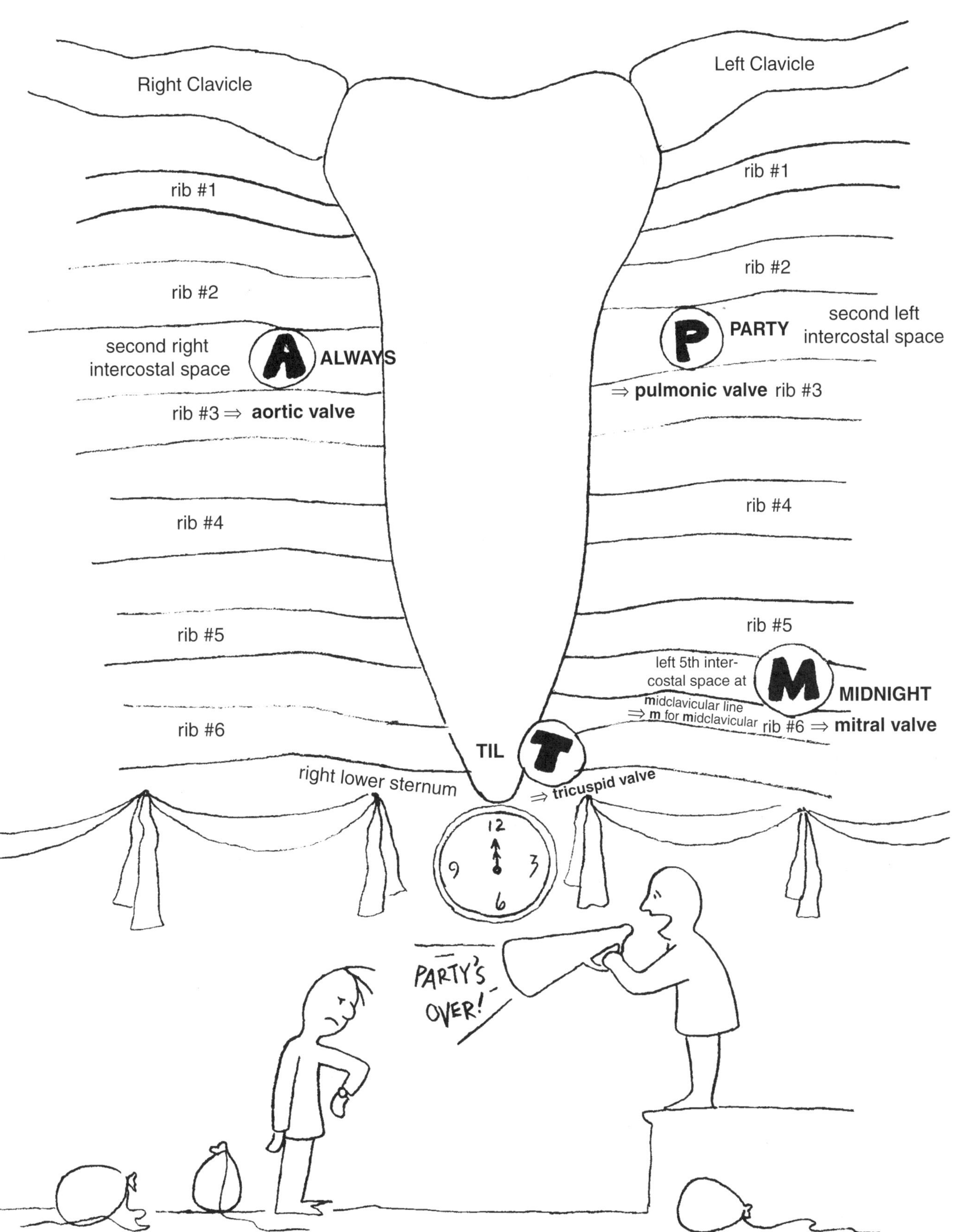
Right Clavicle
Left Clavicle
rib #1
rib #1
rib #2
rib #2
second right intercostal space
A ALWAYS
rib #3 ⇒ aortic valve
P PARTY
second left intercostal space
⇒ pulmonic valve rib #3
rib #4
rib #4
rib #5
rib #5
left 5th intercostal space at midclavicular line ⇒ m for midclavicular
M MIDNIGHT
rib #6 ⇒ mitral valve
rib #6
TIL
T
right lower sternum
⇒ tricuspid valve
12
3
6
9
PARTY'S OVER!

NOTES

CARDIAC MUSCLE

- Sarcomere → contractile component of myocardial cell (Z-Z line)
- Actin → thin filament
- Myosin → thick filament
- Myocardial action potential
  - phases
    - 0 → rapid upstroke; voltage-gated Na^+ channels open; Na^+ enters thus causing depolarization
    - 1 → initial or partial repolarization; Na^+ channels close and voltage-gated K^+ channels open
    - 2 → plateau; voltage-gated Ca^{2+} open allowing calcium in to equal K^+ out
    - 3 → rapid repolarization; increased K^+ efflux as slow K^+ voltage-gated channels open leading to hyperpolarization
    - 4 → resting membrane potential; K^+ in equals K^+ out
- Equilibrium potentials
  - E Na^+ → +65mV E Ca^{2+} → +120mV
  - E K^+ → –90mV E Cl^- → –85mV

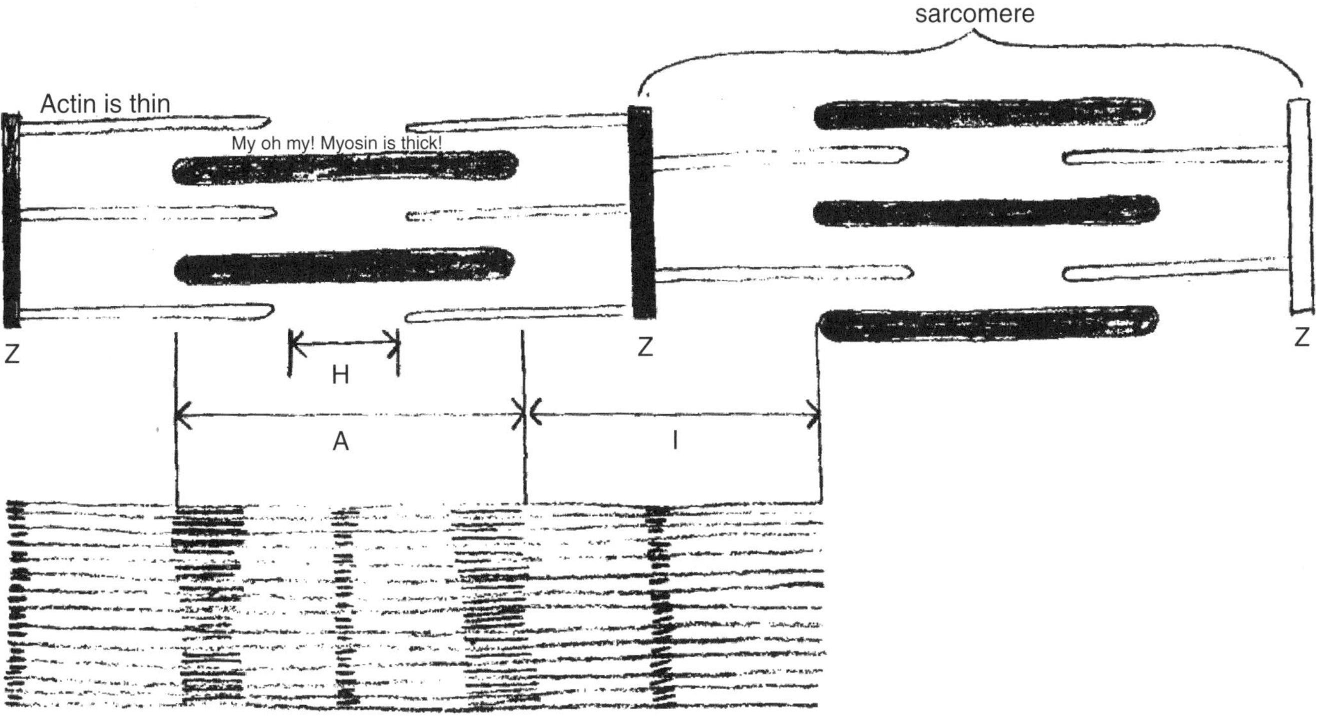
sarcomere
Actin is thin
My oh my! Myosin is thick!
Z
Z
Z
H
A
I

NOTES

CARDIAC MUSCLE CONTRACTION

Action potential (AP) travels down cell membrane → AP continues down T-tubule (which is continuous with cell membrane) → calcium conductance increased (calcium enters cell → inward calcium current) → increased intracellular calcium concentration causes release of more calcium from sarcoplasmic reticulum → calcium binds troponin C → tropomyosin removed from inhibitory site → actin and myosin now free to interact → cross-bridges formed as thick and thin filaments slide past one another → causes contraction (tension intracellular calcium concentration) → active calcium-ATPase pump pumps calcium back into sarcoplasmic reticulum → muscle relaxation

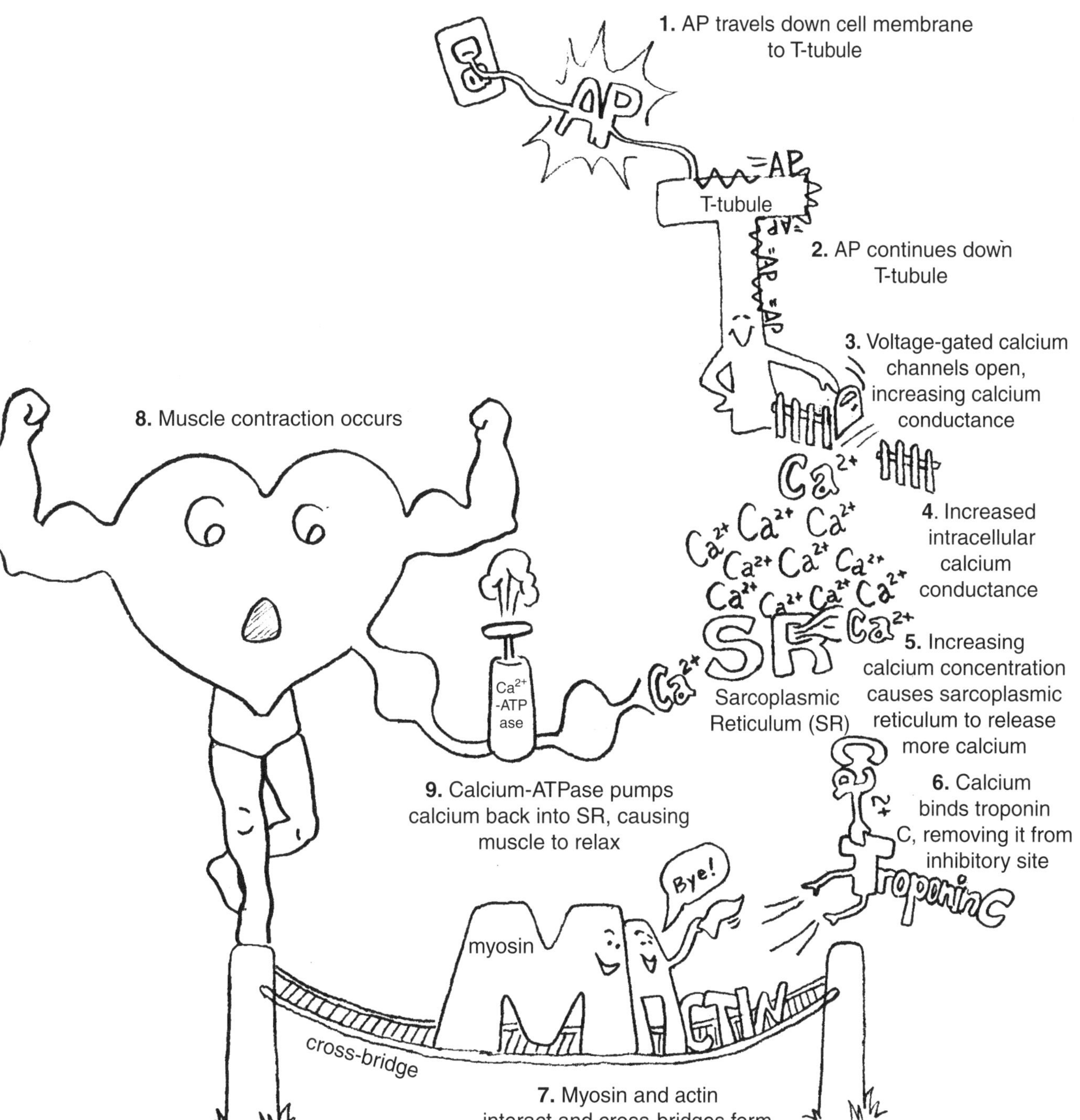
1. AP travels down cell membrane to T-tubule
AP
AP
T-tubule
AP
AP
AP
2. AP continues down T-tubule
3. Voltage-gated calcium channels open, increasing calcium conductance
8. Muscle contraction occurs
Ca2+
4. Increased intracellular calcium conductance
SR
5. Increasing calcium concentration causes sarcoplasmic reticulum to release more calcium
Sarcoplasmic Reticulum (SR)
Ca2+ -ATP ase
6. Calcium binds troponin C, removing it from inhibitory site
9. Calcium-ATPase pumps calcium back into SR, causing muscle to relax
Bye!
TroponinC
myosin
ACTIN
cross-bridge
7. Myosin and actin interact and cross-bridges form

NOTES

PACEMAKER ACTION POTENTIAL (SLOW RESPONSE CELLS)

- Calcium current
- SA (sinoatrial) and AV (atrioventricular) nodes
- Phases 1 and 2 do not exist
- No constant resting membrane potential
- Phase 0
  - Slow upstroke of AP due to inward calcium current
  - No fast sodium channels as in fast response cells
- Phase 3
  - phase in which repolarization occurs
  - increased potassium conductance
  - potassium vacates cell
- Phase 4
  - slow diastolic depolarization
  - potassium conductance decreases
  - sodium conductance increases
  - automaticity or pacemaker activity of SA and AV nodes

SA and AV nodes ⇒ calcium current

*Phases 1 and 2 do not exist

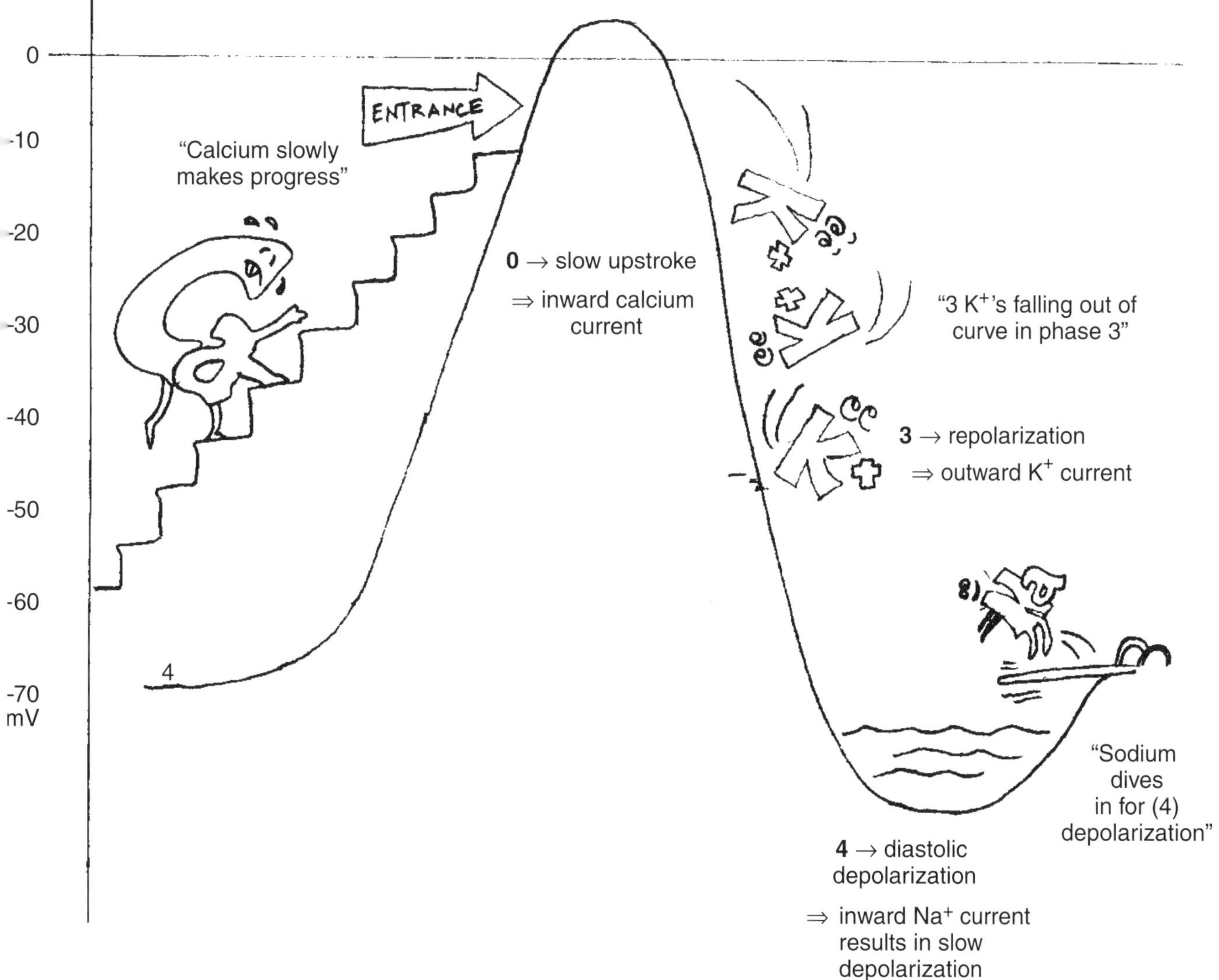

NOTES

⇒ **sodium current**
Atrial, ventricular, internodal, and Purkinje muscle cells

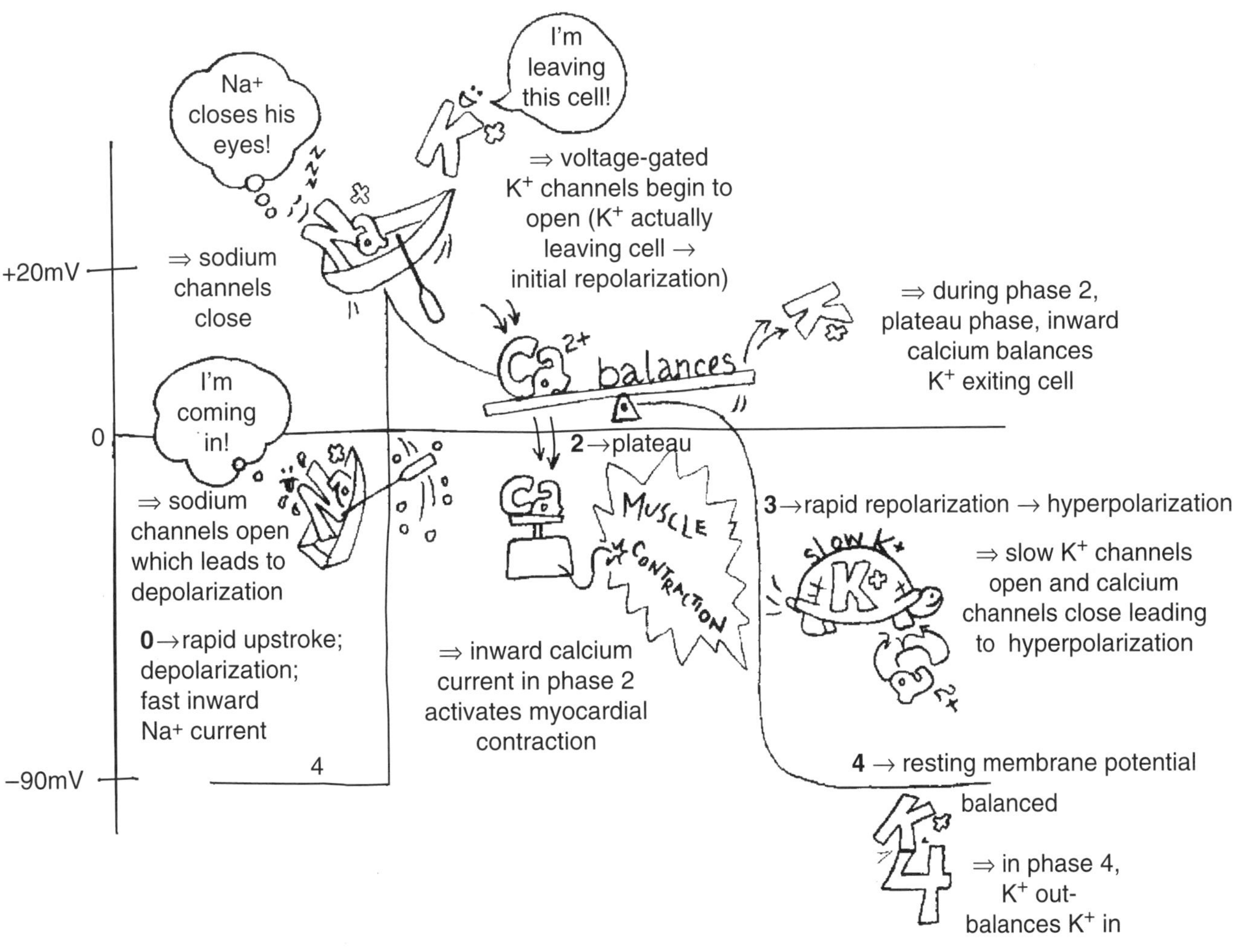
Na^+ closes his eyes!
I'm leaving this cell!
⇒ voltage-gated K^+ channels begin to open (K^+ actually leaving cell → initial repolarization)
+20mV
⇒ sodium channels close
Ca^{2+} balances
⇒ during phase 2, plateau phase, inward calcium balances K^+ exiting cell
I'm coming in!
0
2→plateau
MUSCLE CONTRACTION
3→rapid repolarization → hyperpolarization
⇒ sodium channels open which leads to depolarization
SLOW K^+
⇒ slow K^+ channels open and calcium channels close leading to hyperpolarization
0→rapid upstroke; depolarization; fast inward Na^+ current
⇒ inward calcium current in phase 2 activates myocardial contraction
−90mV
4
4 → resting membrane potential balanced
⇒ in phase 4, K^+ out-balances K^+ in

NOTES

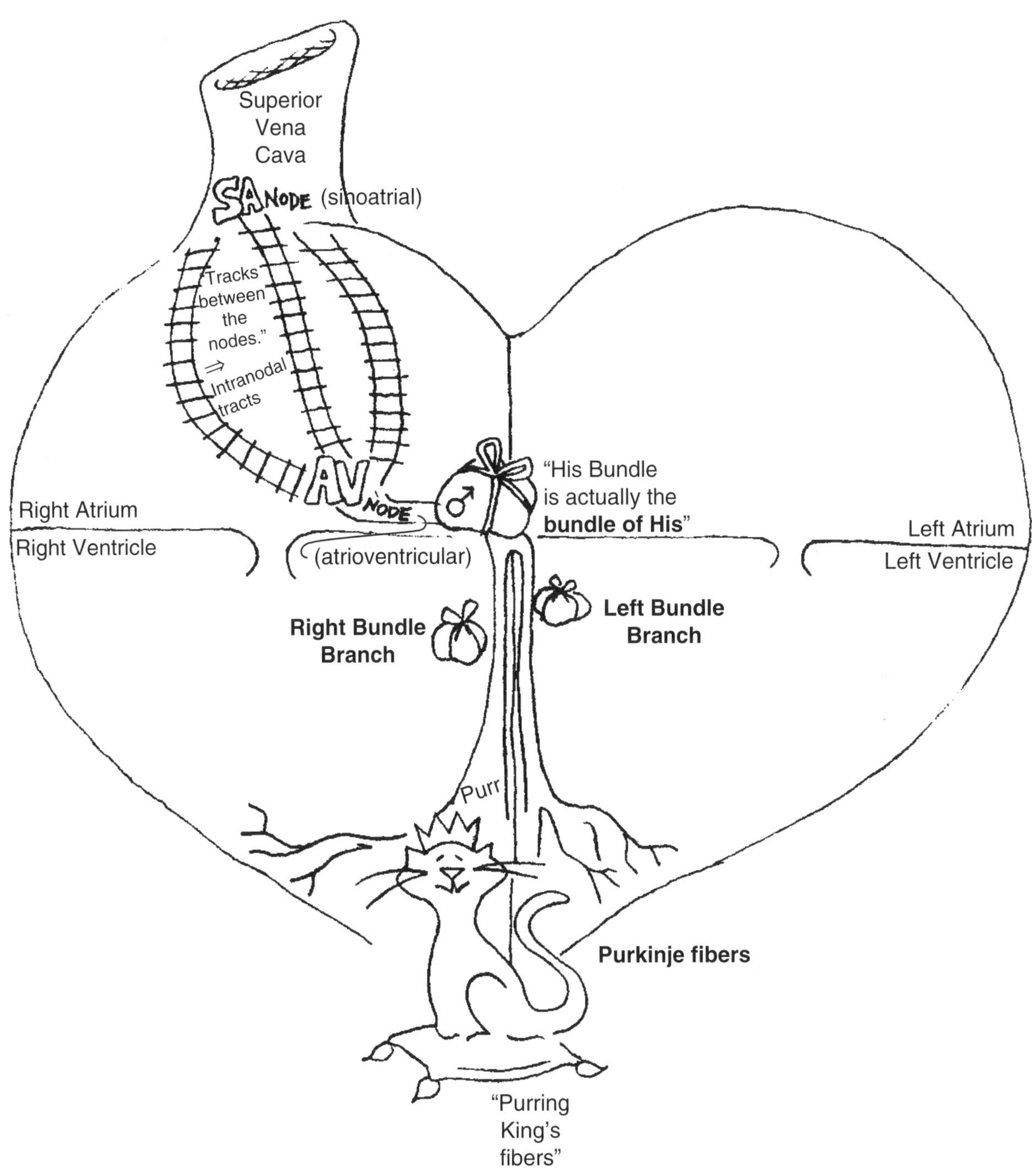
Superior
Vena
Cava
SA NODE (sinoatrial)
"Tracks between the nodes." ⇒ Intranodal tracts
AV NODE
(atrioventricular)
"His Bundle
is actually the
bundle of His"
Right Atrium
Right Ventricle
Left Atrium
Left Ventricle
Right Bundle
Branch
Left Bundle
Branch
Purr
Purkinje fibers
"Purring
King's
fibers"

NOTES

PARASYMPATHETIC AND SYMPATHETIC EFFECTS

PARASYMPATHETIC

- Vagus nerve releases acetylcholine (ACh) that acts on muscarinic cholinergic receptors on the SA and AV nodes but NOT the ventricles
- Decreasing SA node phase 4 depolarization (by decreasing inward sodium current), therefore, decreasing heart rate (negative chronotropic effect)
- Increased PR interval by decreasing conduction velocity (decreased inward calcium current) via AV node (negative dromotropic effect)
    - allows more time for ventricular filling

SYMPATHETIC

- Sympathetics use norepinephrine, which acts on the B1 receptor on the entire heart
- Decreased PR interval by increasing conduction velocity (positive dromotropic effect → increased inward calcium current)
- Increasing SA node phase 4 rate thus increasing heart rate (positive chronotropic effect → increased inward sodium current)

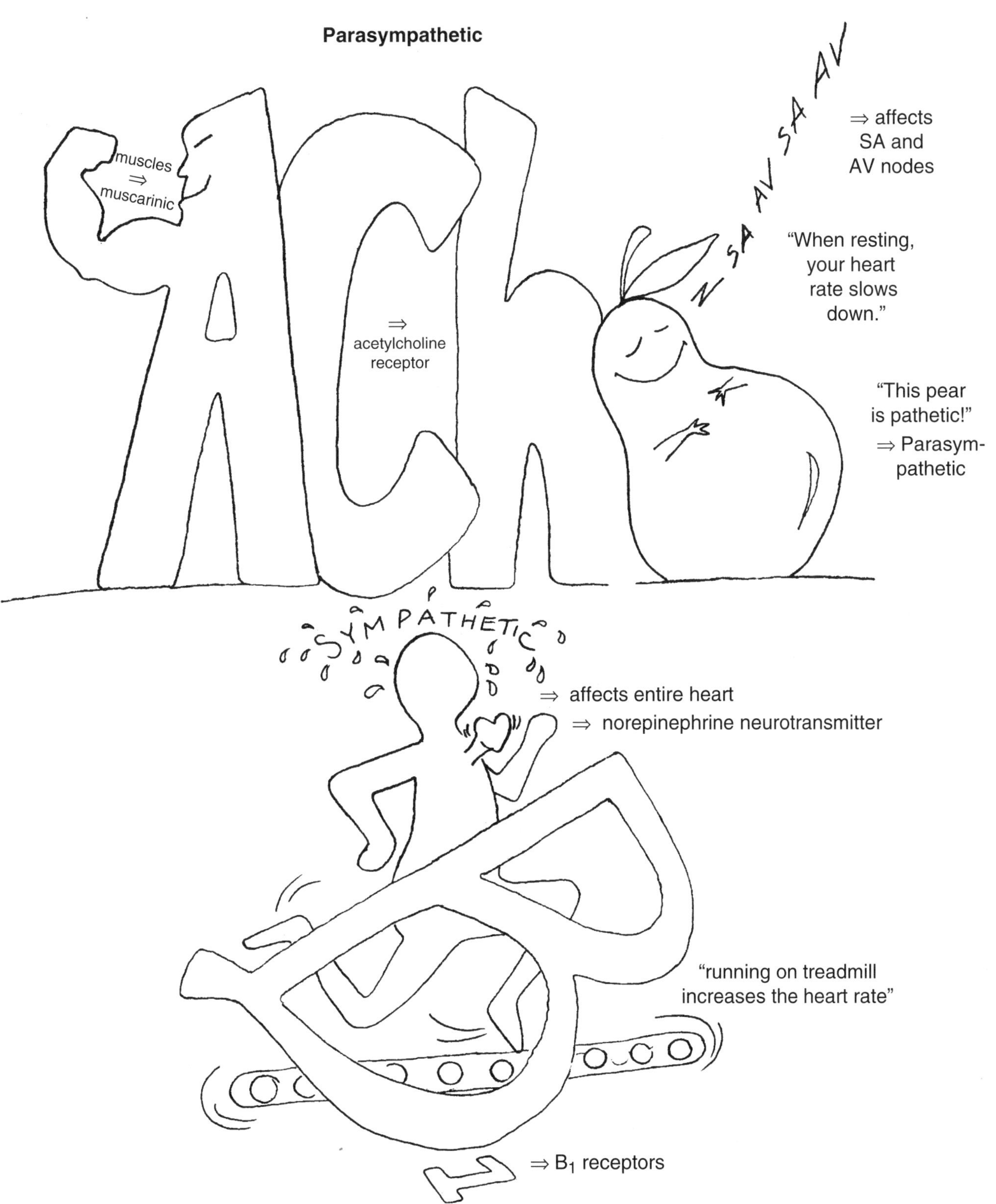
Parasympathetic
muscles
⇒
muscarinic
⇒
acetylcholine
receptor
SA AV SA AV SA AV
⇒ affects
SA and
AV nodes
"When resting,
your heart
rate slows
down."
"This pear
is pathetic!"
⇒ Parasym-
pathetic
SYMPATHETIC
⇒ affects entire heart
⇒ norepinephrine neurotransmitter
"running on treadmill
increases the heart rate"
⇒ B_1 receptors

NOTES

CARDIAC CYCLE

- Seven phases of cardiac cycle
  - atrial systole → aids ventricular filling
  - isovolumetric ventricular contraction → when ventricular > atrial pressure the mitral valve closes; mitral valve closure causes increased ventricular pressure without change in blood volume in ventricle; phase that consumes most oxygen
  - rapid ventricular ejection → most of stroke volume ejected; aortic valve opens when ventricular > aortic pressure (e.g., afterload)
  - slow ventricular ejection
  - isovolumetric ventricular relaxation → ventricular muscle relaxes resulting in decreased ventricular pressure; mitral valve opens when ventricular < atrial pressure
  - rapid and slow ventricular filling → ventricle fills until end diastolic volume (EDV) obtained
- Heart sounds
  - S1 → occurs when mitral and tricuspid valves close
  - S2 → occurs when aortic and pulmonary valves close; inspiration causes splitting of S2
  - S3 → occurs at end of rapid ventricular filling phase when ventricular dilation occurs (as with CHF)
  - S4 → occurs when there is high atrial pressure or stiff ventricle (e.g., with hypertrophic CHF); filling of ventricle during atrial systole
  - S3 and S4 heard when heart abnormalities present
- Jugular venous pulse
  - a wave → contraction of atria causes increased atrial or venous pressure
  - c wave → right ventricular contraction that corresponds to carotid pulse
  - v wave → as tricuspid valve closes the venous return causes increased atrial pressure

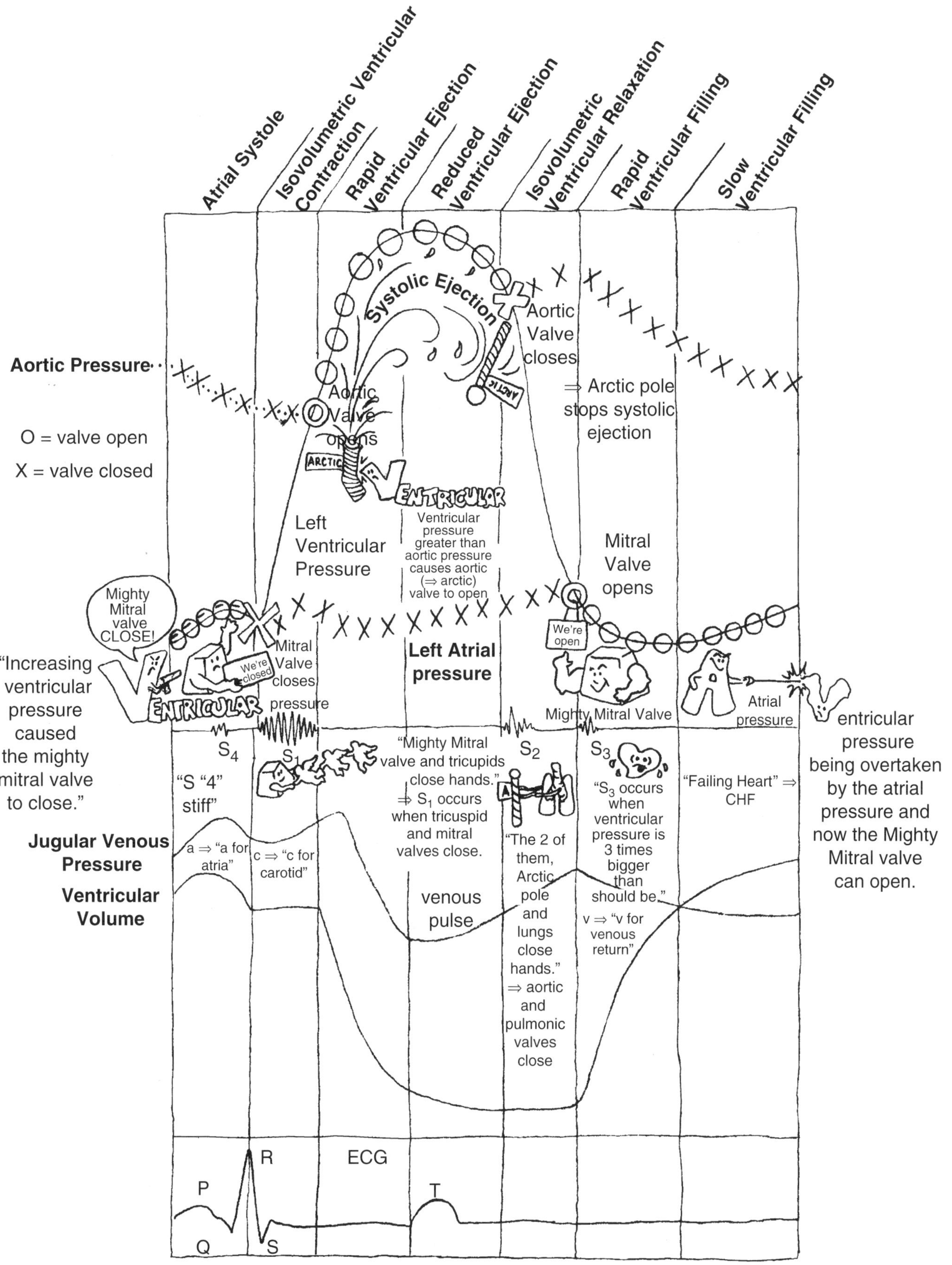

P → atrial depolarization
QRS → ventricular depolarization
T → ventricular repolarization

NOTES

LEFT VENTRICULAR PRESSURE-VOLUME LOOP

- Combination of diastolic and systolic pressure-volume curves
- Cycle explanation
    - A to B → isovolumetric contraction; all valves closed; ventricles begin to contract causing pressure to increase as volume remains the same
    - B to C → ventricular ejection; LV pressure overcomes aortic pressure and leads to ejection of blood from ventricle (stroke volume → pressure-volume loop width)
    - C to D → isovolumetric relaxation; all valves close; ventricle relaxes as volume remains the same
    - D to A → ventricular filling; LV pressure is less than LA pressure, which causes mitral valve to open allowing ventricular filling to occur
- Increased contractility → ↑ stroke volume
- Increased preload → ↑ stroke volume
- Increased afterload → ↓ stroke volume

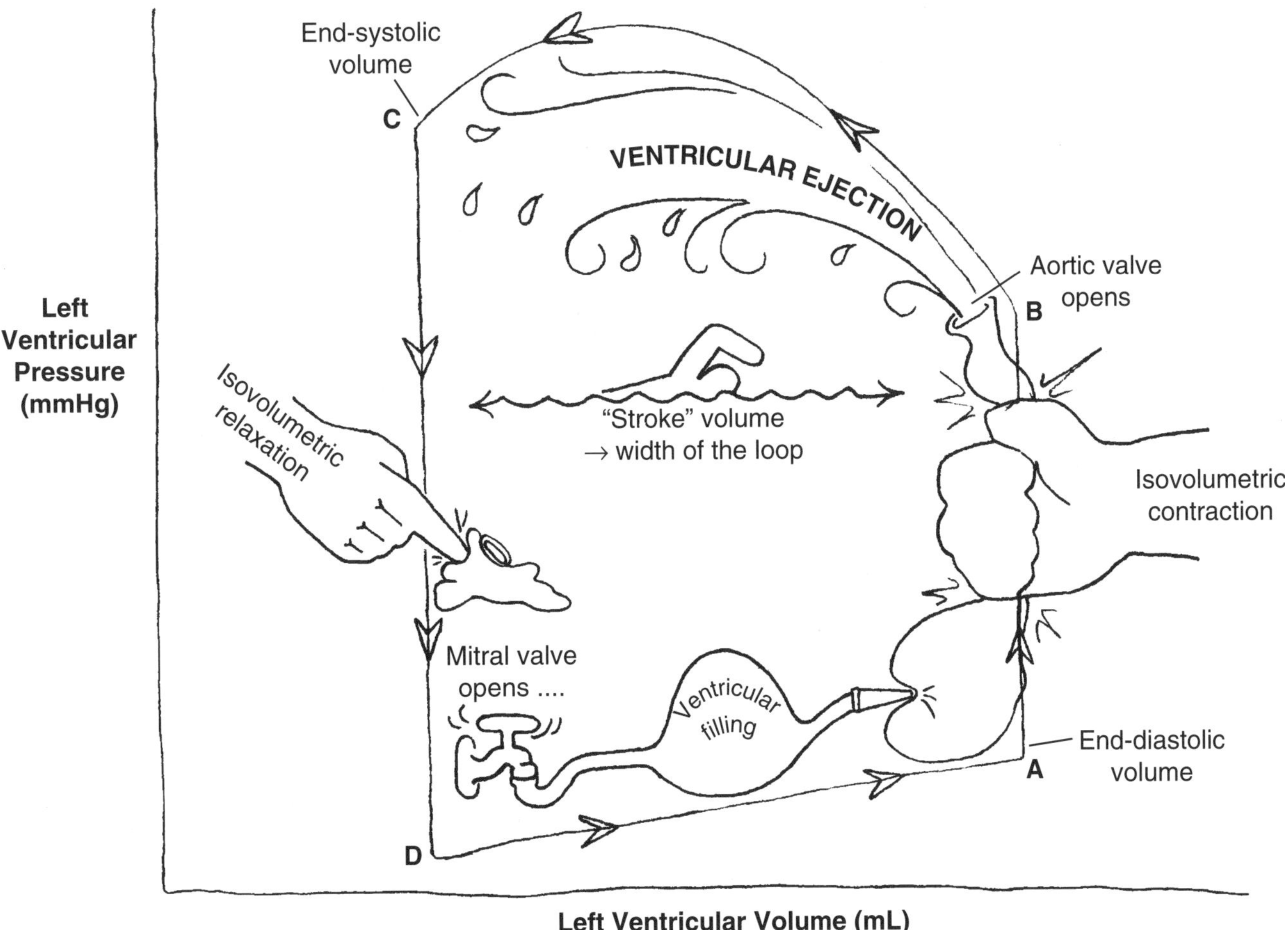
End-systolic
volume
C
VENTRICULAR EJECTION
Aortic valve
opens
B
Left
Ventricular
Pressure
(mmHg)
Isovolumetric
relaxation
"Stroke" volume
→ width of the loop
Isovolumetric
contraction
Mitral valve
opens ....
Ventricular
filling
End-diastolic
volume
A
D
Left Ventricular Volume (mL)

NOTES

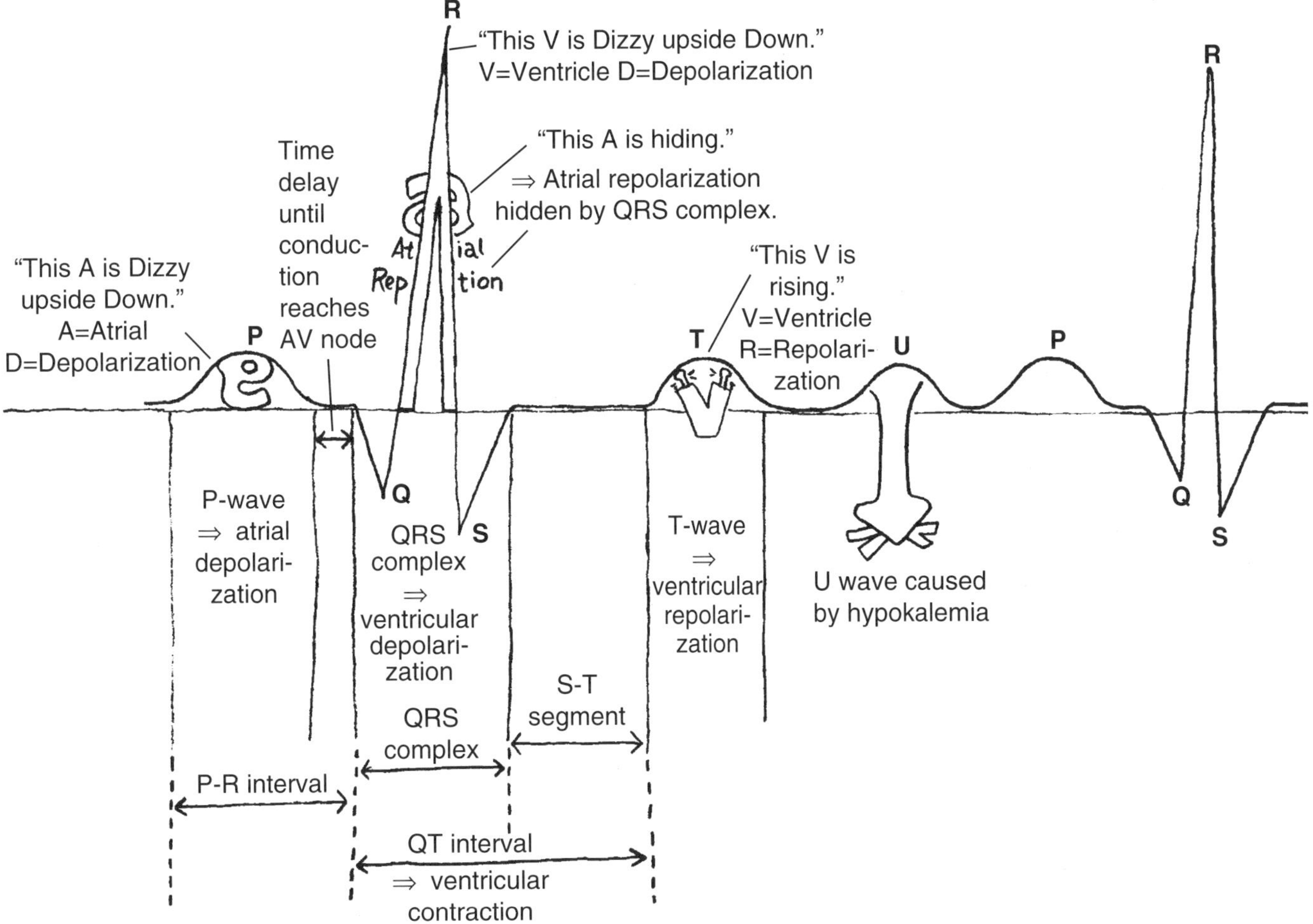
Start at top of heart with depolarization of atrium then ventricles.
Then repolarization must occur in the same order.
R
"This V is Dizzy upside Down."
V=Ventricle D=Depolarization
"This A is hiding."
⇒ Atrial repolarization
hidden by QRS complex.
Time delay until conduc-tion reaches AV node
Atrial Repolarization
"This A is Dizzy upside Down."
A=Atrial
D=Depolarization
P
"This V is rising."
V=Ventricle
R=Repolari-zation
T
U
P
R
Q
S
Q
S
P-wave ⇒ atrial depolari-zation
QRS complex ⇒ ventricular depolari-zation
T-wave ⇒ ventricular repolari-zation
U wave caused by hypokalemia
S-T segment
QRS complex
P-R interval
QT interval
⇒ ventricular contraction

NOTES

CONGENITAL HEART DISEASE

- Abnormalities of heart or great vessels
- Cause of congenital malformations: genetic factors and environmental factors
- Malformation categories: left-to-right shunt, right-to-left shunt, and obstruction
- Right-to-left shunts: cyanosis occurs due to decreased pulmonary blood flow and poorly oxygenated blood enters the systemic circulation (cyanotic congenital heart disease); examples include tetralogy of Fallot, transposition of the great vessels, persistent truncus arteriosus, tricuspid atresia, and total anomalous pulmonary venous connection
- Tetralogy of Fallot: four characteristics are VSD, subpulmonary stenosis, aorta that overrides VSD, and right ventricular hypertrophy; degree of difficulty depends on severity of subpulmonary stenosis; heart is boot-shaped
- Transposition of great arteries: aorta arises from right ventricle and pulmonary artery originates from the left ventricle; incompatible with life unless some form of shunt is present (e.g., VSD) that allows adequate blood mixing
- Truncus arteriosus: separation failure of aorta and pulmonary artery; single artery receives blood from both ventricles
- Tricuspid atresia: complete occlusion of tricuspid valve; VSD is also present
- Total anomalous pulmonary venous connection: no pulmonary veins join the left atrium directly; instead pulmonary veins are connected to superior vena cava or inferior vena cava; therefore, blood from lungs returns to right side of heart; patent foramen ovale or an ASD is always present
- Left-to-right shunt: ASD, ventricular septal defect (VSD), patent ductus arteriosus (PDA), and AV septal defects (AVSD)
- Pulmonary blood flow is increased, and therefore, cyanosis is not present; increased pulmonary pressure results in pulmonary hypertension that causes right ventricular hypertrophy and possible failure; eventually pulmonary pressure reaches systemic levels and the shunt is reversed to right-to-left, thereby sending unoxygenated blood into the systemic circulation (late cyanotic congenital heart disease or Eisenmenger syndrome)
- Atrial septal defect (ASD): abnormal opening in atrial septum (not a patent foramen ovale, which does NOT allow mixing of blood)
- Ventricular septal defect (VSD): most common congenital cardiac anomaly; Swiss-cheese septum (multiple VSDs in muscular septum)
- Patent ductus arteriosus (PDA): persistence of connection between pulmonary artery and aorta; a machine-like, continuous harsh murmur is heard
- Atrioventricular septal defect (AVSD): superior and inferior endocardial cushions do not fuse adequately; associated with Down's syndrome
- Obstructive congenital anomalies
    - coarctation of aorta—narrowing of the aorta; women with Turner's syndrome have this disease; two forms are infantile (constriction proximal to PDA) and adult (distal to PDA); hypertension in upper extremities and weak pulse in lower, resulting in claudication; murmur is heard throughout systole; associated with rib notching
    - pulmonary stenosis and atresia: obstruction of pulmonary valve → right ventricular hypertrophy
    - aortic stenosis and atresia: can be valvular, subvalvular, and supravalvular (thickening of ascending aortic wall associated with Williams syndrome); systolic murmur and thrill heard

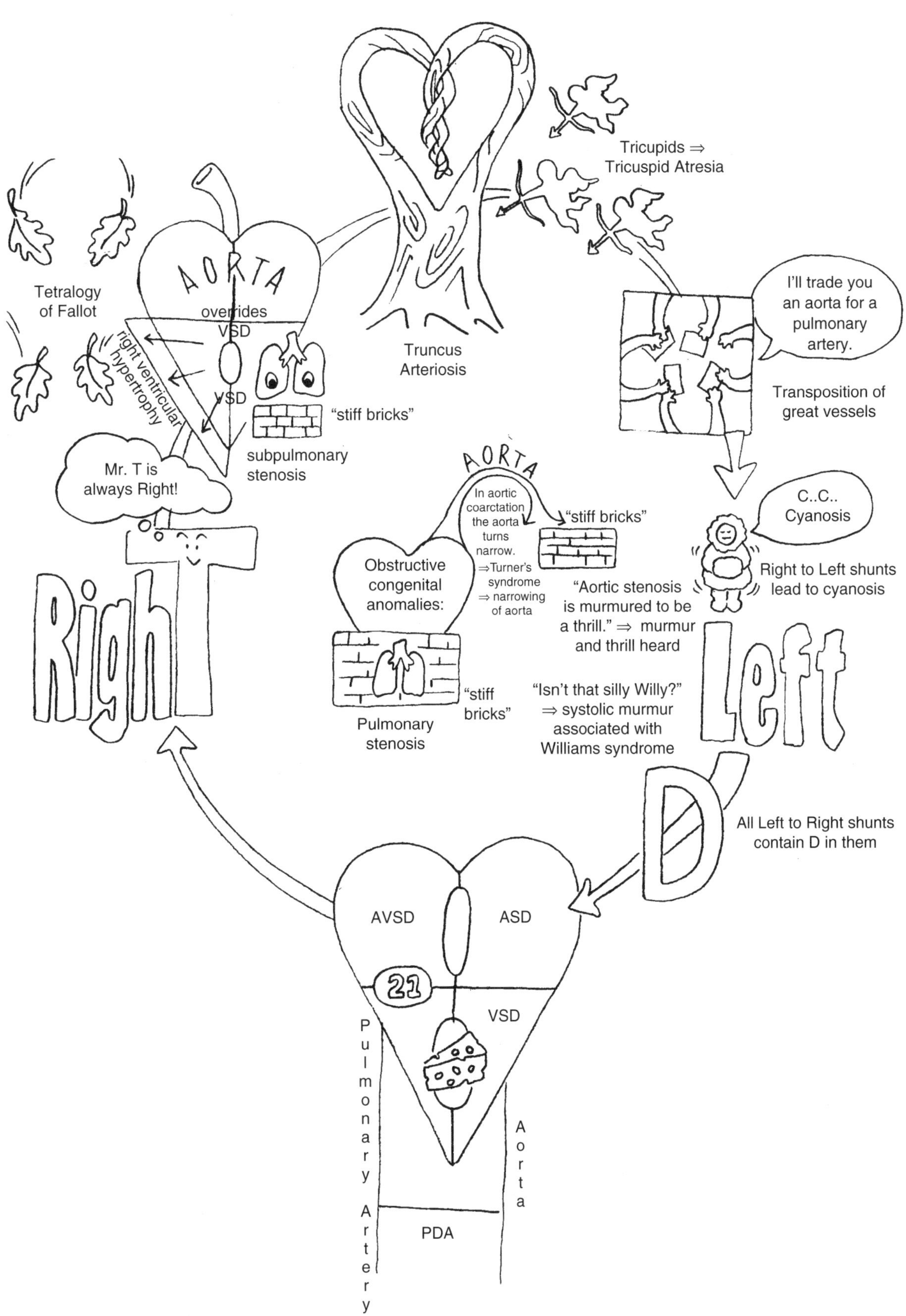
Tricupids ⇒ Tricuspid Atresia
Truncus Arteriosis
I'll trade you an aorta for a pulmonary artery.
Transposition of great vessels
AORTA
Tetralogy of Fallot
overrides VSD
right ventricular hypertrophy
VSD
"stiff bricks"
subpulmonary stenosis
Mr. T is always Right!
RighT
AORTA
In aortic coarctation the aorta turns narrow. ⇒Turner's syndrome ⇒ narrowing of aorta
"stiff bricks"
Obstructive congenital anomalies:
"stiff bricks"
Pulmonary stenosis
"Aortic stenosis is murmured to be a thrill." ⇒ murmur and thrill heard
"Isn't that silly Willy?" ⇒ systolic murmur associated with Williams syndrome
C.C.. Cyanosis
Right to Left shunts lead to cyanosis
Left
D
All Left to Right shunts contain D in them
AVSD
ASD
21
VSD
Pulmonary Artery
Aorta
PDA

NOTES

MYOCARDIAL INFARCTION

Two types:

- Transmural infarct—the entire thickness of vascular wall is affected
- Subendocardial infarct—inner one-third of myocardium affected because it is most susceptible to ischemia; caused by diffuse coronary atherosclerosis or global borderline perfusion

Early damage (within 20–40 minutes) is reversible

Almost all transmural infarcts involve the left ventricle; the right ventricle is rarely infarcted alone

Reperfusion injury can occur with the generation of free oxygen radicals; necrosis with contraction bands occurs when irreversibly damaged myocytes are reperfused and the cell's membranes are exposed to a high plasma calcium concentration; myocytes reperfused may be stunned, which depresses function

Clinical Features

- Patients present with rapid, weak pulse, diaphoresis, dyspnea, or pulmonary edema; ECG changes include formation of Q waves

Laboratory tests measure intracellular macromolecules concentrations released from damaged myocytes (creatine kinase → CK, of which CKMB is specific for the heart, and troponin I and troponin T)

Complications

- Contractile dysfunction
- Arrhythmias
- Myocardial rupture: most commonly the ventricular free wall → leads to cardiac tamponade; second most common is the ventricular septum → leads to left-to-right shunt; third most common is the papillary muscle → leads to mitral regurgitation; occurs 3–7 days postmyocardial infarction
- Pericarditis
- Right ventricular infarction
- Infarct extension or expansion
- Mural thrombosis
- Ventricular aneurysm
- Papillary muscle dysfunction
- Progressive heart failure

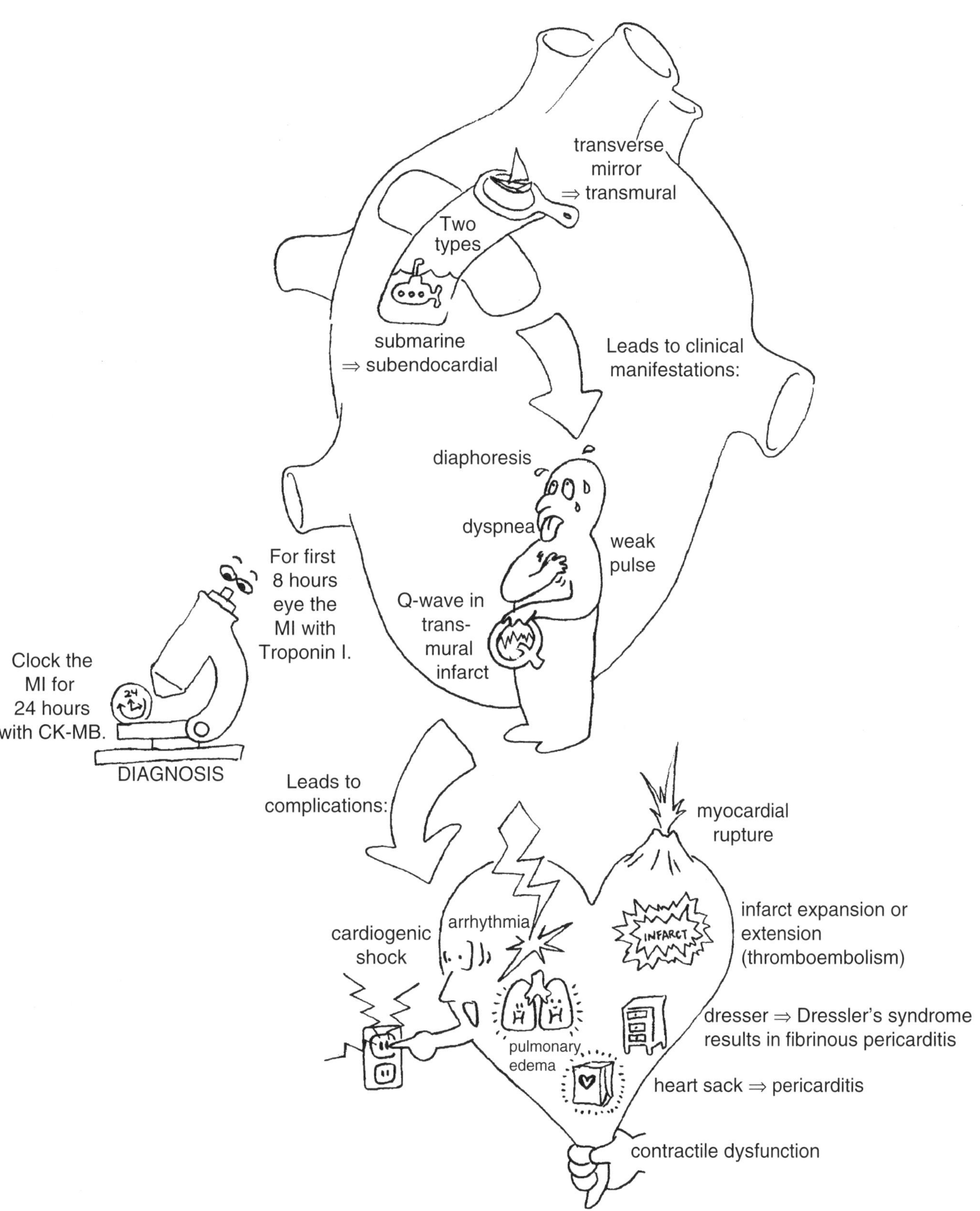
transverse
mirror
⇒ transmural
Two
types
submarine
⇒ subendocardial
Leads to clinical
manifestations:
diaphoresis
dyspnea
weak
pulse
Q-wave in
trans-
mural
infarct
For first
8 hours
eye the
MI with
Troponin I.
Clock the
MI for
24 hours
with CK-MB.
24
DIAGNOSIS
Leads to
complications:
myocardial
rupture
arrhythmia
cardiogenic
shock
INFARCT
infarct expansion or
extension
(thromboembolism)
pulmonary
edema
dresser ⇒ Dressler's syndrome
results in fibrinous pericarditis
heart sack ⇒ pericarditis
contractile dysfunction

NOTES

CONGESTIVE HEART FAILURE

General

- Defined as impaired cardiac function, leaves heart unable to maintain a cardiac output capable of meeting the body's metabolic demands
- CHF consequence of systolic dysfunction → decreased myocardial contractile function or diastolic dysfunction → heart does not sufficiently relax during diastole for proper filling
- Compensatory mechanisms: hypertrophy, ventricular dilation, blood volume expansion, and tachycardia

Causes of Right-Sided Heart Failure

- Number one cause is left-sided heart failure
- Pulmonary embolus

Leads to

- Decreased forward venous flow
- Liver congestion (a.k.a. nutmeg liver)
- Peripheral edema
- CNS and renal congestion

Causes of Left-Sided Heart Failure

- Hypertension
- Ischemic heart disease

Clinical Features

- Paroxysmal nocturnal dyspnea (patient needs many pillows to sleep without experiencing dyspnea)
- Orthopnea
- Dyspnea on exertion
- Other manifestations: histologically → heart failure cells in lungs; decreased CNS perfusion; decreased renal perfusion → increased renin production and release

Causes of left-sided heart failure:

hypertension

ischemic heart disease

Causes of right-sided heart failure:

#1 is left-sided heart failure and also –

pulmonary embolus

#1 cause of right-sided heart failure is left-sided heart failure

LEFT

RIGHT

knocks out forward venous flow

venous flow

Leads to:

cardiac dilation

I can't breathe!

heart failure cells

I can't breathe at night or lying down!

dyspnea on exertion

pulmonary edema

paroxysmal nocturnal dyspnea and orthopnea

Liver congestion

nutmeg liver

right-sided failure also causes:

CNS and RENAL congestion

right-sided failure also causes:

peripheral edema

Left-sided also causes:

decreased CNS perfusion & decreased renal perfusion

Leads to: increased RENIN release

NOTES

RESPIRATORY TRACT

- The respiratory tract conducts air to the lungs where gaseous exchange occurs. It is separated into air-conducting and respiratory (where gas exchange occurs) divisions.
- Upper respiratory tract includes the nasal cavity, pharynx, and larynx. The lower respiratory tract includes the trachea, bronchi, and bronchial tree.
- Beginning at the larynx, the respiratory tract is cartilaginous; the cartilage is then replaced by smooth muscle beginning at the bronchioles.
- The conchae are bony structures in the nasal cavity that increase the surface area, increase moisture, and warm the air that is conducted through the nasal passages.
- The pharynx consists mostly of skeletal muscle (the constrictor muscles) and fibrous tissue. It resides posterior and inferior to the nasal cavity and posterior to the oral cavity. It ends at the larynx and esophagus.
- The larynx produces sound for speech. The epiglottis covers the laryngeal opening during swallowing to prevent aspiration.
- The lobes of the lungs are encased in visceral pleura that eventually reflect off the lungs to become the parietal pleura that lines the inner wall of the thorax. The visceral and parietal pleura are separated only by a serous fluid. The potential space between these two pleura is called the "pleural cavity."

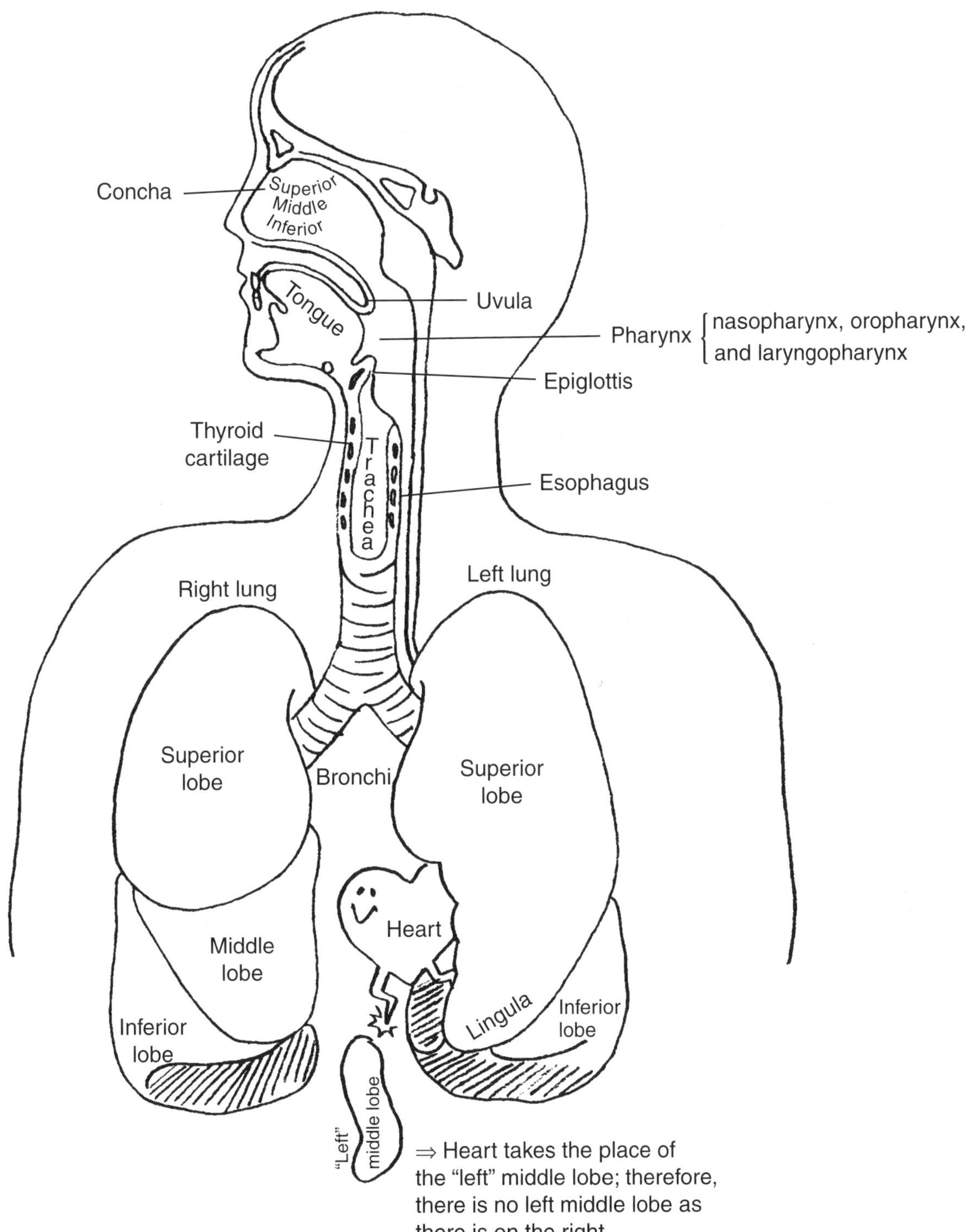

⇒ Heart takes the place of the "left" middle lobe; therefore, there is no left middle lobe as there is on the right.

NOTES

LOWER RESPIRATORY TRACT

- The lower respiratory tract consists of the trachea, bronchi, and bronchial tree. The lungs are divided into separate bronchopulmonary segments each served by its own segmental bronchus, artery, vein, and lymphatics.
- The segmental or tertiary bronchus branches into bronchioles that consist of smooth muscle rather than cartilage.
- The bronchioles then branch into even smaller terminal bronchioles that mark the end of the purely air-conducting system.
- The terminal bronchioles then branch into the respiratory bronchioles that contain occasional alveolar sacs on their walls. The respiratory bronchiole terminates as an alveolar duct that opens into alveolar sacs where gaseous exchange occurs in the alveolar cells.
- The alveolar air cells are made of simple squamous epithelium. Each alveolus is surrounded by capillaries that originate in the pulmonary arterioles and, in turn, mark the beginning of pulmonary venules.
- Gas exchange (oxygen for carbon dioxide) occurs via the alveolar-blood barrier. This barrier consists of the capillary endothelial lining, basement membrane, and alveolar epithelium.

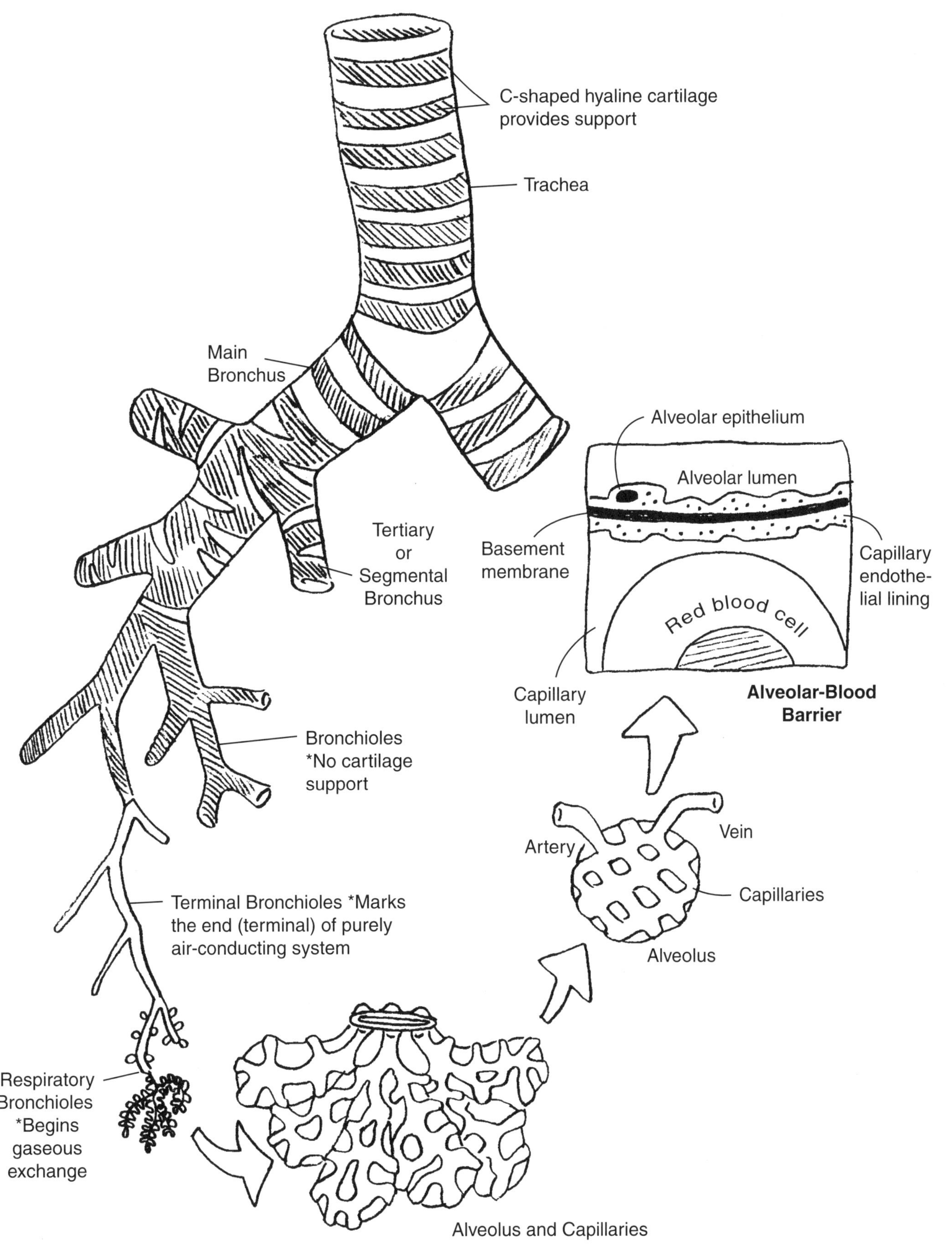
C-shaped hyaline cartilage provides support
Trachea
Main Bronchus
Tertiary or Segmental Bronchus
Bronchioles *No cartilage support
Terminal Bronchioles *Marks the end (terminal) of purely air-conducting system
Respiratory Bronchioles *Begins gaseous exchange
Alveolus and Capillaries
Artery
Vein
Capillaries
Alveolus
Alveolar epithelium
Alveolar lumen
Basement membrane
Capillary endothelial lining
Red blood cell
Capillary lumen
Alveolar-Blood Barrier

NOTES

MECHANICS OF RESPIRATION

- Respiration consists of inspiration and expiration. Air movement occurs secondary to the inverse relationship of pressure and volume (if one goes up, the other must go down).
- 500 mL of air is moved with each breath.
- The flattening contraction of the diaphragm is responsible primarily for most of the inspiratory effort and secondarily for contraction of the external intercostal muscles that elevate the ribs. These actions collectively increase the intrathoracic volume that causes a decrease in pressure. At this point the internal thoracic pressure is lower than the outer atmospheric pressure, which forces air to enter the respiratory tract.
- Expiration provides the relaxation of the diaphragm and external intercostals. The contraction of the internal intercostals and the natural elastic recoil of the lungs also aid in exhalation. Collectively, these actions decrease the intrathoracic volume and thus increase the pressure. At this point the intrathoracic pressure is greater than the external atmospheric pressure, which forces air to exit the respiratory tract.

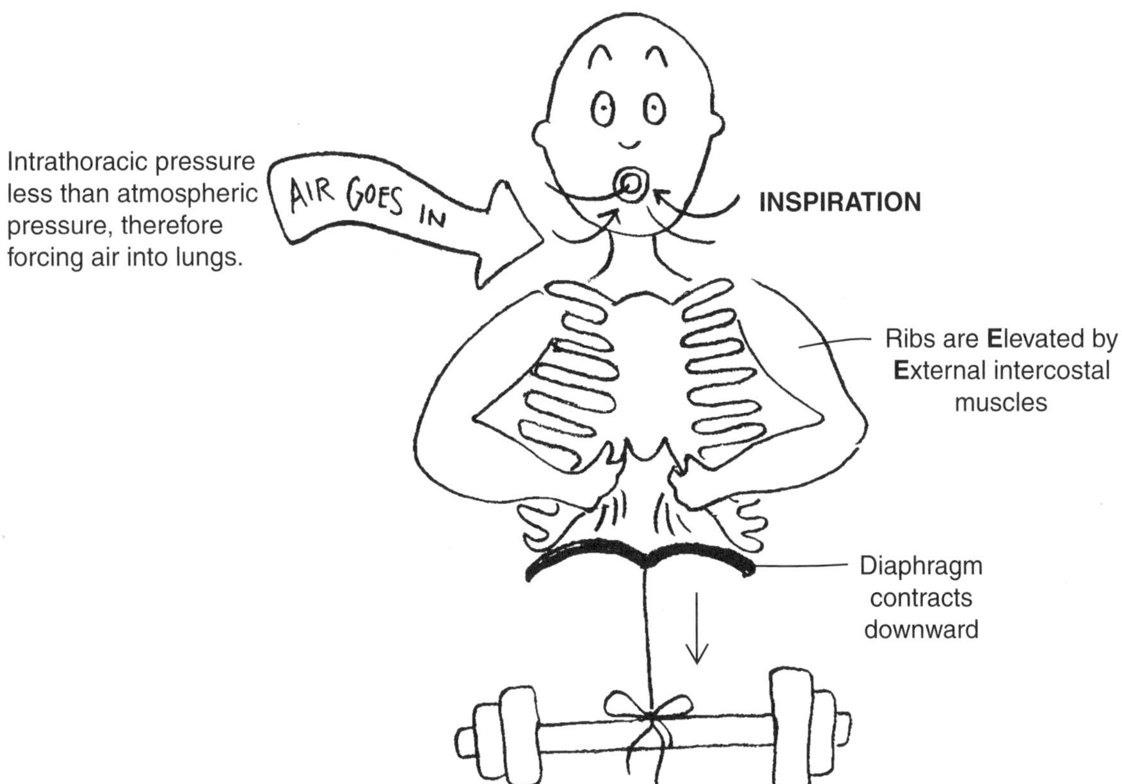
Intrathoracic pressure less than atmospheric pressure, therefore forcing air into lungs.
AIR GOES IN
INSPIRATION
Ribs are **E**levated by **E**xternal intercostal muscles
Diaphragm contracts downward

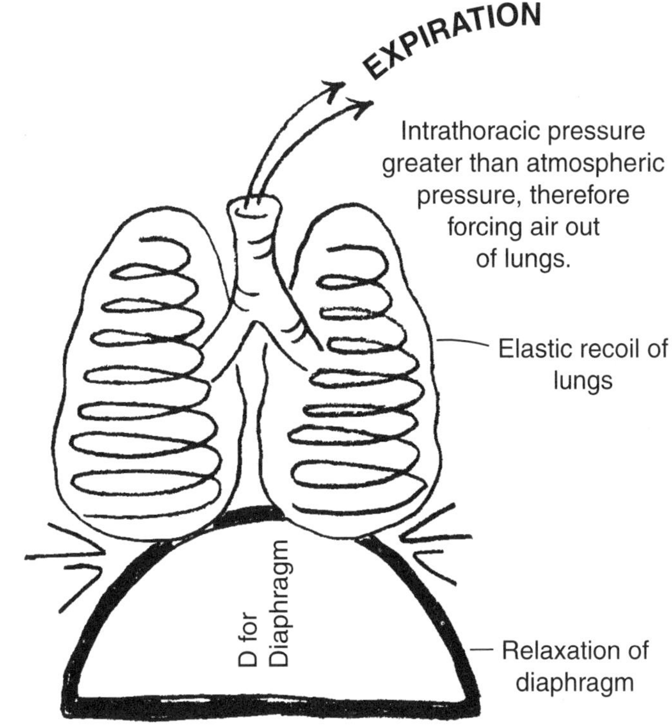
EXPIRATION
Intrathoracic pressure greater than atmospheric pressure, therefore forcing air out of lungs.
Elastic recoil of lungs
D for Diaphragm
Relaxation of diaphragm

NOTES

CO_2 TRANSPORT

- Transported in venous blood in three forms:
  - HCO_3^- → hydration of CO_2 in RBCs; 90%
  - carbaminohemoglobin → CO_2 bound to hemoglobin
  - dissolved CO_2
- HCO_3^- transport of CO_2
  - CO_2 from tissues diffuses into RBCs → CO_2 combines with H_2O → forms H_2CO_3, which dissociates into H+ and HCO_3^-
  - chloride shift causes HCO_3^- to exit the RBC in exchange for Cl^- ion. This allows the HCO_3^- to be transported in the plasma to the lungs where reverse reactions occur (see illustration) allowing CO_2 to be exhaled.
  - H^+ ion from the dissociation of H_2CO_3 is buffered by deoxyhemoglobin in the RBC.

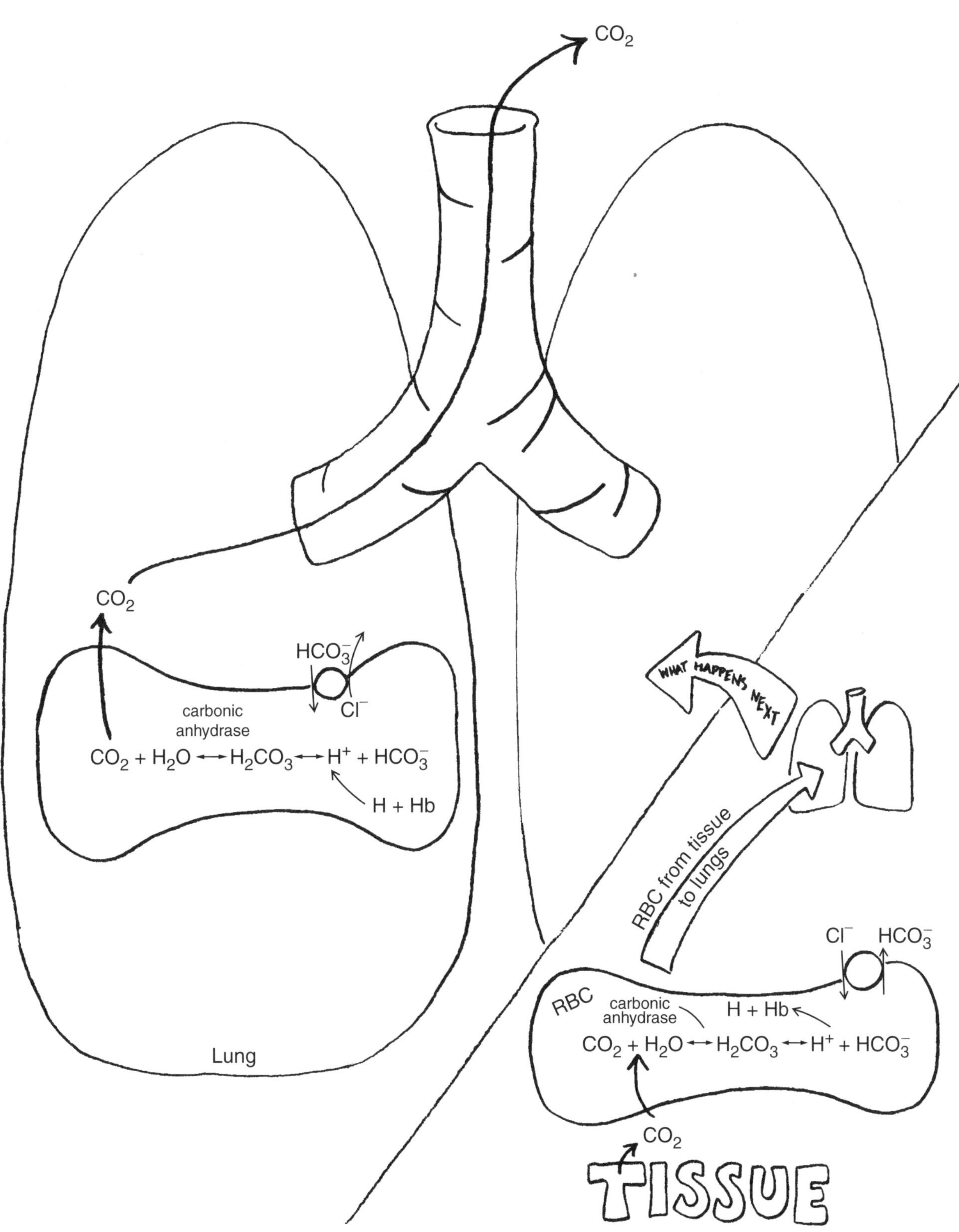
CO_2
CO_2
HCO_3^-
Cl^-
carbonic
anhydrase
$CO_2 + H_2O \leftrightarrow H_2CO_3 \leftrightarrow H^+ + HCO_3^-$
H + Hb
Lung
WHAT HAPPENS NEXT
RBC from tissue
to lungs
Cl^-
HCO_3^-
RBC
carbonic
anhydrase
H + Hb
$CO_2 + H_2O \leftrightarrow H_2CO_3 \leftrightarrow H^+ + HCO_3^-$
CO_2
TISSUE

NOTES

HEMOGLOBIN-OXYGEN DISSOCIATION CURVE

- Dalton's law of partial pressure: partial pressure = total pressure × fractional gas concentration
- In dry air the partial pressure is:
  - PO_2 = 760 mm Hg (atmospheric pressure) × 0.21 (fractional concentration of oxygen) = 160 mm Hg
- The air we inhale is humidified in the nasal cavity and trachea, resulting in a need to correct the PO_2.
  - PO_2 = (760 mm Hg – 47 mm Hg partial pressure of H_2O) × 0.21 = 150 mm Hg
- Alveolar air is approximately 100 mm Hg → decreased secondarily to diffusion of oxygen to pulmonary arterial blood
- Arterial blood partial pressure of oxygen is approximately 100 mm Hg because the pulmonary capillary blood equilibrates with the alveolar air
- Diffusion rates of oxygen and carbon dioxide depend on pressure gradients through the alveolar-blood barrier
- Oxygen is carried in the blood as a dissolved form and bound to hemoglobin (Hgb)
- Adult hemoglobin (four subunits → $\alpha_2\beta_2$) dramatically increases the blood's capacity to carry oxygen; Hgb contains an iron element (heme) that—when in the ferrous state (Fe_2^+)—binds oxygen; when in the methemoglobin state (Fe_3^+) does not bind oxygen.
- Fetal hemoglobin (four subunits → $\alpha_2\beta_2$) possesses a higher affinity for oxygen than adult hemoglobin because it does not bind as well to 2,3-DPG; the oxygen from the mother's blood will therefore more readily transfer to the fetus' blood during pregnancy
- When bound to oxygen hemoglobin forms oxyhemoglobin; the hemoglobin-oxygen dissociation curve illustrates the percentage of hemoglobin saturated with oxygen at a specific partial pressure of oxygen in the blood
  - Hgb is 100% saturated at a PO_2 of 100 mm Hg
  - Hgb is 75% saturated at a PO_2 of 40 mm Hg
  - Hgb is 50% saturated at a PO_2 of 25 mm Hg (also known as the P_{50}—the point at which oxygen binds to two of the four heme groups of the hemoglobin)
- Sigmoid shape of curve secondary to positive cooperativity property of hemoglobin; each successive oxygen molecule bound to hemoglobin increases the affinity for the next oxygen molecule to bind; hemoglobin will therefore have the highest affinity for the fourth and final oxygen molecule
- The flat portion of the curve illustrates that a large deficit of hemoglobin's ability to carry oxygen or a change in atmospheric concentration of oxygen may be tolerated before it becomes a problem
- Shifts to right on the curve mean a decrease in the affinity of Hgb for oxygen; unloading of oxygen to tissues is increased; examples: decrease in pH, increase in temperature, and increase in 2,3-DPG)
- Shifts to the left indicate an increase in the affinity of Hgb for oxygen; unloading of oxygen to tissues is decreased; the opposite circumstances apply here: increase in pH, decrease in temperature, and decrease in 2,3-DPG)
- Carbon monoxide decreases the oxygen content in blood by directly competing for sites on the hemoglobin molecule; hemoglobin's affinity for CO is 200 times that of oxygen

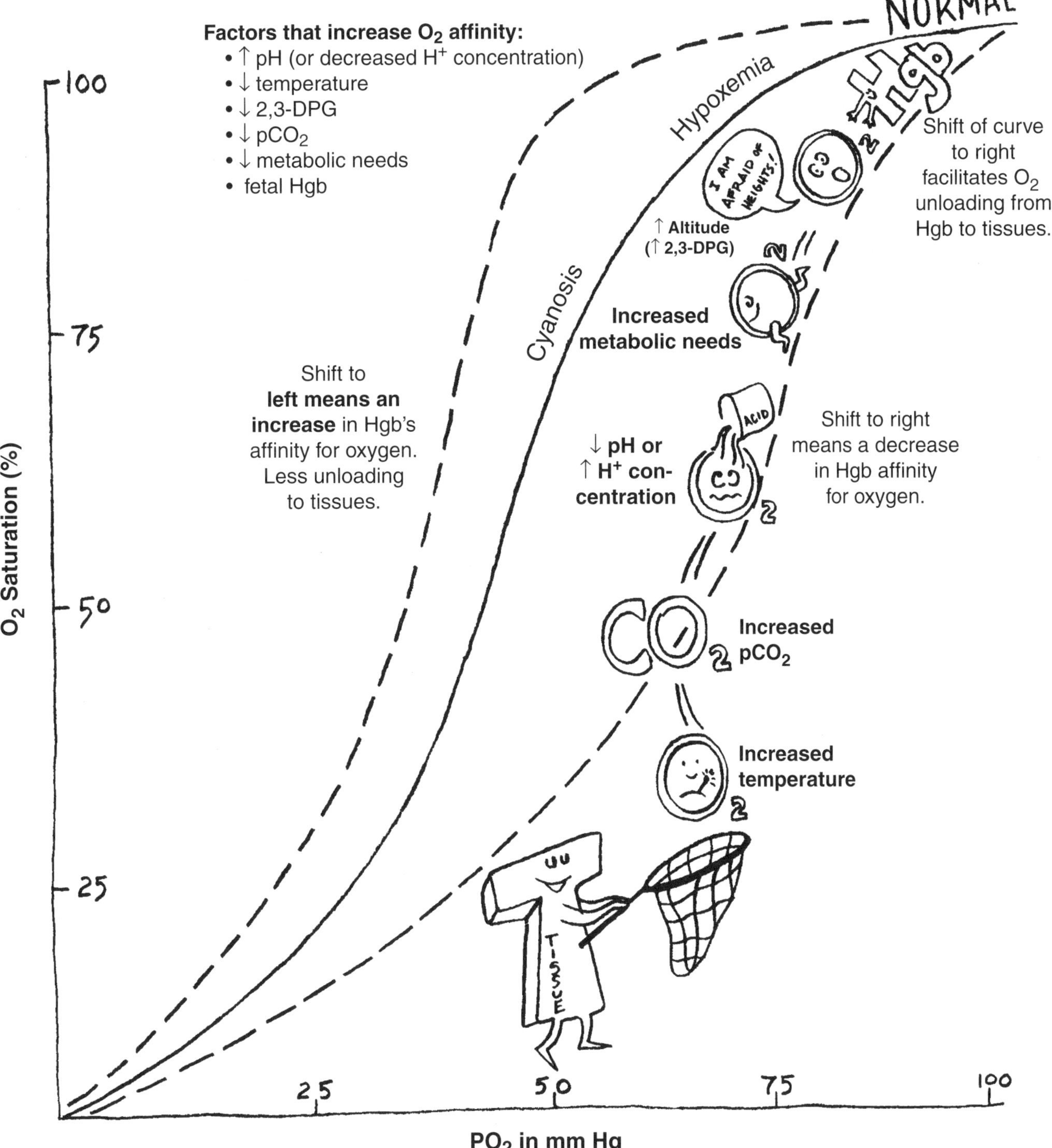
NORMAL
Factors that increase O_2 affinity:
• ↑ pH (or decreased H^+ concentration)
• ↓ temperature
• ↓ 2,3-DPG
• ↓ pCO_2
• ↓ metabolic needs
• fetal Hgb
Hypoxemia
Cyanosis
Hgb
I AM AFRAID OF HEIGHTS!
↑ Altitude
(↑ 2,3-DPG)
Shift of curve to right facilitates O_2 unloading from Hgb to tissues.
Increased metabolic needs
Shift to left means an increase in Hgb's affinity for oxygen. Less unloading to tissues.
ACID
↓ pH or ↑ H^+ concentration
Shift to right means a decrease in Hgb affinity for oxygen.
Increased pCO_2
Increased temperature
TISSUE
100
75
50
25
O_2 Saturation (%)
25
50
75
100
PO_2 in mm Hg

NOTES

V/Q MISMATCH

- V/Q ratio → ratio of alveolar ventilation (V) to pulmonary blood flow (Q)
- Normally equal to 0.8
- In airway obstruction the ventilation decreases; therefore no gas exchange, resulting in a V/Q ratio equal to 0 (0/Q = 0)
- In blood flow obstruction the perfusion of the lung is decreased; V/Q ratio therefore equals infinity (∞) (V/0 = ∞)
- Ratios vary according to anatomical locations in lung:
    - at apex, perfusion is the least secondary to gravity and ventilation is the greatest; the V/Q ratio is therefore highest (>1.0) at the apex; gas exchange is more efficient
    - at the base, perfusion is the greatest secondary to gravity and ventilation is the least; the V/Q ratio is therefore lowest (<0.8) at the base; gas exchange is less efficient.

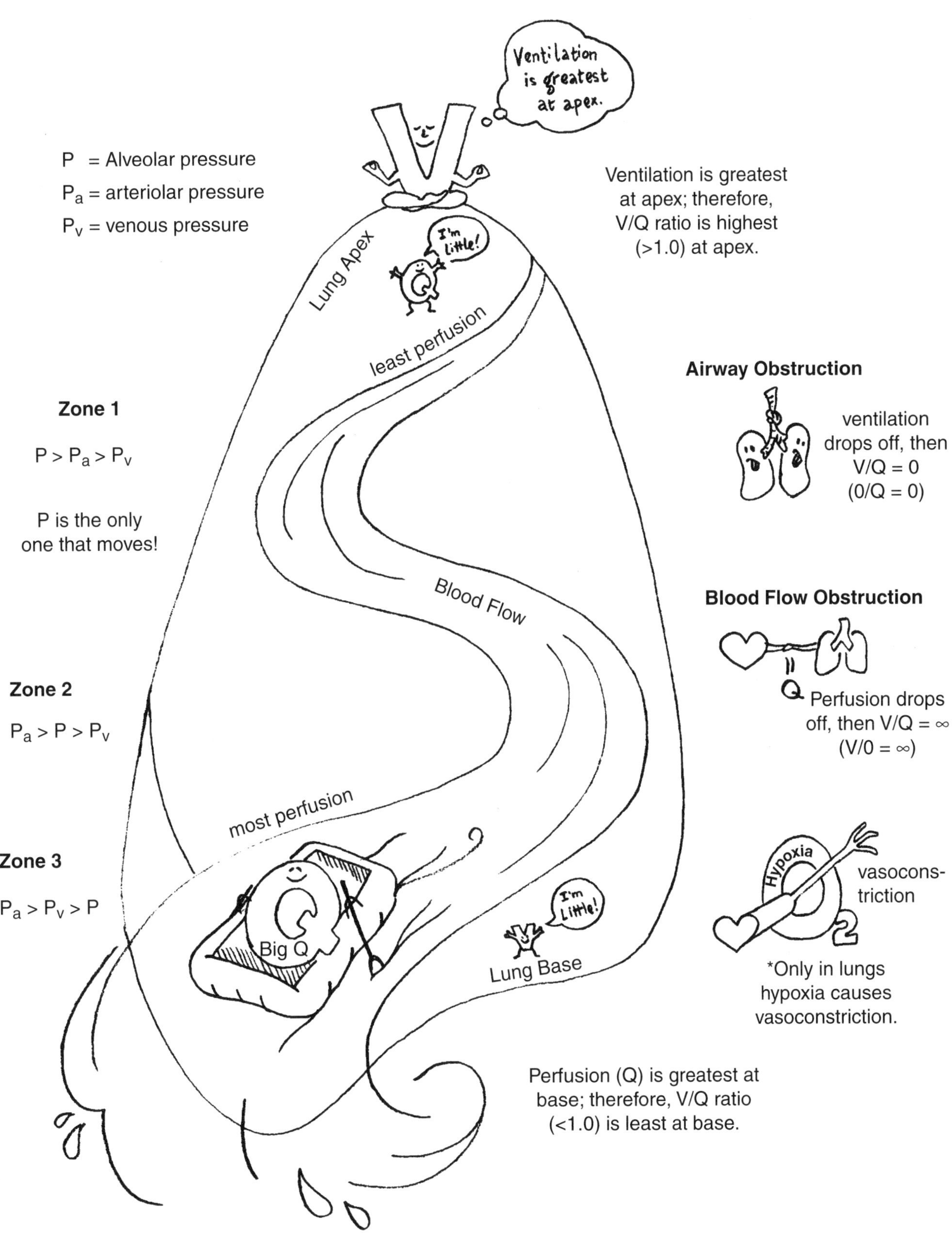
Ventilation is greatest at apex.
P = Alveolar pressure
P_a = arteriolar pressure
P_v = venous pressure
Ventilation is greatest at apex; therefore, V/Q ratio is highest (>1.0) at apex.
Lung Apex
I'm Little!
least perfusion
Airway Obstruction
ventilation drops off, then V/Q = 0 (0/Q = 0)
Zone 1
$P > P_a > P_v$
P is the only one that moves!
Blood Flow
Blood Flow Obstruction
Q
Perfusion drops off, then V/Q = ∞ (V/0 = ∞)
Zone 2
$P_a > P > P_v$
most perfusion
Zone 3
$P_a > P_v > P$
Big Q
I'm Little!
Lung Base
Hypoxia
vasoconstriction
O_2
*Only in lungs hypoxia causes vasoconstriction.
Perfusion (Q) is greatest at base; therefore, V/Q ratio (<1.0) is least at base.

NOTES

WHAT PRODUCT DO THE LUNGS MAKE?

- Surfactant: reduces surface tension in alveoli and prevents their collapse
- Histamine
- Angiotensin converting enzyme: ACE converts angiotensin I to angiotensin II; it also inactivates bradykinin; therefore, when ACE inhibitors are used to control blood pressure, bradykinin is in its active form; a side effect would be a cough
- Kallikrein: activates bradykinin
- Prostaglandins: important in augmenting inflammatory reactions

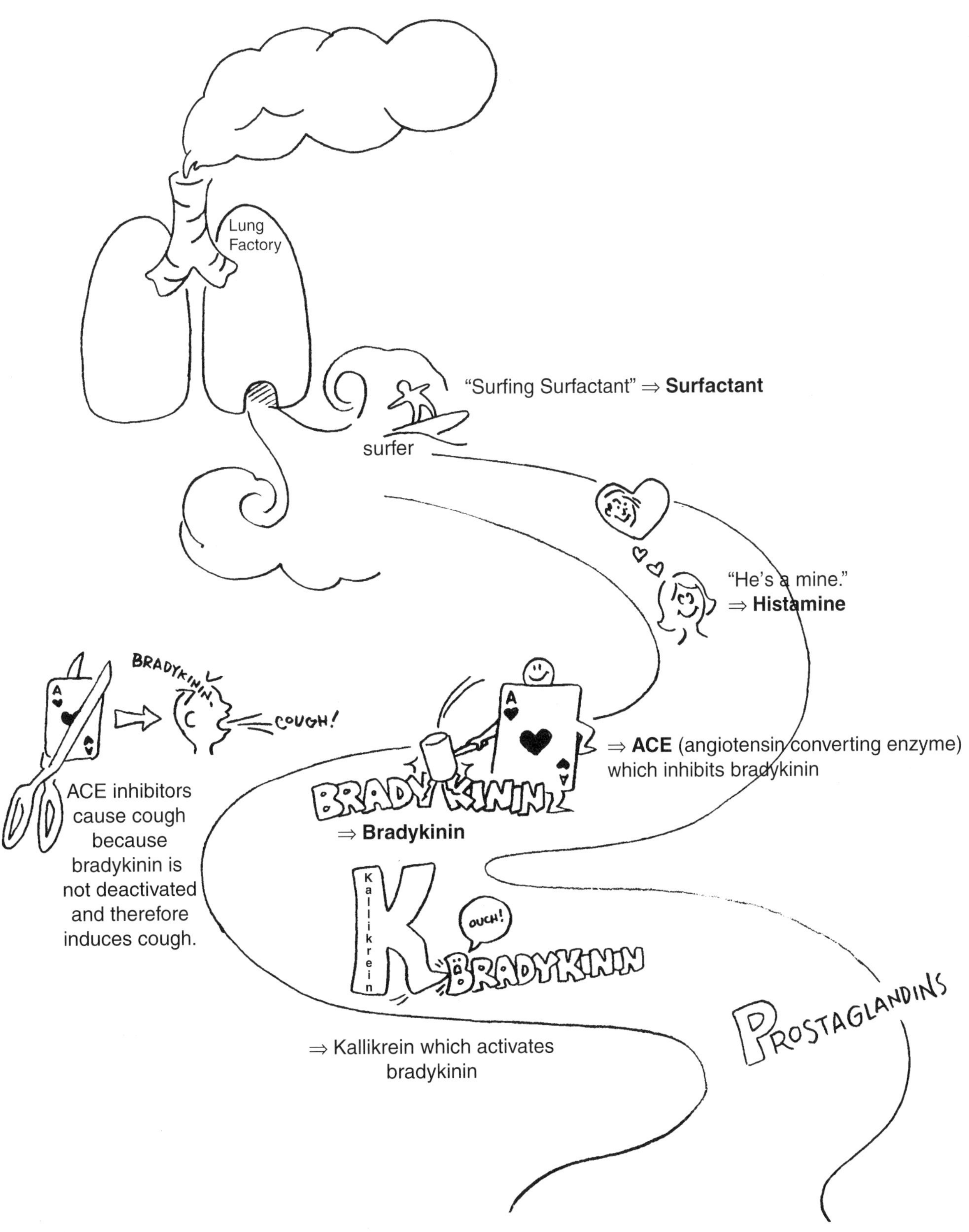
Lung Factory
"Surfing Surfactant" ⇒ **Surfactant**
surfer
"He's a mine."
⇒ **Histamine**
⇒ **ACE** (angiotensin converting enzyme) which inhibits bradykinin
BRADYKININ
⇒ **Bradykinin**
BRADYKININ
COUGH!
ACE inhibitors cause cough because bradykinin is not deactivated and therefore induces cough.
Kallikrein
OUCH!
BRADYKININ
⇒ Kallikrein which activates bradykinin
PROSTAGLANDINS

NOTES

CHANGES THAT OCCUR AT HIGH ALTITUDE

- Increased ventilation → leads to an increase in CO_2 expiration → respiratory alkalosis results → leads to renal compensation in the form of increased bicarbonate excretion
- Hypoxia causes three responses:
    - pulmonary vasoconstriction → leads to increased pressure in pulmonary artery → increased pressure in right ventricle; therefore → leads to right ventricular hypertrophy
    - increased 2,3-DPG causes increased unloading of oxygen from Hgb to tissues
    - increased erythropoietin results in increased RBC production; therefore → increased Hgb and hematocrit

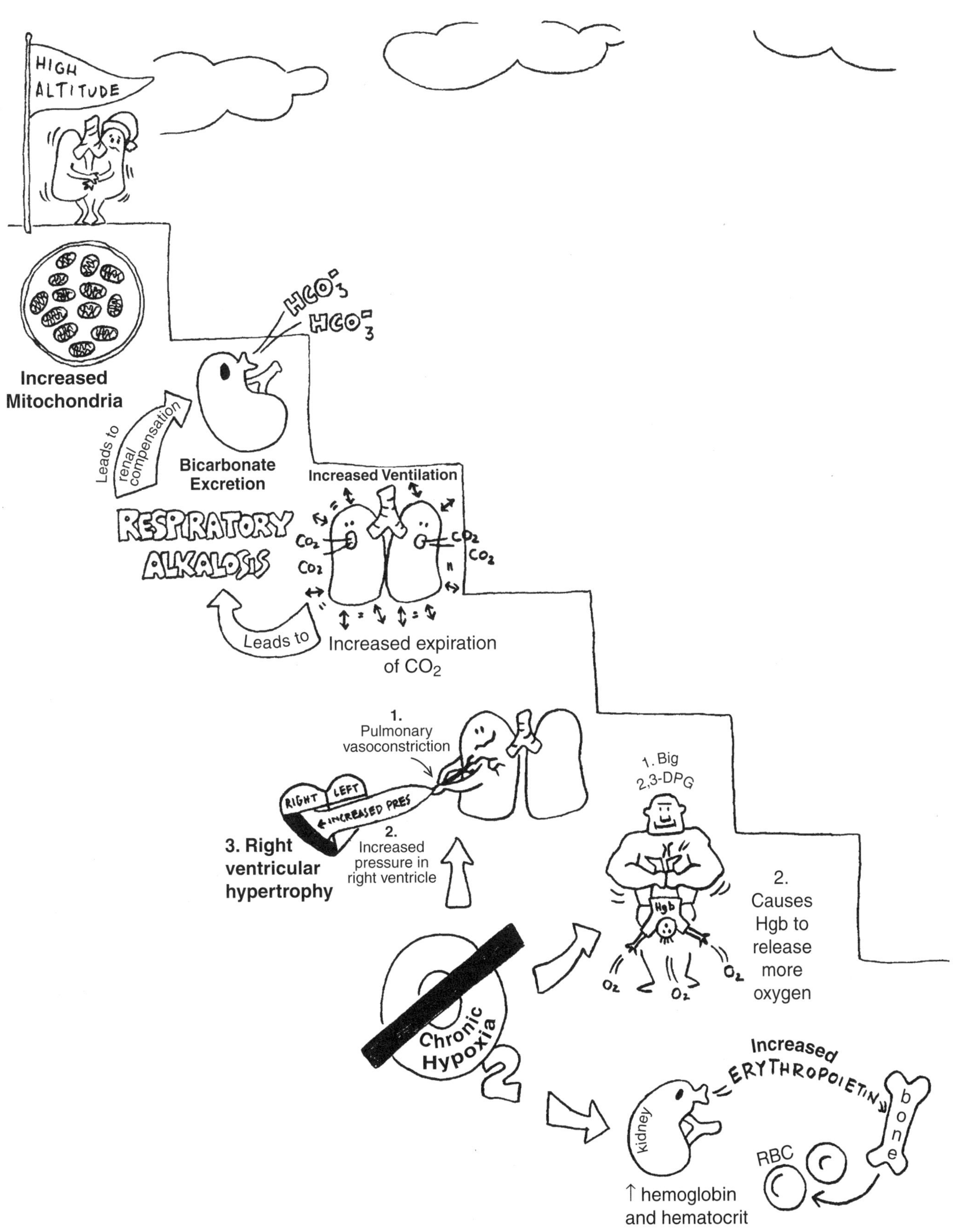
HIGH ALTITUDE
Increased Mitochondria
HCO_3^-
HCO_3^-
Leads to renal compensation
Bicarbonate Excretion
Increased Ventilation
RESPIRATORY ALKALOSIS
CO_2
CO_2
CO_2
CO_2
Leads to
Increased expiration of CO_2
1. Pulmonary vasoconstriction
RIGHT
LEFT
INCREASED PRES
2. Increased pressure in right ventricle
3. Right ventricular hypertrophy
1. Big 2,3-DPG
Hgb
2. Causes Hgb to release more oxygen
O_2
O_2
O_2
Chronic Hypoxia
Increased ERYTHROPOIETIN
kidney
bone
RBC
↑ hemoglobin and hematocrit

NOTES

LUNG VOLUMES

- Total lung capacity
- Vital capacity
- Inspiratory capacity
- Functional reserve capacity
- Inspiratory reserve volume
- Tidal volume
- Expiratory reserve volume
- Residual volume

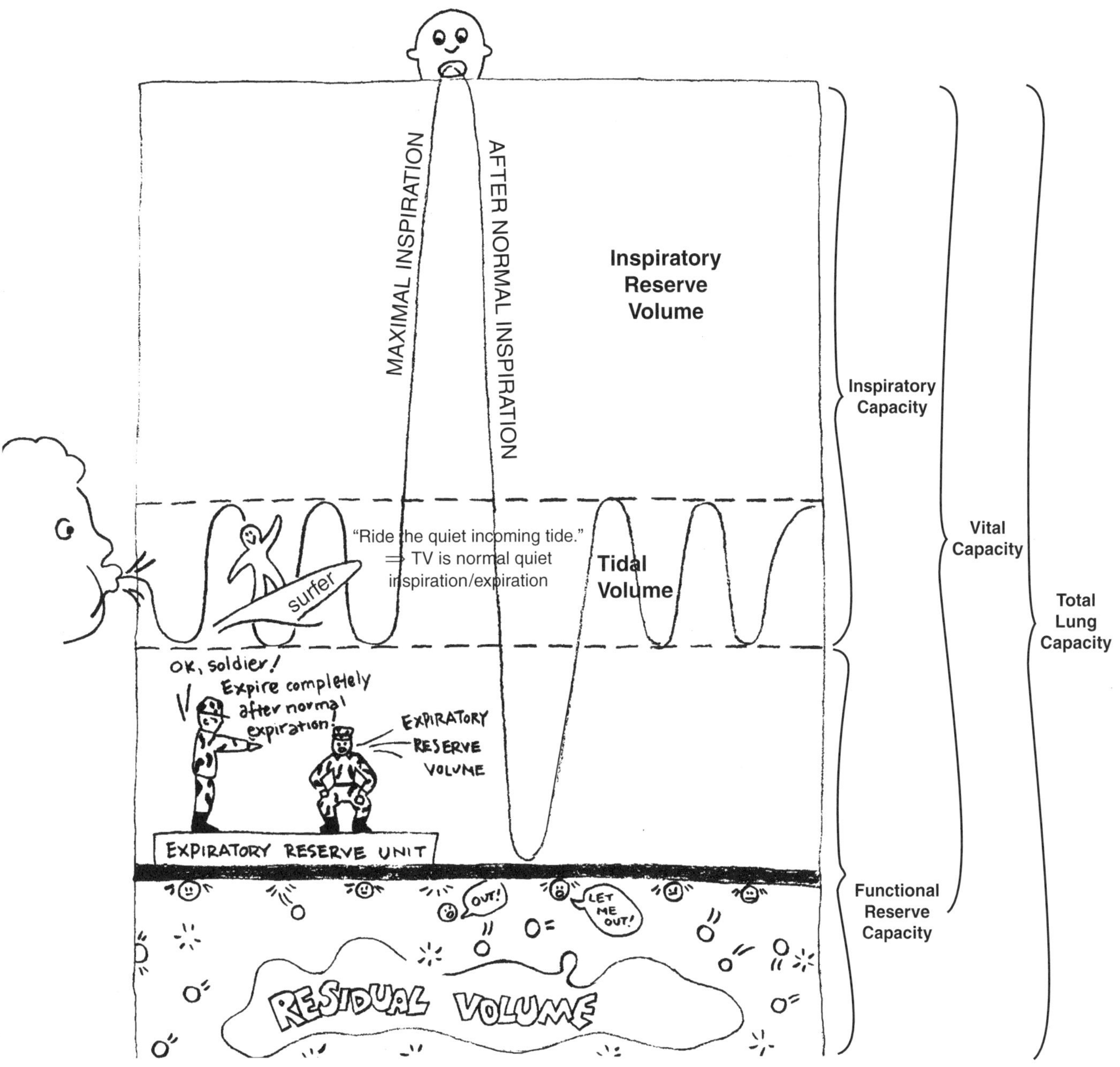
MAXIMAL INSPIRATION
AFTER NORMAL INSPIRATION
Inspiratory Reserve Volume
"Ride the quiet incoming tide."
⟹ TV is normal quiet inspiration/expiration
surfer
Tidal Volume
OK, soldier!
Expire completely after normal expiration!
EXPIRATORY RESERVE VOLUME
EXPIRATORY RESERVE UNIT
OUT!
LET ME OUT!
RESIDUAL VOLUME
Inspiratory Capacity
Vital Capacity
Total Lung Capacity
Functional Reserve Capacity

NOTES

See Table 6.1 in Appendix.

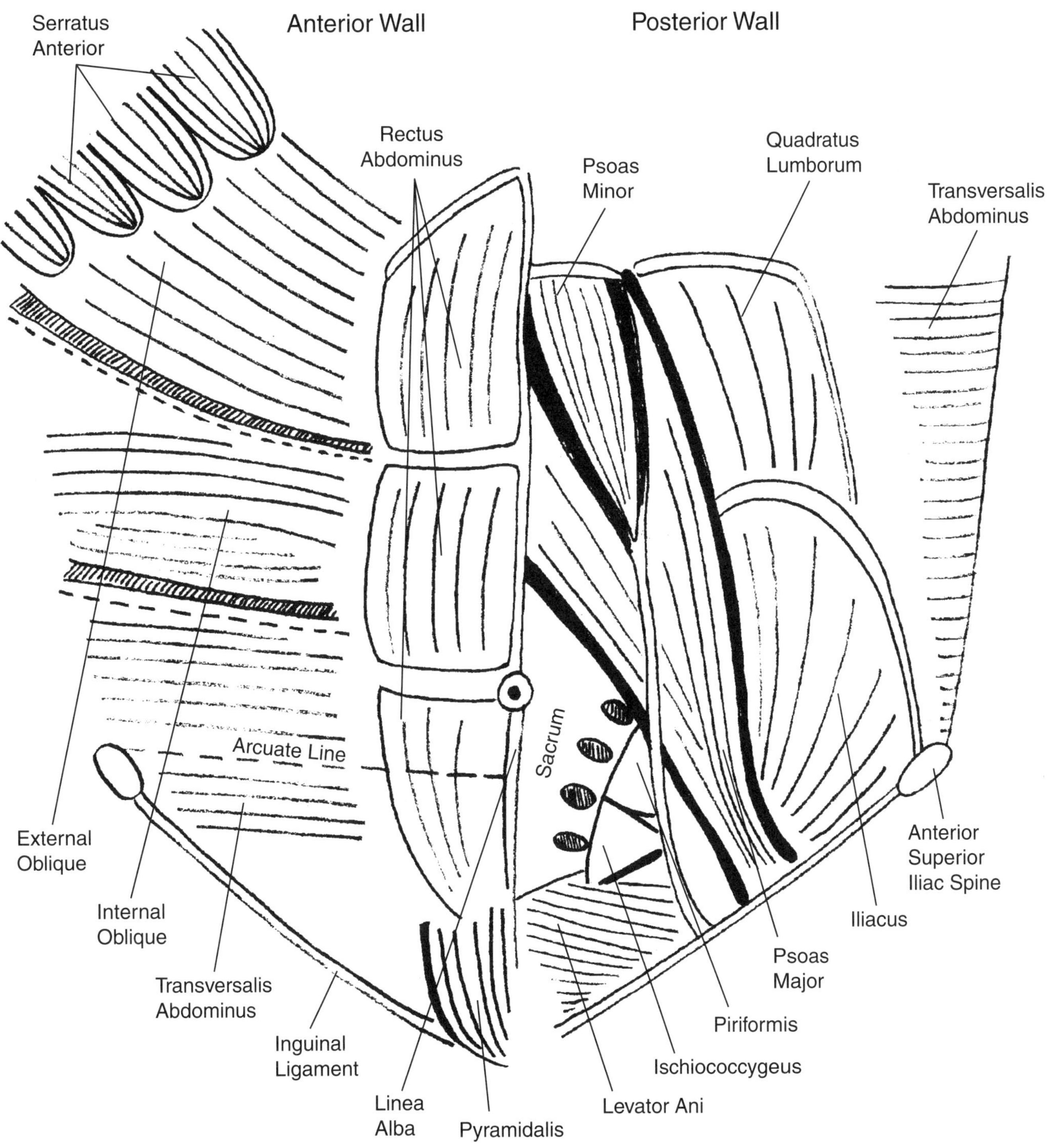
Anterior Wall
Posterior Wall
Serratus Anterior
Rectus Abdominus
Psoas Minor
Quadratus Lumborum
Transversalis Abdominus
Sacrum
Arcuate Line
External Oblique
Internal Oblique
Transversalis Abdominus
Inguinal Ligament
Linea Alba
Pyramidalis
Levator Ani
Ischiococcygeus
Piriformis
Psoas Major
Iliacus
Anterior Superior Iliac Spine

See Table 6.1 in Appendix.

RECTUS SHEATH

Arcuate Line (Linea Semicircularis)

- Semicircular line is located directly below the level of the iliac crest
- This marks the end of the posterior layer of the rectus sheath

Above the Arcuate Line

- Anterior layer of the rectus sheath contains the aponeuroses of the external and internal oblique muscles
- Posterior layer of rectus sheath contains the aponeuroses of the internal oblique and transversus abdominus muscles

Below the Arcuate Line

- Anterior layer of the rectus sheath contains the aponeuroses of the external oblique, internal oblique, and transversus abdominus muscles
- Posterior to the rectus abdominus muscle is transversalis fascia

Above the Arcuate Line

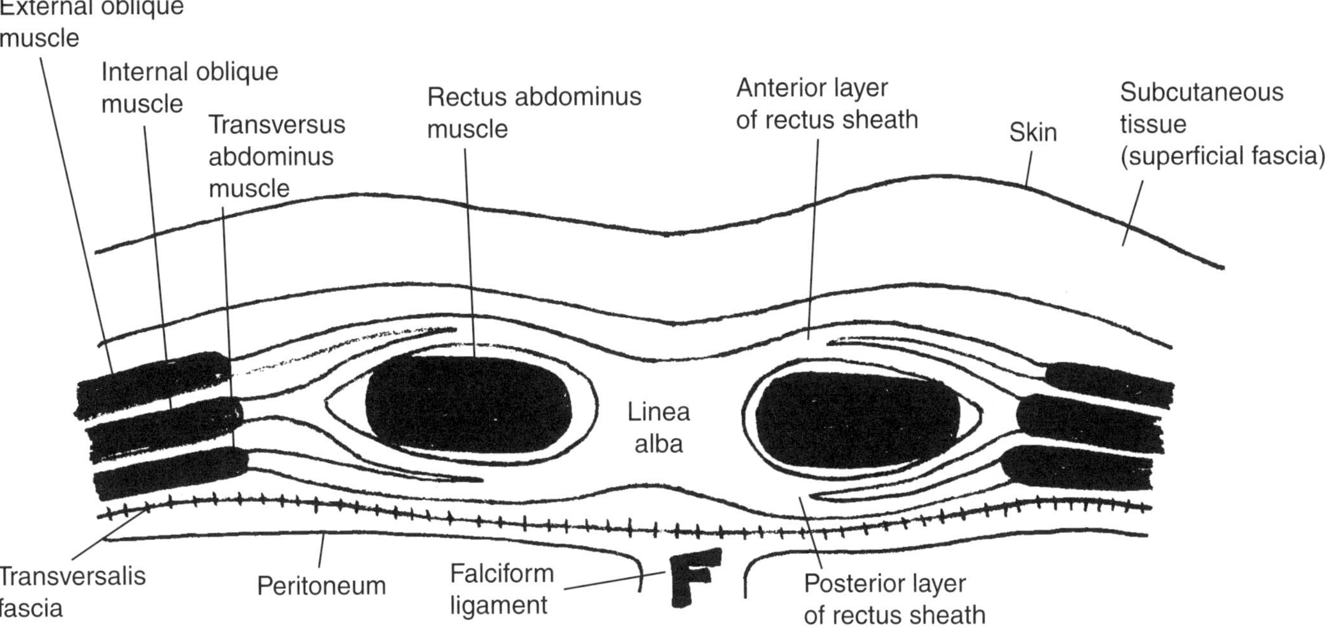

Below the Arcuate Line

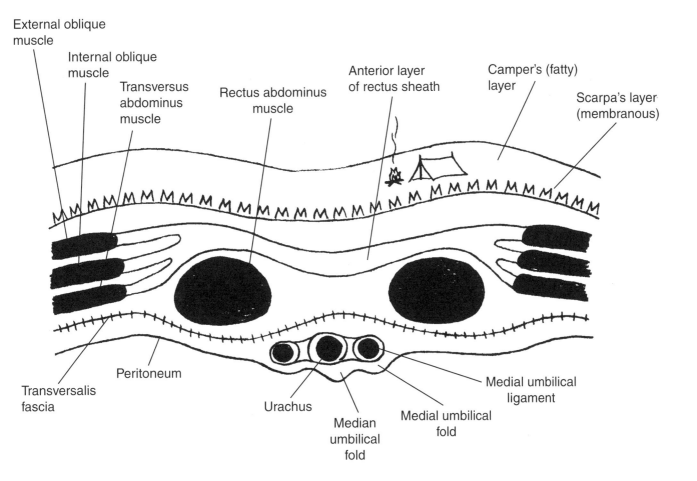

External oblique muscle
Internal oblique muscle
Transversus abdominus muscle
Rectus abdominus muscle
Anterior layer of rectus sheath
Camper's (fatty) layer
Scarpa's layer (membranous)
Peritoneum
Transversalis fascia
Urachus
Median umbilical fold
Medial umbilical fold
Medial umbilical ligament

NOTES

See Table 6.1 in Appendix.

INGUINAL REGION

Hesselbach's Inguinal Triangle

- Bounded by the inguinal ligament, lateral border of the rectus abdominus, and the inferior epigastric vessels
- Common site of a direct inguinal hernia

Superficial (External) Inguinal Ring

- Located in the aponeurosis of the external oblique muscle, lateral to the pubic tubercle
- The spermatic cord and the round ligament of the uterus pass through the superficial inguinal ring

Deep (Internal) Inguinal Ring

- Located in the transversalis fascia, lateral to the inferior epigastric vessels
- An extension of the processus vaginalis

Direct Hernia

- Protrusion through Hesselbach's triangle
- Only passes through the superficial inguinal ring
- Protrudes through the abdominal wall medial to the inferior epigastric vessels

Indirect Hernia

- Most common hernia in men
- Passes through the superficial and deep inguinal rings
- Passes into the deep inguinal ring lateral to the inferior epigastric vessels and into the scrotum

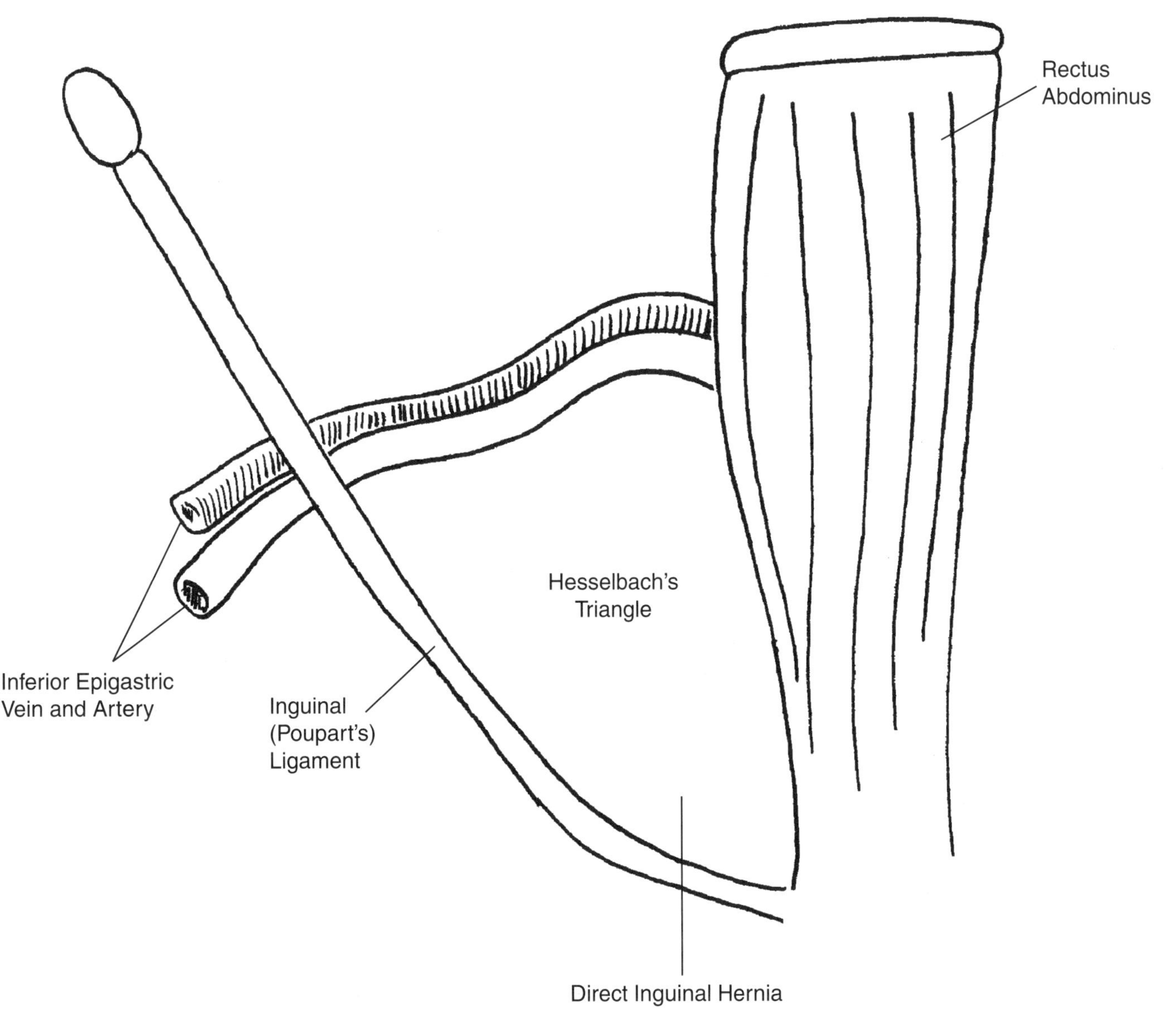
Rectus
Abdominus
Hesselbach's
Triangle
Inferior Epigastric
Vein and Artery
Inguinal
(Poupart's)
Ligament
Direct Inguinal Hernia

NOTES

See Table 6.1 in Appendix.

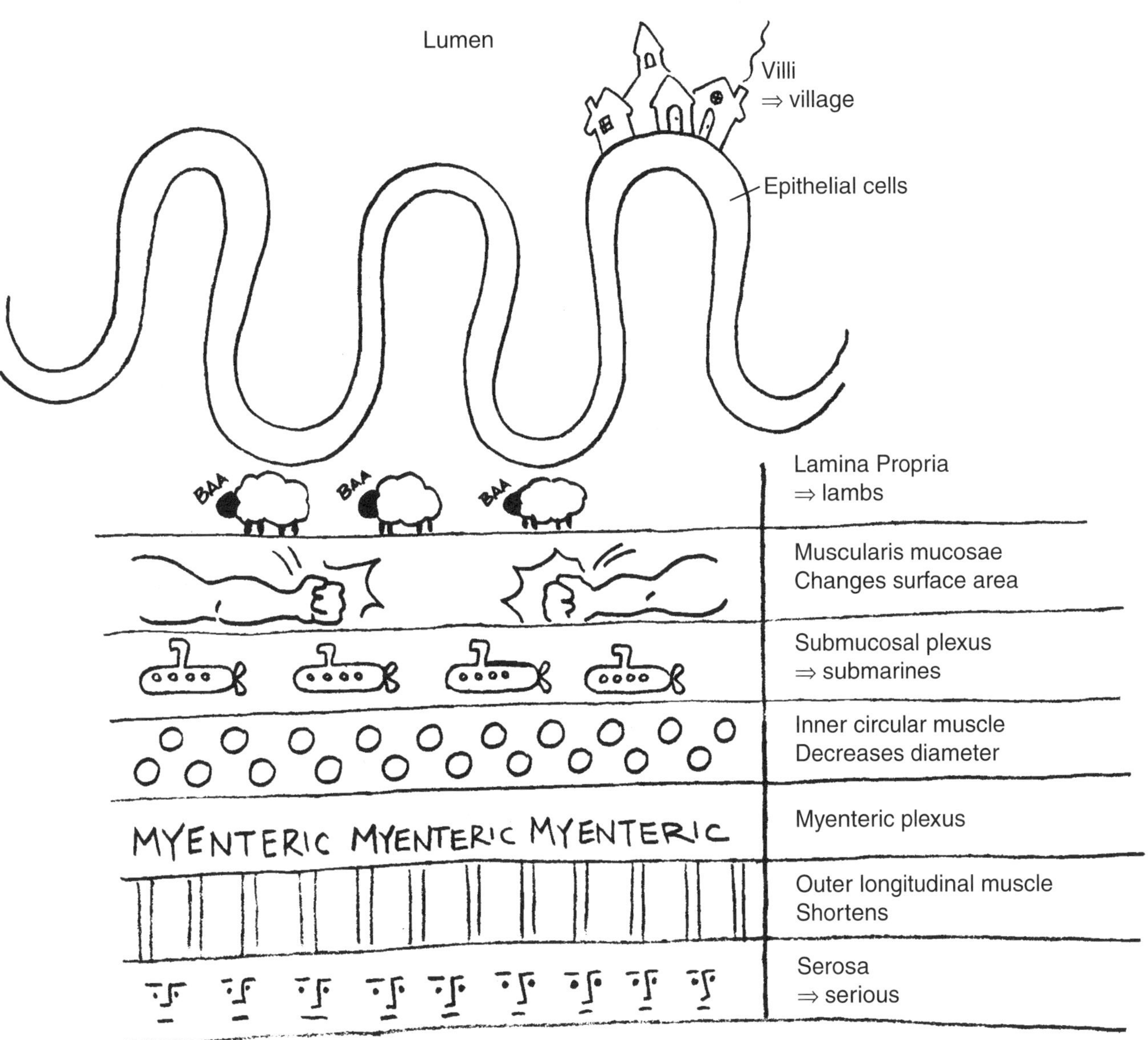

- **S**ubmucosal Plexus (Meissner's)
  Controls **S**ecretions
- **M**yenteric Plexus (Auerbach's)
  Controls **M**otility

NOTES

See Table 6.1 in Appendix.

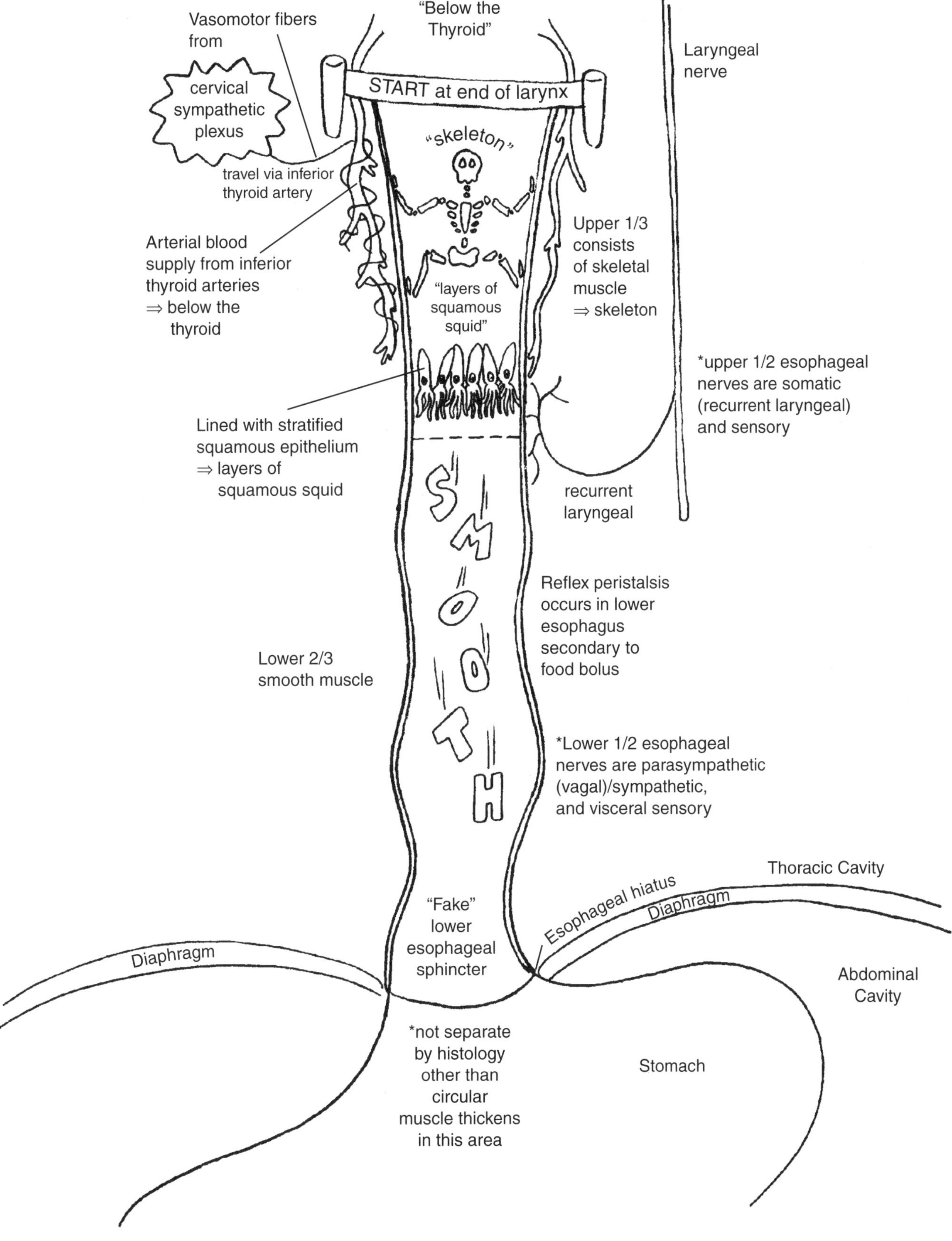
"Below the Thyroid"
Vasomotor fibers from
cervical sympathetic plexus
travel via inferior thyroid artery
START at end of larynx
Laryngeal nerve
"skeleton"
Arterial blood supply from inferior thyroid arteries ⇒ below the thyroid
Upper 1/3 consists of skeletal muscle ⇒ skeleton
"layers of squamous squid"
*upper 1/2 esophageal nerves are somatic (recurrent laryngeal) and sensory
Lined with stratified squamous epithelium ⇒ layers of squamous squid
recurrent laryngeal
SMOOTH
Reflex peristalsis occurs in lower esophagus secondary to food bolus
Lower 2/3 smooth muscle
*Lower 1/2 esophageal nerves are parasympathetic (vagal)/sympathetic, and visceral sensory
Thoracic Cavity
Esophageal hiatus
Diaphragm
"Fake" lower esophageal sphincter
Diaphragm
Abdominal Cavity
*not separate by histology other than circular muscle thickens in this area
Stomach

NOTES

See Table 6.1 in Appendix.

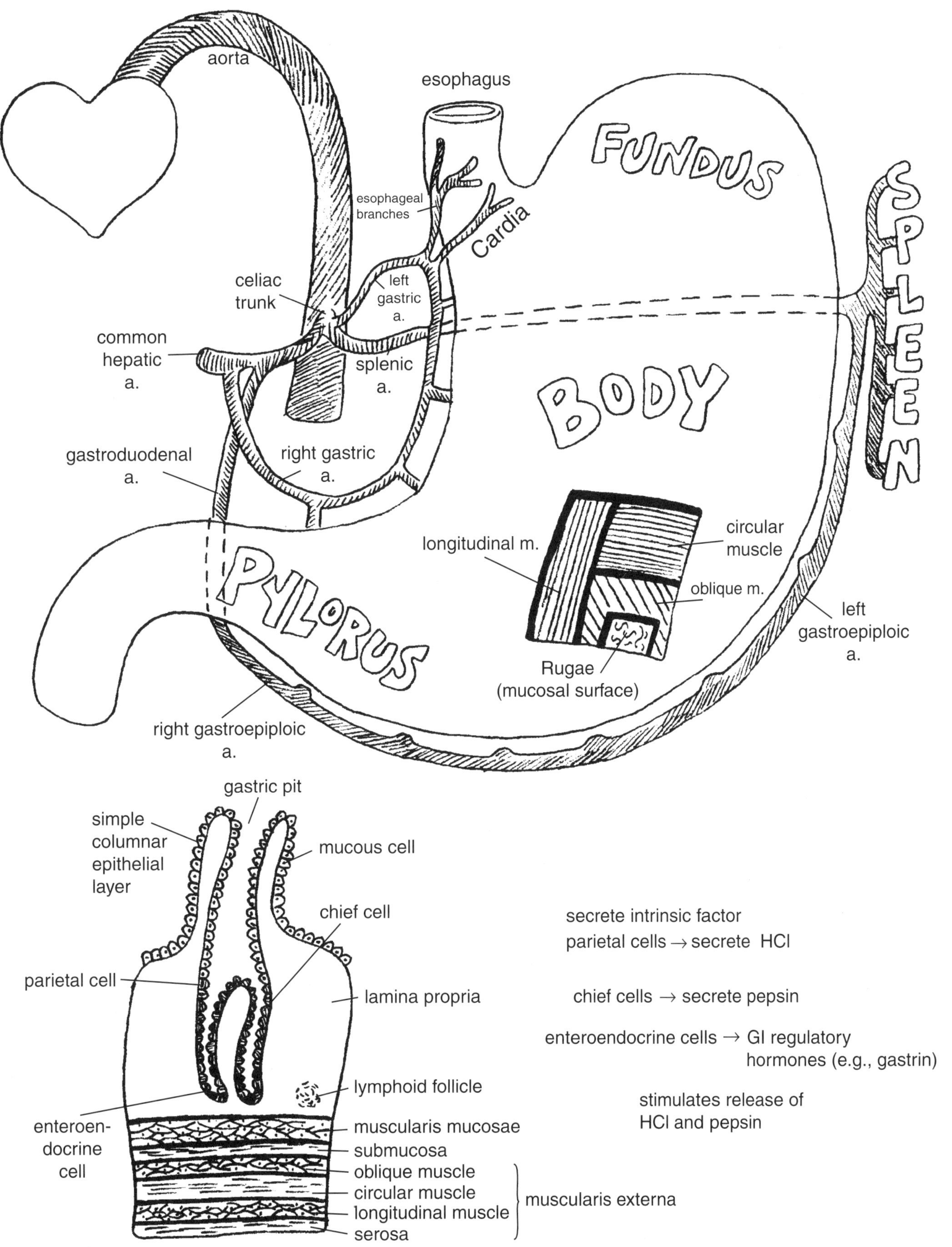

secrete intrinsic factor
parietal cells → secrete HCl

chief cells → secrete pepsin

enteroendocrine cells → GI regulatory hormones (e.g., gastrin)

stimulates release of HCl and pepsin

NOTES

See Table 6.1 in Appendix.

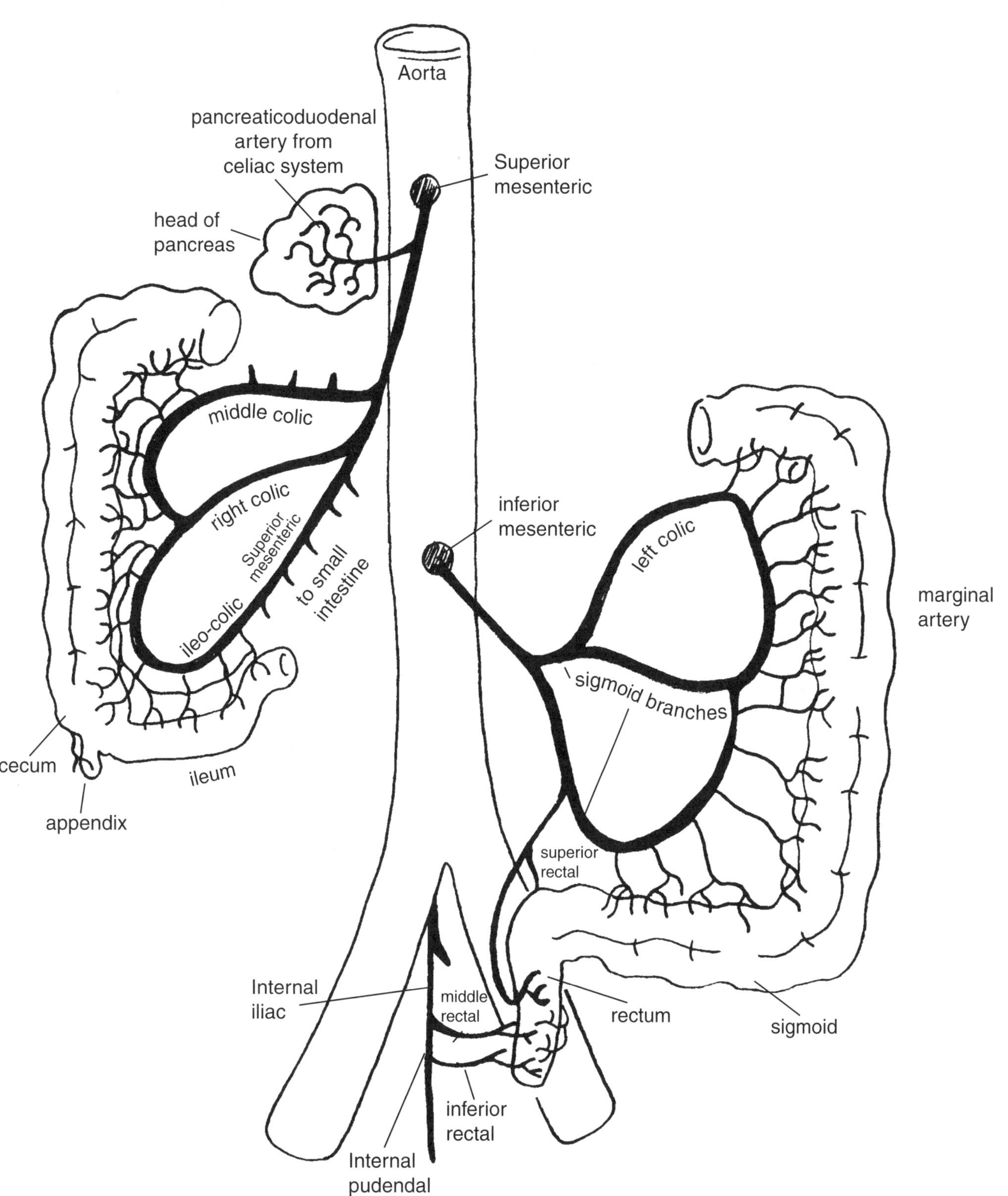
Aorta
pancreaticoduodenal artery from celiac system
Superior mesenteric
head of pancreas
middle colic
right colic
Superior mesenteric
ileo-colic
to small intestine
inferior mesenteric
left colic
marginal artery
sigmoid branches
cecum
appendix
ileum
superior rectal
Internal iliac
middle rectal
rectum
sigmoid
inferior rectal
Internal pudendal

NOTES

ANATOMY OF THE SMALL INTESTINE

Duodenum

- The duodenum is the shortest segment of the small intestine and surrounds the head of the pancreas
- The superior duodenum is also called the duodenal cap
- The descending duodenum contains the major papilla where the accessory pancreatic duct opens
- The transverse duodenum is posterior to the superior mesenteric vessels
- The ascending duodenum is kept in position by the ligament of Treitz

Jejunum

- Plicae circulares (circular folds) are long and compact
- Longer straight arteries than the ileum
- Fewer anastomotic loops (arcades) than the ileum
- Jejunum consists of the proximal two-fifths of the small intestine

Ileum

- Peyer's patches (lymphoid tissue)
- Shorter straight arteries than the jejunum
- More anastomotic loops than the jejunum
- Ileum consists of the distal three-fifths of the small intestine

See Table 6.1 in Appendix.

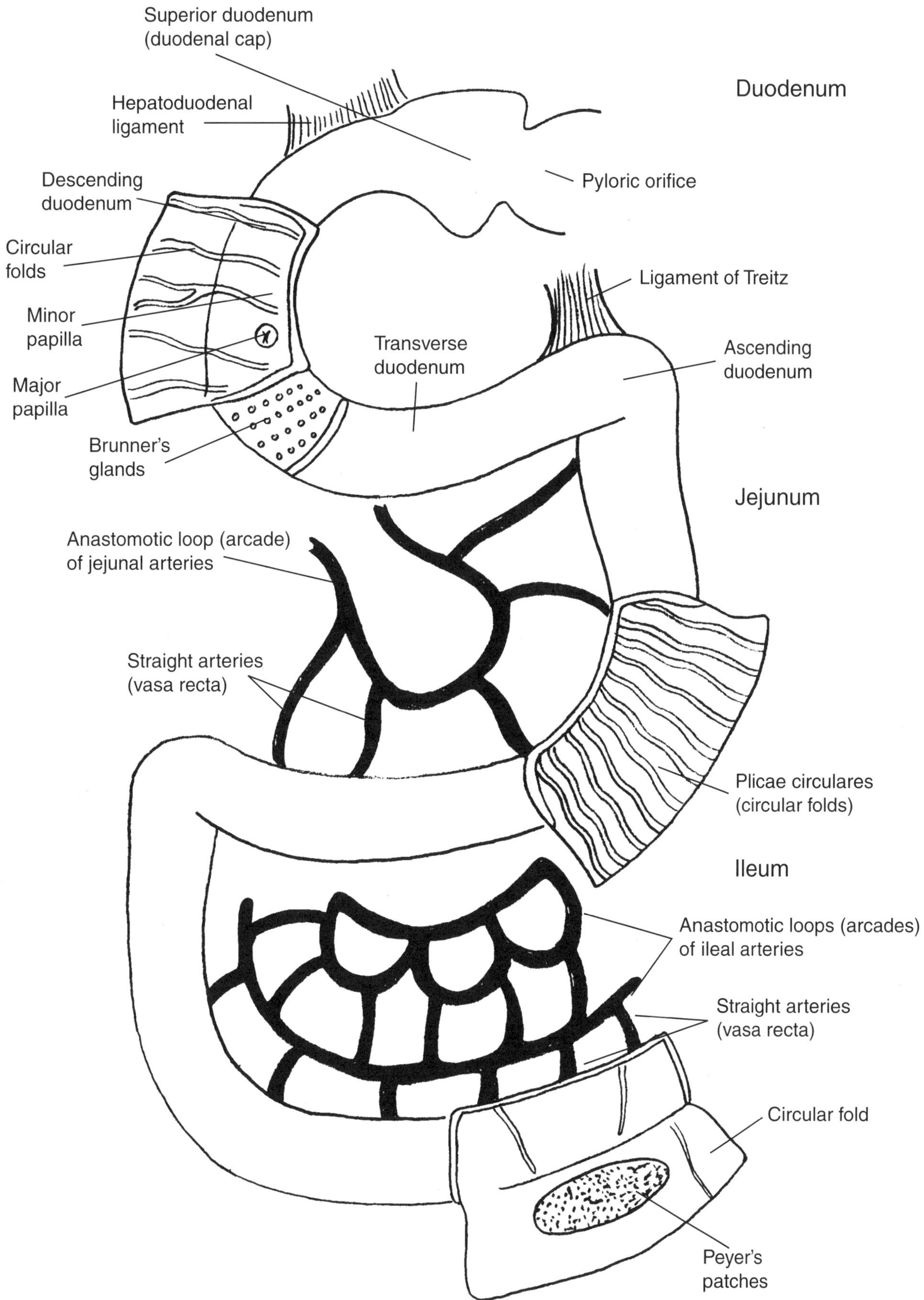
Superior duodenum
(duodenal cap)
Duodenum
Hepatoduodenal
ligament
Descending
duodenum
Pyloric orifice
Circular
folds
Ligament of Treitz
Minor
papilla
Transverse
duodenum
Ascending
duodenum
Major
papilla
Brunner's
glands
Jejunum
Anastomotic loop (arcade)
of jejunal arteries
Straight arteries
(vasa recta)
Plicae circulares
(circular folds)
Ileum
Anastomotic loops (arcades)
of ileal arteries
Straight arteries
(vasa recta)
Circular fold
Peyer's
patches

NOTES

ANATOMY OF THE LARGE INTESTINE

- Large intestine is approximately 1.5 m long
- Ascending and descending colon are retroperitoneal
- Transverse and sigmoid colon have mesentery, the transverse mesocolon, and sigmoid mesocolon
- Haustra are sacculations caused by the teniae coli that are shorter than the gut
- Teniae coli are three narrow, longitudinal muscular bands
- Epiploic appendages are sacs of fat located along the teniae
- Teniae spread to become a continuous muscle layer at the rectosigmoid junction

See Table 6.1 in Appendix.

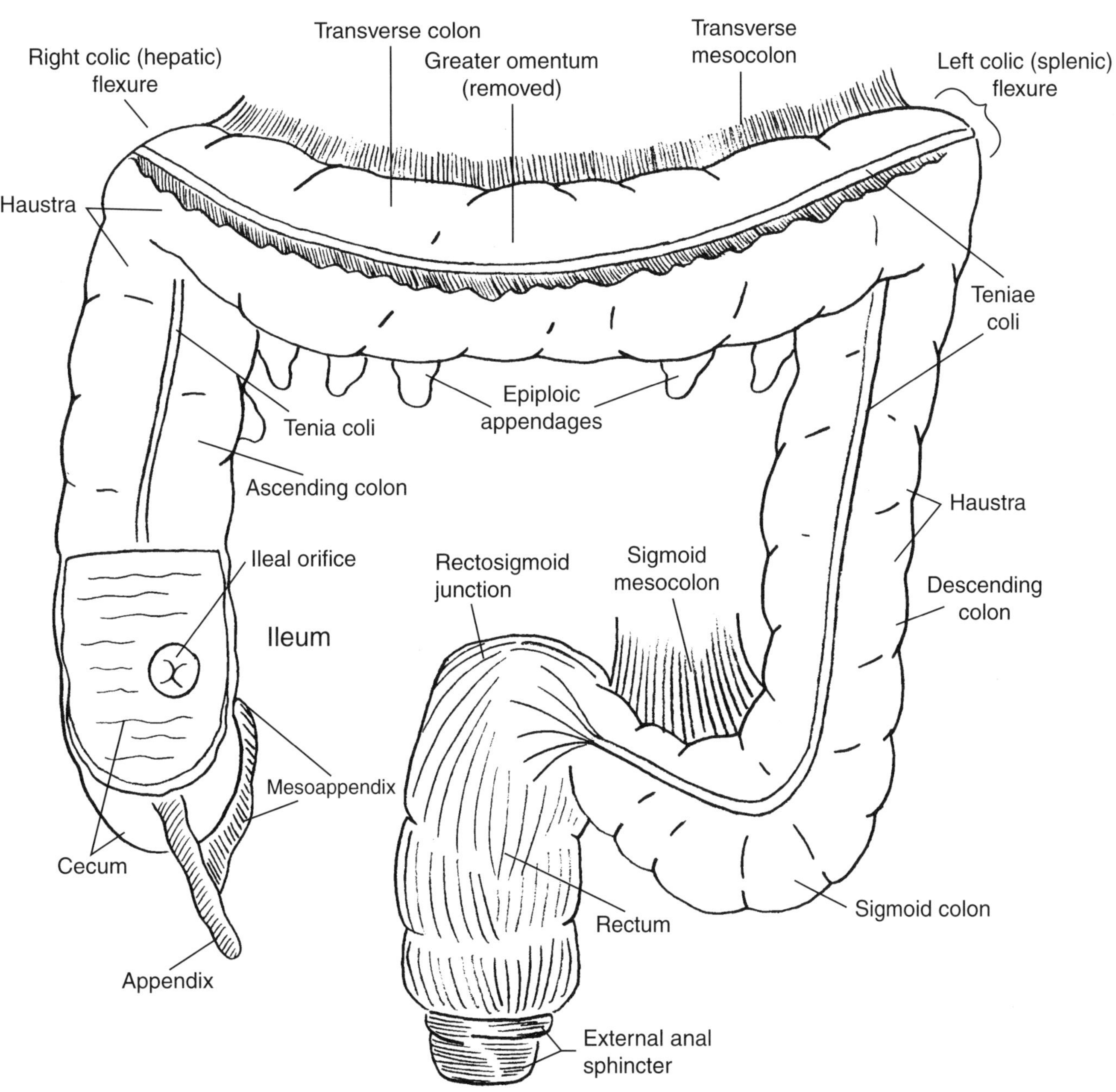
Transverse colon
Right colic (hepatic) flexure
Greater omentum (removed)
Transverse mesocolon
Left colic (splenic) flexure
Haustra
Teniae coli
Tenia coli
Epiploic appendages
Ascending colon
Haustra
Ileal orifice
Ileum
Rectosigmoid junction
Sigmoid mesocolon
Descending colon
Mesoappendix
Cecum
Appendix
Rectum
Sigmoid colon
External anal sphincter

See Table 7.1 in Appendix.

ANATOMY OF THE LIVER

- Right and left lobes are separated by the gallbladder fossa and the inferior vena cava
- Caudate lobe is the medial superior segment of the left lobe
- Quadrate lobe is the medial inferior segment of the left lobe
- Coronary ligament connects the liver and diaphragm and bounds the bare area of the liver
- Triangular ligament
- Falciform ligament attaches the liver to the diaphragm
- Round ligament (ligamentum teres) is the fetal remnant of the umbilical vein
- Ligamentum venosum is the fetal remnant of the ductus venosus
- Hepatoduodenal ligament is composed of lesser omentum that connects the porta hepatis and the duodenum
- Hepatogastric ligament is composed of lesser omentum that extends between the ligamentum venosum and the lesser curvature of the stomach
- Porta hepatis (portal fissure) is a fissure where the portal vein and hepatic artery enter and the hepatic ducts leave the liver
- Portal triad enters the liver at the porta hepatis and includes the portal vein, hepatic artery, and hepatic ducts
- Right and left hepatic ducts drain the right and left lobes of the liver and join to form the common hepatic duct

Anterior View

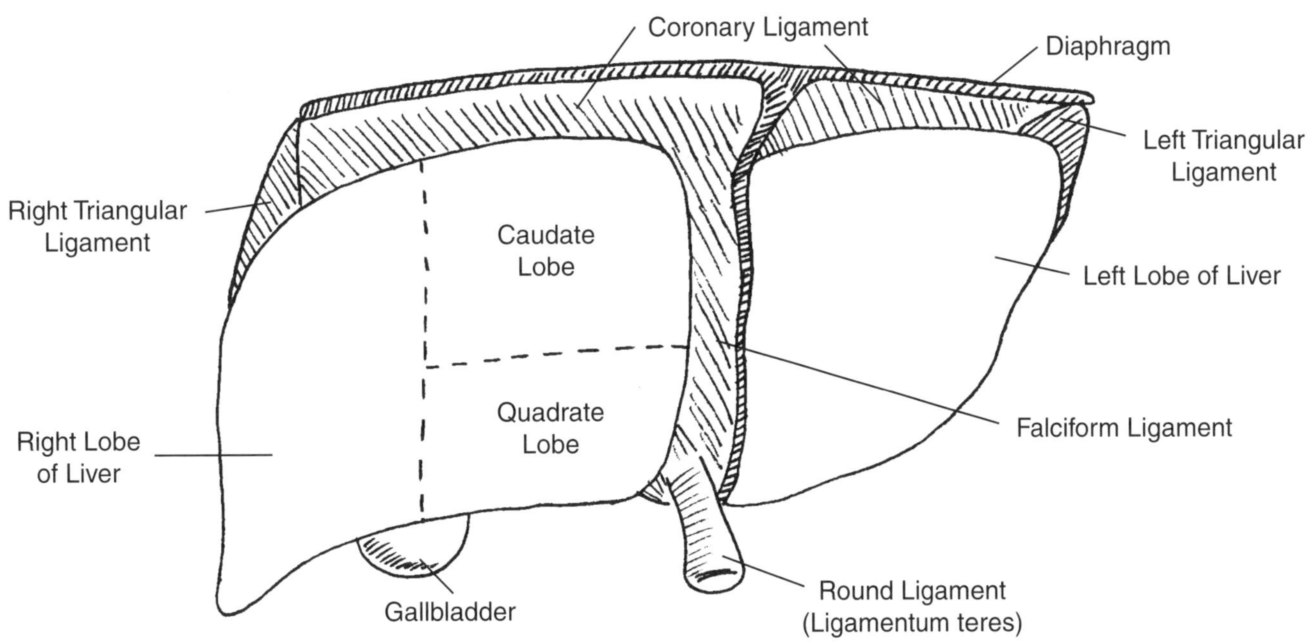
Coronary Ligament
Diaphragm
Left Triangular Ligament
Right Triangular Ligament
Caudate Lobe
Left Lobe of Liver
Quadrate Lobe
Falciform Ligament
Right Lobe of Liver
Gallbladder
Round Ligament (Ligamentum teres)

Visceral Surface

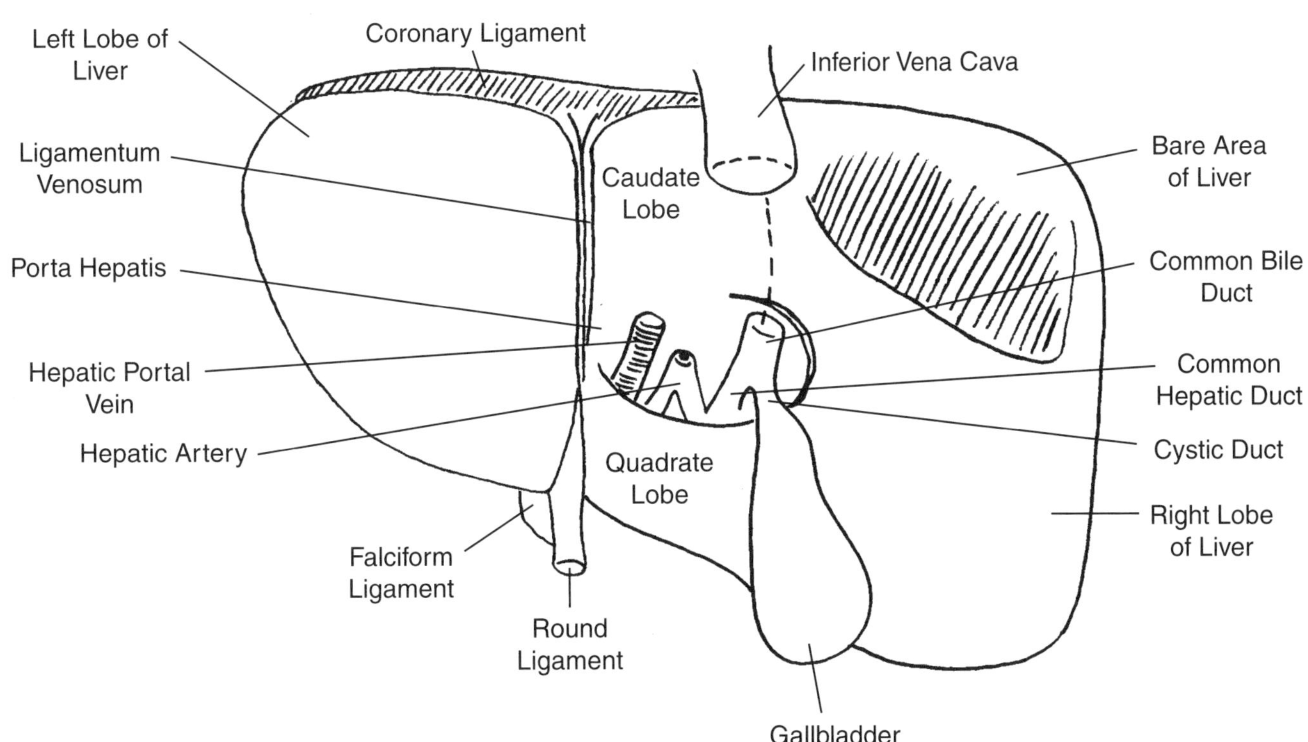
Left Lobe of Liver
Coronary Ligament
Inferior Vena Cava
Ligamentum Venosum
Caudate Lobe
Bare Area of Liver
Porta Hepatis
Common Bile Duct
Hepatic Portal Vein
Common Hepatic Duct
Hepatic Artery
Cystic Duct
Quadrate Lobe
Right Lobe of Liver
Falciform Ligament
Round Ligament
Gallbladder

NOTES

See Table 7.1 in Appendix.

BILIRUBIN

bilirubin ⇒ belly rubbin'

Red blood cells containing hemoglobin are destroyed and engulfed by macrophages in the liver, spleen, and bone marrow

RBCs contain hemoglobin ⇒ RBC holding heme on a globe

Bilirubin is a product of heme breakdown

- Direct bilirubin is conjugated and water soluble
  conjugated ⇒ holding hands
  water soluble ⇒ in water
- Indirect bilirubin is unconjugated and fat soluble
  unconjugated ⇒ broken in half
  fat soluble ⇒ butter
- Accumulation of bilirubin leads to jaundice

Removal and excretion of bilirubin

1. Bilirubin is removed from blood by the liver
2. Glucuronyl transferase conjugates glucuronate with bilirubin
   glucuronate ⇒ glue
3. Conjugated bilirubin is then excreted into bile
4. Bacteria in the colon convert bilirubin to urobilinogen
5. Some urobilinogen is circulated to the liver and excreted in urine
6. Excretion as stercobilin in feces
   stercobilin ⇒ stereo

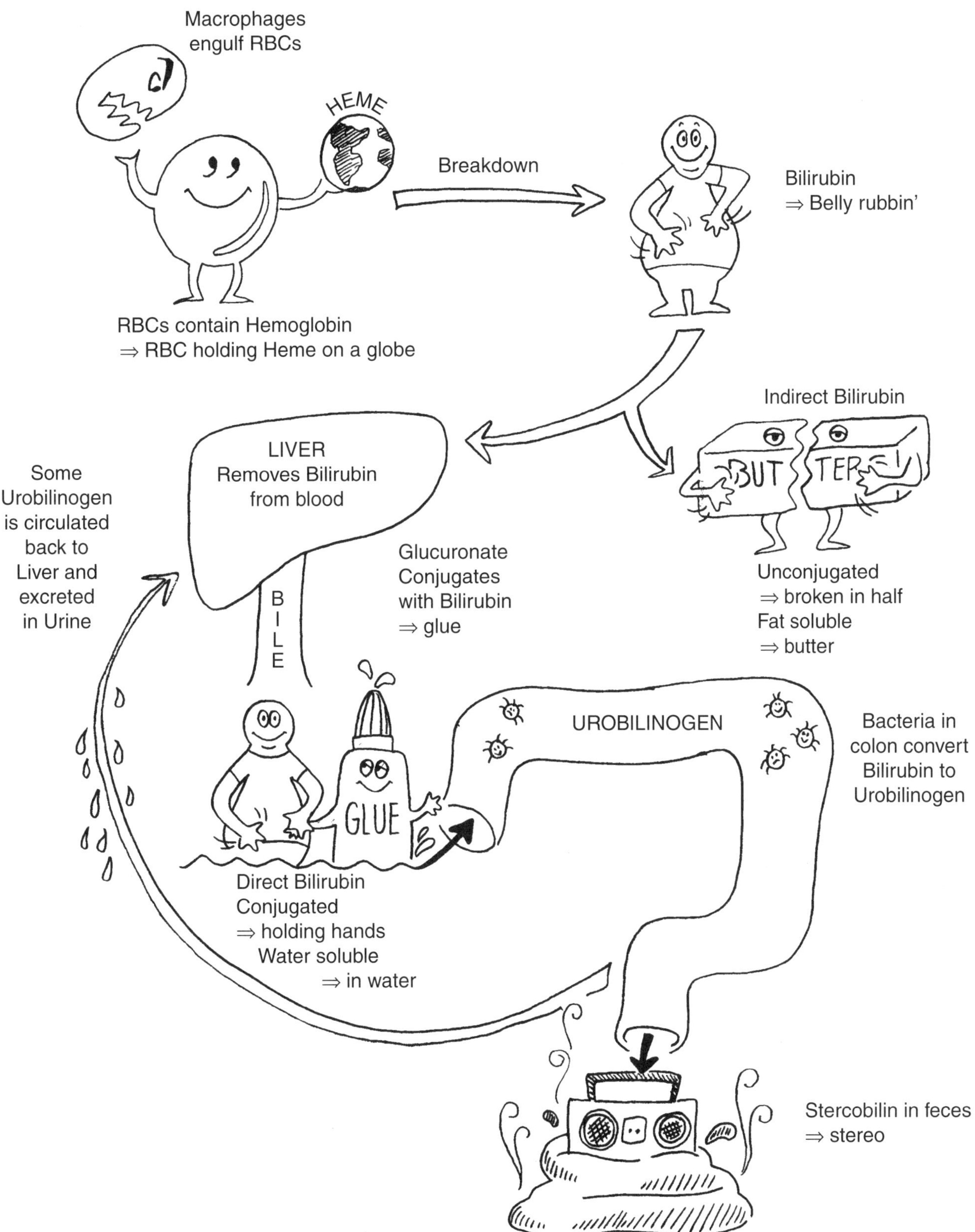
Macrophages
engulf RBCs
HEME
Breakdown
Bilirubin
⇒ Belly rubbin'
RBCs contain Hemoglobin
⇒ RBC holding Heme on a globe
Indirect Bilirubin
BUT
TER
Unconjugated
⇒ broken in half
Fat soluble
⇒ butter
LIVER
Removes Bilirubin
from blood
Some
Urobilinogen
is circulated
back to
Liver and
excreted
in Urine
Glucuronate
Conjugates
with Bilirubin
⇒ glue
BILE
GLUE
UROBILINOGEN
Bacteria in
colon convert
Bilirubin to
Urobilinogen
Direct Bilirubin
Conjugated
⇒ holding hands
Water soluble
⇒ in water
Stercobilin in feces
⇒ stereo

NOTES

GALLBLADDER ANATOMY

- The gallbladder is located between the right and quadrate lobes of the inferior liver
- The fundus is the rounded wide end usually located at the ninth costal cartilage
- The neck of the gallbladder is narrow
- The cystic duct contains spiral valves and connects the neck to the common hepatic duct
- The infundibulum of the gallbladder (Hartmann's pouch) is located where the neck and cystic duct join
  Hartman ⇒ heart man
- Calot's triangle (cystohepatic triangle) contains the cystic artery and is formed by the inferior border of the liver, the cystic duct, and the common hepatic duct

See Table 7.1 in Appendix.

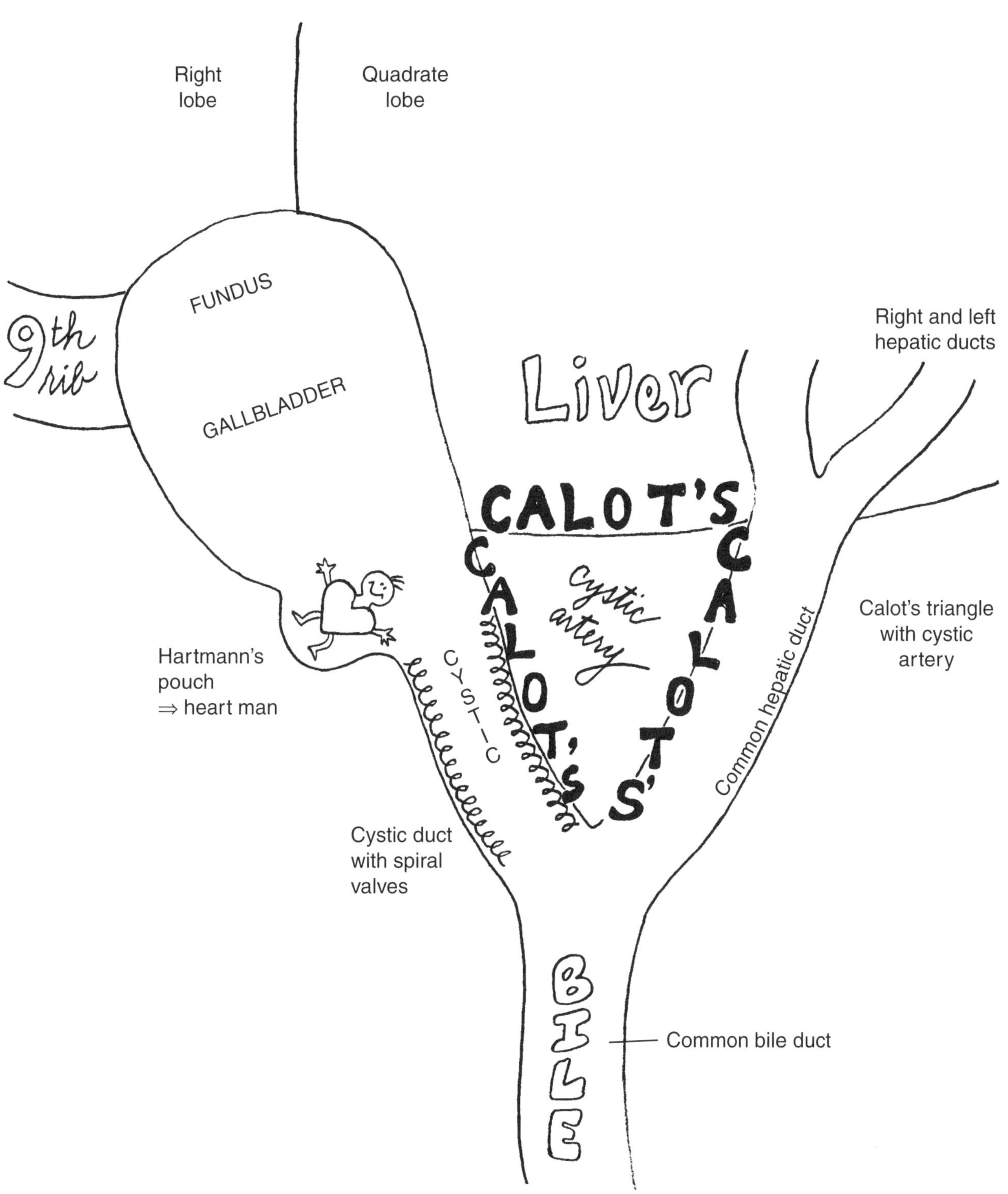
Right
lobe
Quadrate
lobe
FUNDUS
9th
rib
GALLBLADDER
Right and left
hepatic ducts
Liver
CALOT'S
CALOT'S
CALOT'S
cystic
artery
Hartmann's
pouch
⇒ heart man
CYSTIC
Common hepatic duct
Calot's triangle
with cystic
artery
Cystic duct
with spiral
valves
BILE
Common bile duct

NOTES

BILE SECRETION

⇒ "On the River Bile"

- Bile secreted by hepatocytes and storec in the gallbladder
- Bile contains bile salts, phospholipids, cholesterol, and bilirubin
  bile salts ⇒ salt shaker
  bilirubin ⇒ belly rubbin'
  phospholipids and cholesterol ⇒ butter
- Bile acids are synthesized from cholesterol by hepatocytes
  ⇒ butter → acid on Bile River
- Bile salts form by the conjugation of bile acids and glycine or taurine
- Bile salts are amphipathic (hydrophobic and hydrophilic)
  amphipathic ⇒ one hand in water, one hand away from water
- CCK (cholecystokinin) leads to contraction of the gallbladder and relaxation of the sphincter of Oddi
- Bile acids are recirculated to the liver
- Sodium-bile acid cotransporter is located in the terminal ileum that recirculates bile acids to the liver

See Table 7.1 in Appendix.

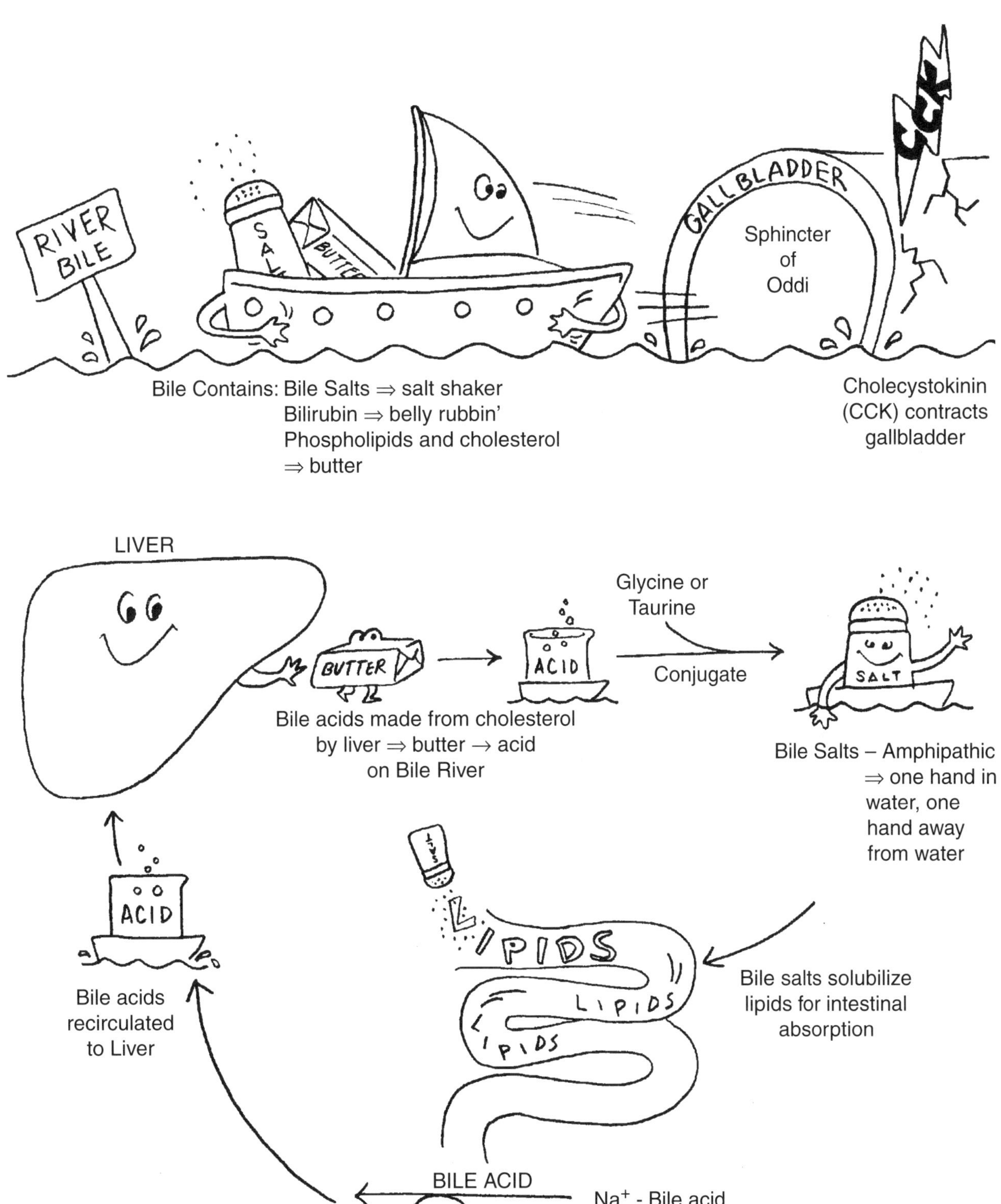
RIVER BILE
SALT
BUTTER
GALLBLADDER
Sphincter of Oddi
CCK
Bile Contains: Bile Salts ⇒ salt shaker
Bilirubin ⇒ belly rubbin'
Phospholipids and cholesterol ⇒ butter
Cholecystokinin (CCK) contracts gallbladder
LIVER
BUTTER
ACID
Glycine or Taurine
Conjugate
SALT
Bile acids made from cholesterol by liver ⇒ butter → acid on Bile River
Bile Salts – Amphipathic ⇒ one hand in water, one hand away from water
LIPIDS
LIPIDS
LIPIDS
Bile salts solubilize lipids for intestinal absorption
ACID
Bile acids recirculated to Liver
BILE ACID
Na+ - Bile acid cotransporter
Na+

NOTES

ANATOMY OF THE PANCREAS

- Pancreas lies retroperitoneally posterior to the stomach
  retroperitoneal ⇒ parrot
- Head of the pancreas lies in the C-shaped curve of the duodenum
- Uncinate process is a projection from the lower part of the head and extends behind the superior mesenteric artery
- Neck of the pancreas lies over the superior mesenteric vessels and behind pylorus of the stomach
  pylorus ⇒ pie

Body of the Pancreas

- Tail of the pancreas is located near the hilum of the spleen
  hilum ⇒ hills
- Main pancreatic duct (duct of Wirsung) begins in the tail and runs through the pancreas to join the bile duct and form the hepatopancreatic ampulla
  Wirsung ⇒ "we sung"
- Hepatopancreatic ampulla (ampulla of Vater) opens into the descending duodenum at the major duodenal papilla
  ampulla of Vater ⇒ amp
- Hepatopancreatic sphincter (sphincter of Oddi) controls the flow of bile and pancreatic secretions
- Accessory pancreatic duct (duct of Santorini) begins in the uncinate process and empties into the minor duodenal papilla located above the major papilla
  Santorini ⇒ magician

See Table 7.1 in Appendix.

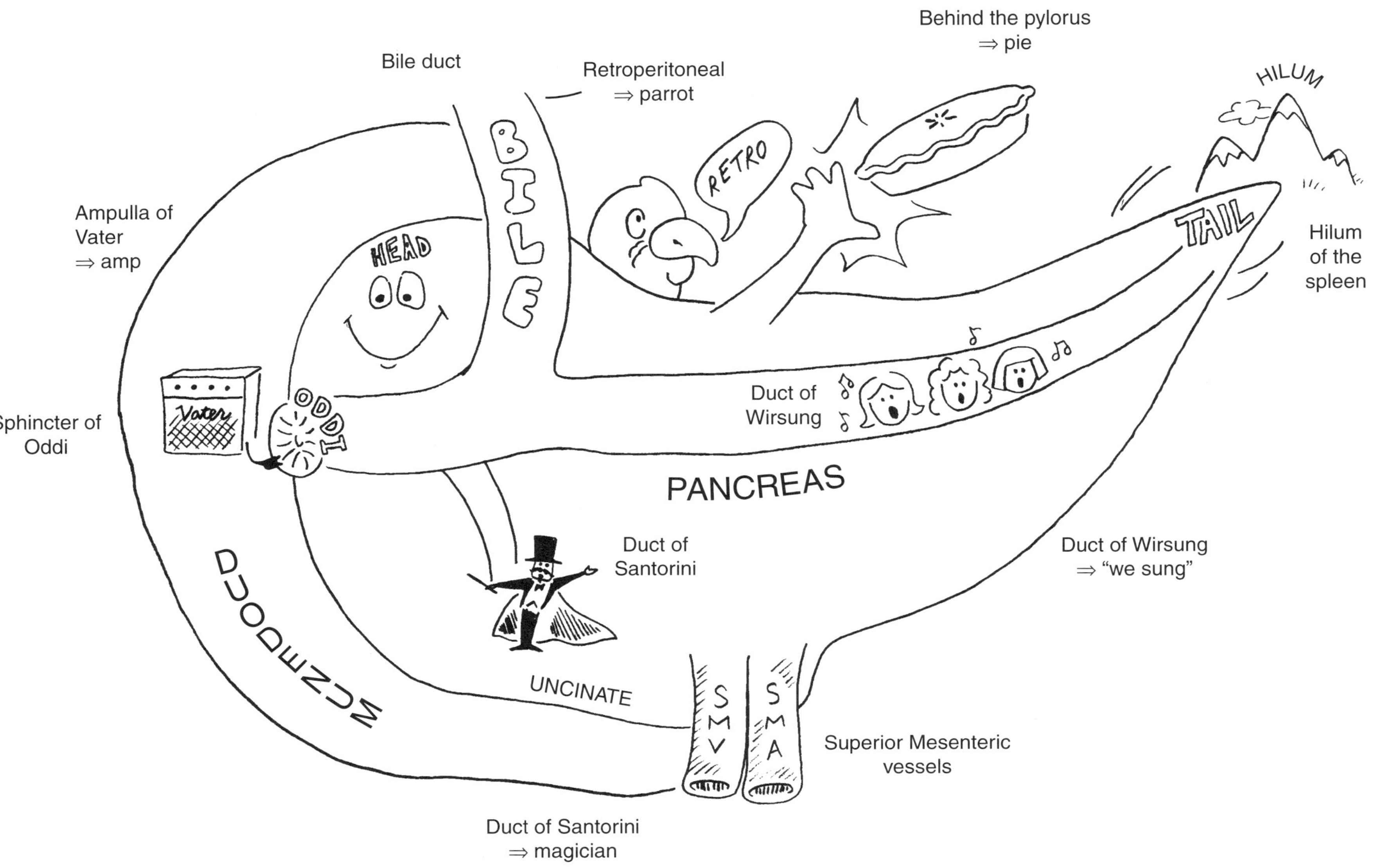
Bile duct
Retroperitoneal
⇒ parrot
Behind the pylorus
⇒ pie
HILUM
BILE
RETRO
Ampulla of
Vater
⇒ amp
HEAD
TAIL
Hilum
of the
spleen
Sphincter of
Oddi
Vater
ODDI
Duct of
Wirsung
PANCREAS
Duct of
Santorini
Duct of Wirsung
⇒ "we sung"
DUODENUM
UNCINATE
SMV
SMA
Superior Mesenteric
vessels
Duct of Santorini
⇒ magician

NOTES

EXOCRINE PANCREAS

- Isotonic
- Higher HCO_3^- concentration than in plasma
- Equivalent Na^+ and K^+ concentrations as plasma
- HCO_3^- neutralizes acidic chyme
- α-amylase digests starches
  amylase ⇒ Amy
- Lipase and phospholipase A digest fat
  lipase ⇒ lips
- Trypsin and chymotrypsin are proteases that digest protein
  trypsin ⇒ trip   protein ⇒ steak
- Trypsinogen is converted to trypsin (active) by enterokinase
  ⇒ leg tripping
- Acinar cells produce Na^+, Cl^-, and enzymes and are stimulated by ACh and CCK
- Ductal cells secrete HCO_3^- and absorb Cl^- by a Cl^-—HCO_3^- exchange
  ductal cells ⇒ duck

See Table 7.1 in Appendix.

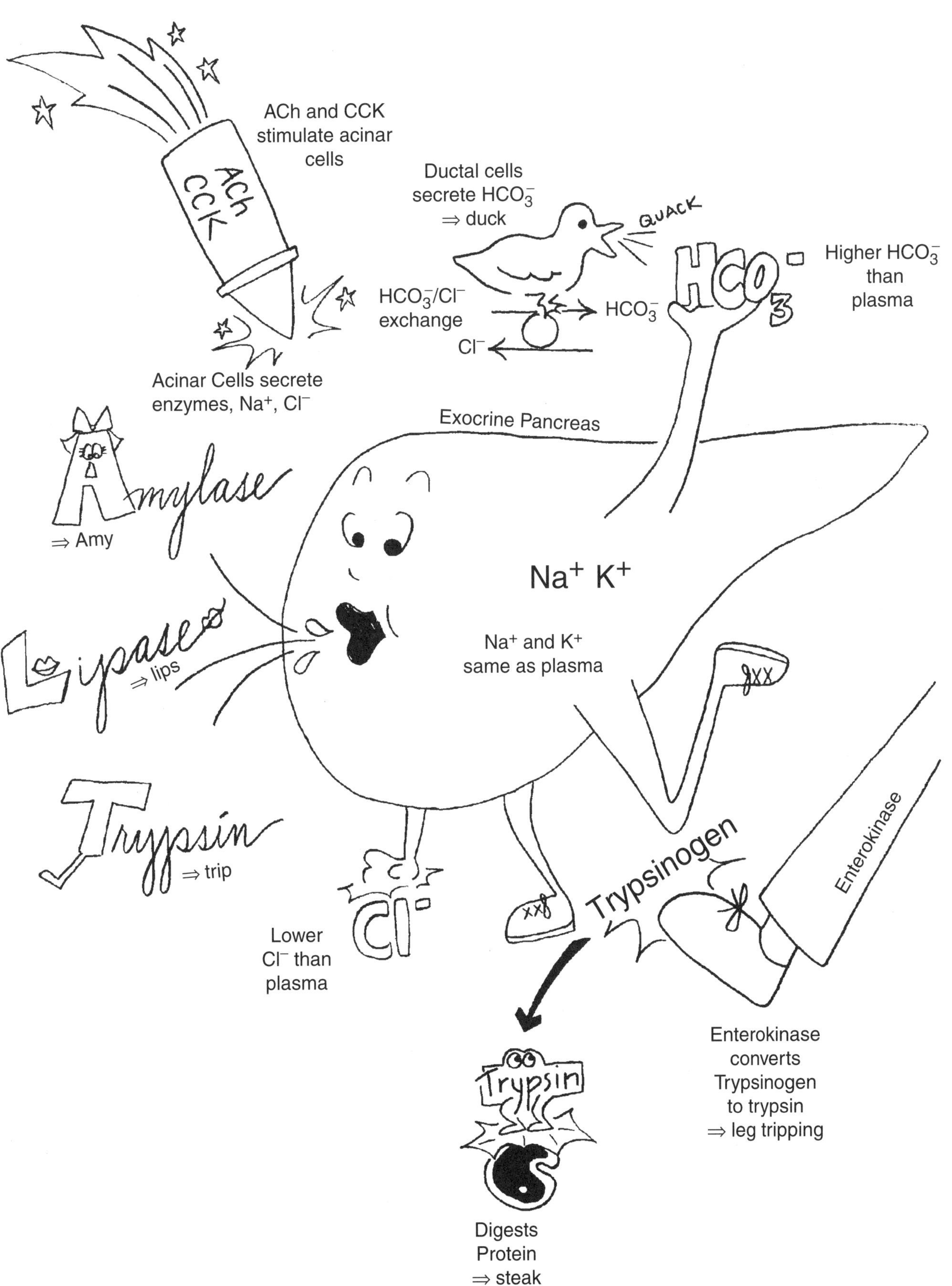
ACh and CCK stimulate acinar cells
ACh CCK
Ductal cells secrete HCO_3^- ⇒ duck
QUACK
HCO_3^-
Higher HCO_3^- than plasma
HCO_3^-/Cl^- exchange
HCO_3^-
Cl^-
Acinar Cells secrete enzymes, Na^+, Cl^-
Exocrine Pancreas
Amylase
⇒ Amy
Na^+ K^+
Na^+ and K^+ same as plasma
Lipase
⇒ lips
Trypsin
⇒ trip
Enterokinase
Trypsinogen
Cl^-
Lower Cl^- than plasma
Enterokinase converts Trypsinogen to trypsin ⇒ leg tripping
Trypsin
Digests Protein ⇒ steak

NOTES

REGULATION OF PANCREATIC SECRETIONS

- CCK (cholecystokinin) is secreted by the I cells of the duodenum and stimulates acinar cells to increase secretion of amylase, lipase, and proteases
  amylase ⇒ Amy
  lipase ⇒ lips
  protease ⇒ protein = steak
  - second messenger is IP_3 and Ca^{2+}
- Secretin is secreted by the S cells of the duodenum in response to H^+
  - secretin stimulates ductal cells to increase HCO_3^- that neutralizes the gastrin H^+ secretion
  - second messenger is cAMP
- ACh stimulates acinar cell secretion of enzymes
- Both ACh and CCK potentiate secretin to stimulate HCO_3^- secretion

See Table 7.1 in Appendix.

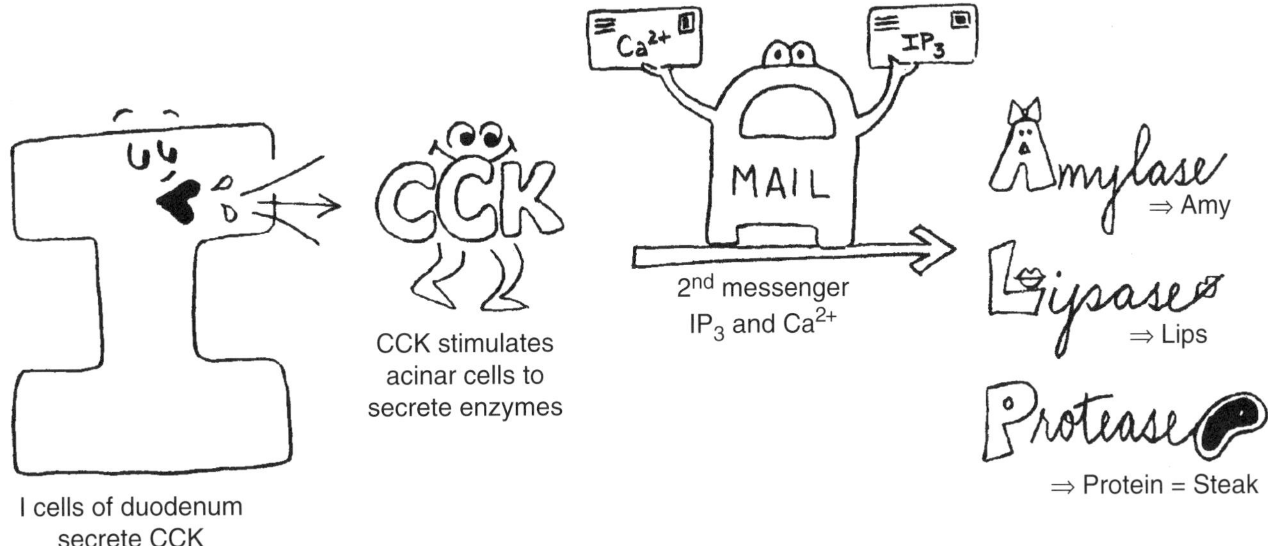

I cells of duodenum secrete CCK
⇒ I spitting out CCK

CCK stimulates acinar cells to secrete enzymes

2nd messenger
IP_3 and Ca^{2+}

⇒ Amy

⇒ Lips

⇒ Protein = Steak

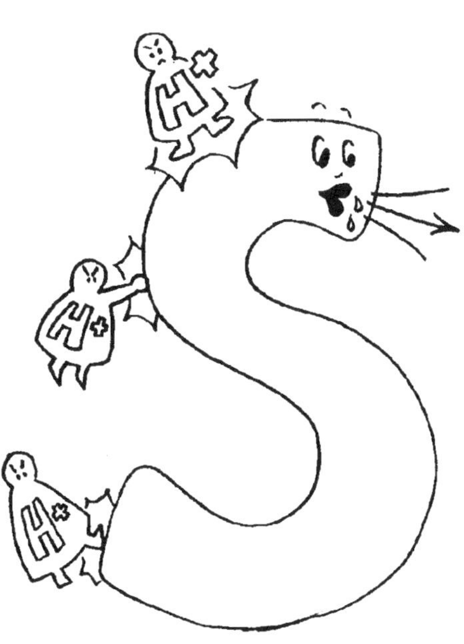

S cells of duodenum secrete secretin
⇒ S spitting out secretin
S cells respond to H^+
⇒ H^+ hitting S

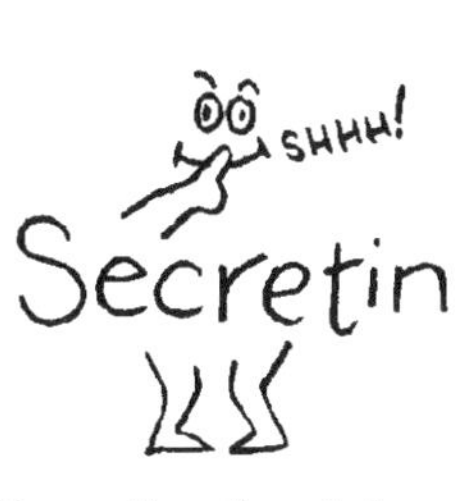

Secretin stimulates ductal cells to increase HCO_3^-

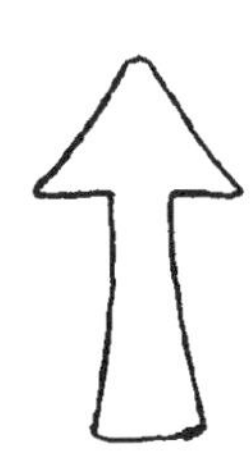

ACh and CCK potentiate secretin

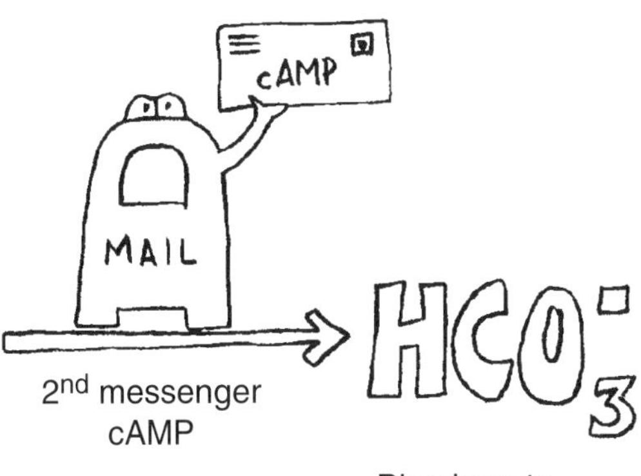

2nd messenger
cAMP

Bicarbonate

NOTES

ANATOMY OF THE SPLEEN

The spleen is a lymphatic organ located at ribs 9–11 and covered with peritoneum except at the hilum

hilum ⇒ hills

peritoneum ⇒ parrot

- Splenic artery and vein enter and leave the spleen at the hilum
- Capsule of the spleen consists of fibroelastic connective tissue
  capsule ⇒ cap
- Gastrosplenic ligament connects the spleen to the greater curvature of the stomach
  gastrosplenic ligament ⇒ stomach-grabbing spleen
- Splenorenal ligament connects the spleen and the left kidney
  splenorenal ligament ⇒ spleen-grabbing kidney

See Table 7.1 in Appendix.

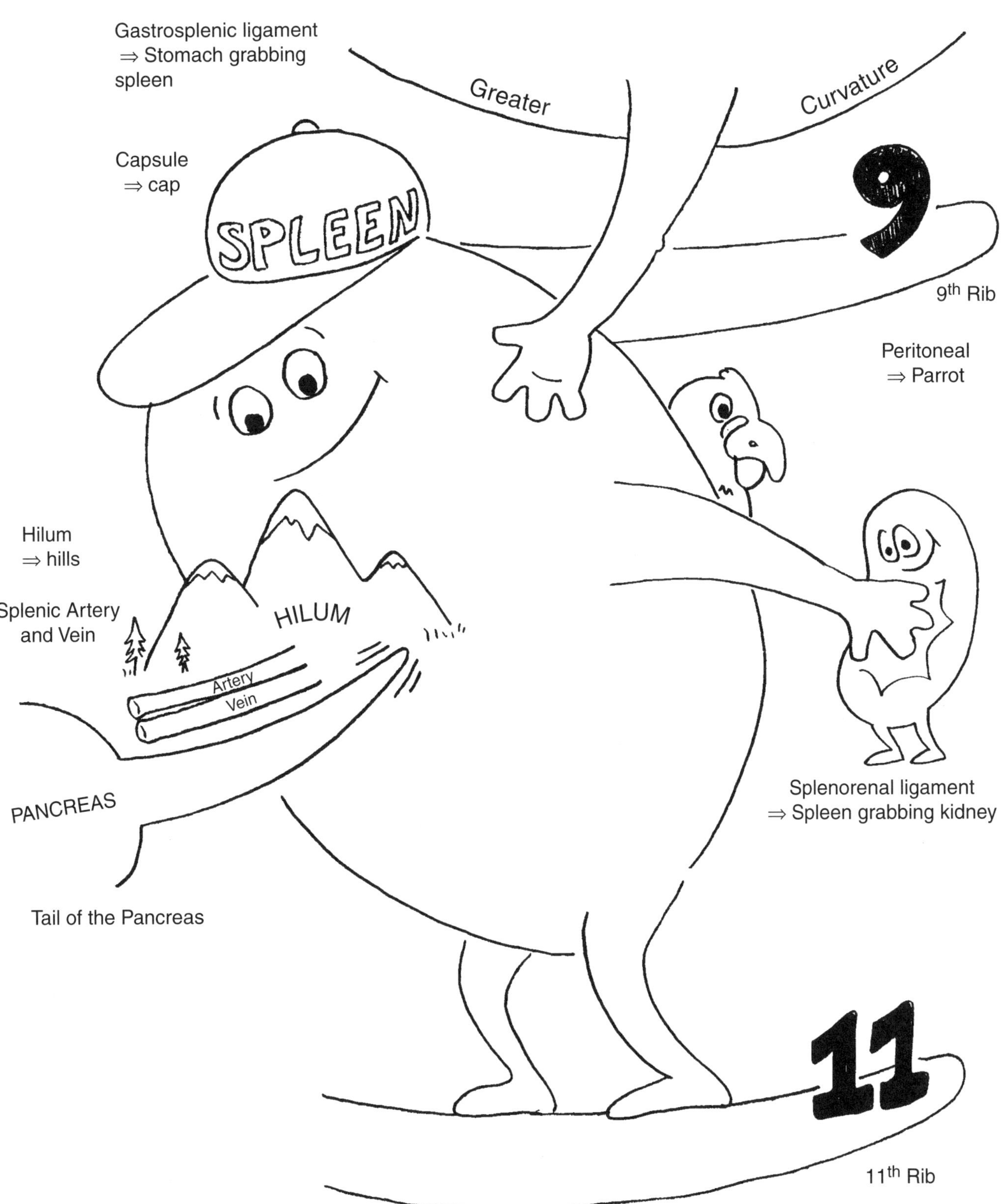
Gastrosplenic ligament
⇒ Stomach grabbing spleen
Greater Curvature
Capsule
⇒ cap
SPLEEN
9
9th Rib
Peritoneal
⇒ Parrot
Hilum
⇒ hills
HILUM
Splenic Artery and Vein
Artery
Vein
PANCREAS
Tail of the Pancreas
Splenorenal ligament
⇒ Spleen grabbing kidney
11
11th Rib

NOTES

SINUSOIDS OF SPLEEN

- Red pulp contains venous sinuses, arterial channels, and T cells
- White pulp contains B cells
- PALS (periarterial lymphoid sheath) contains T cells
  ⇒ "T cells are pals"
- Germinal center is a pale area of lymphopoietic cells in the center of lymphatic nodules
  germinal centers ⇒ germs

See Table 7.1 in Appendix.

Red Pulp contains T cells
White Pulp contains B cells

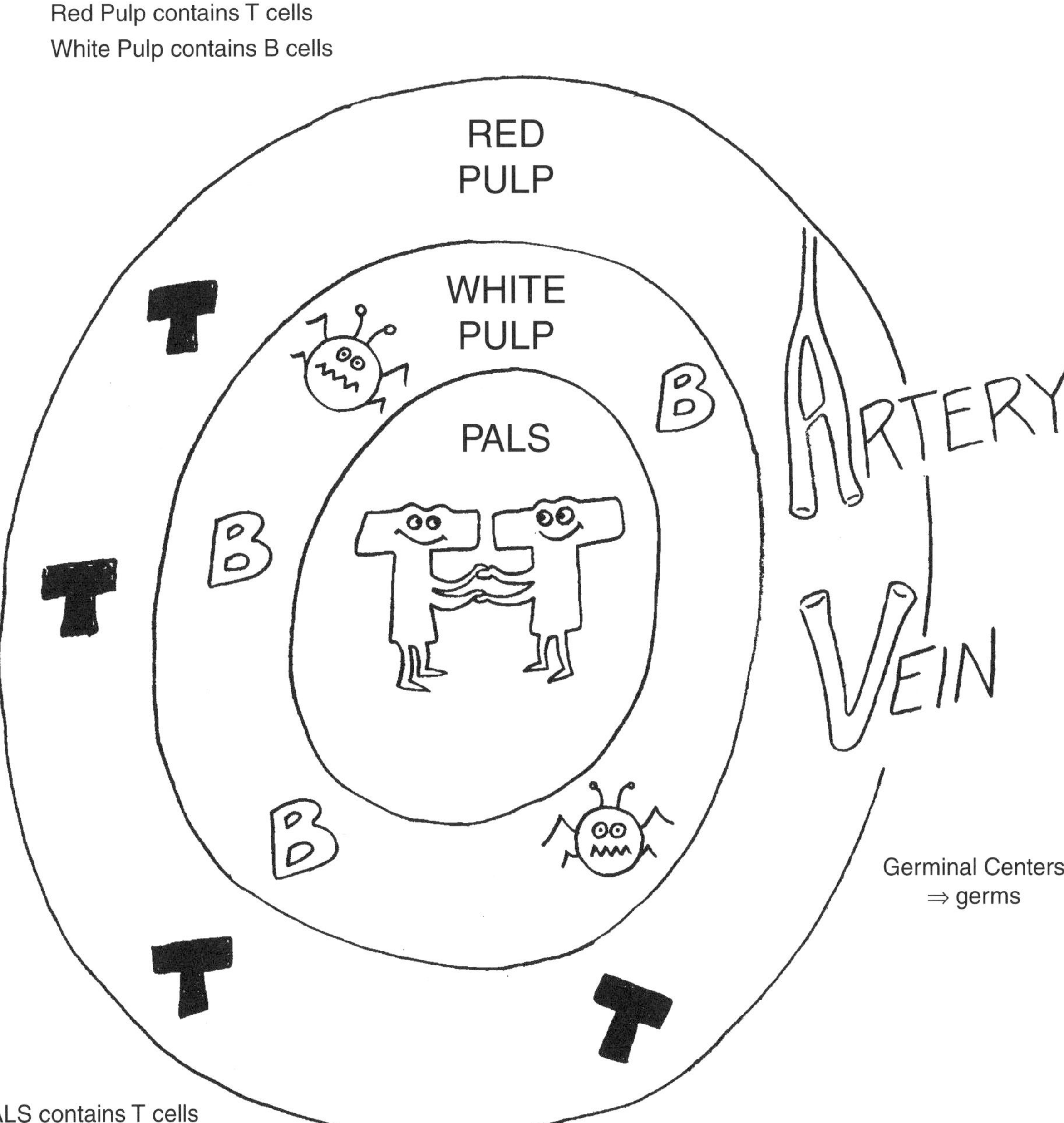

Germinal Centers
⇒ germs

PALS contains T cells
⇒ "T cells are pals"

NOTES

RENAL ANATOMY

- Kidney is retroperitoneal; right kidney lies lower than left
- Each kidney contains a medulla and cortex and 1.5 million nephrons
- Nephrons are the functional unit of the kidney
- Cortex contains the nephron's glomerulus, proximal and distal convoluted tubules
- Medulla consists of 8–12 renal pyramids that contain the nephron's ascending and descending loops and the collecting tubule or duct

Ureter

- Extends from kidney to bladder
- Muscular tube

Adrenal glands

- Located on the superior aspect of the kidneys

Blood Supply

- Renal arteries originate at the aorta; give rise to ureteric and inferior suprarenal arteries
- Divides into superior, anterior, inferior, and posterior segmental branches; then further divides into lobar → to interlobar → to arcuate → to interlobular arteries

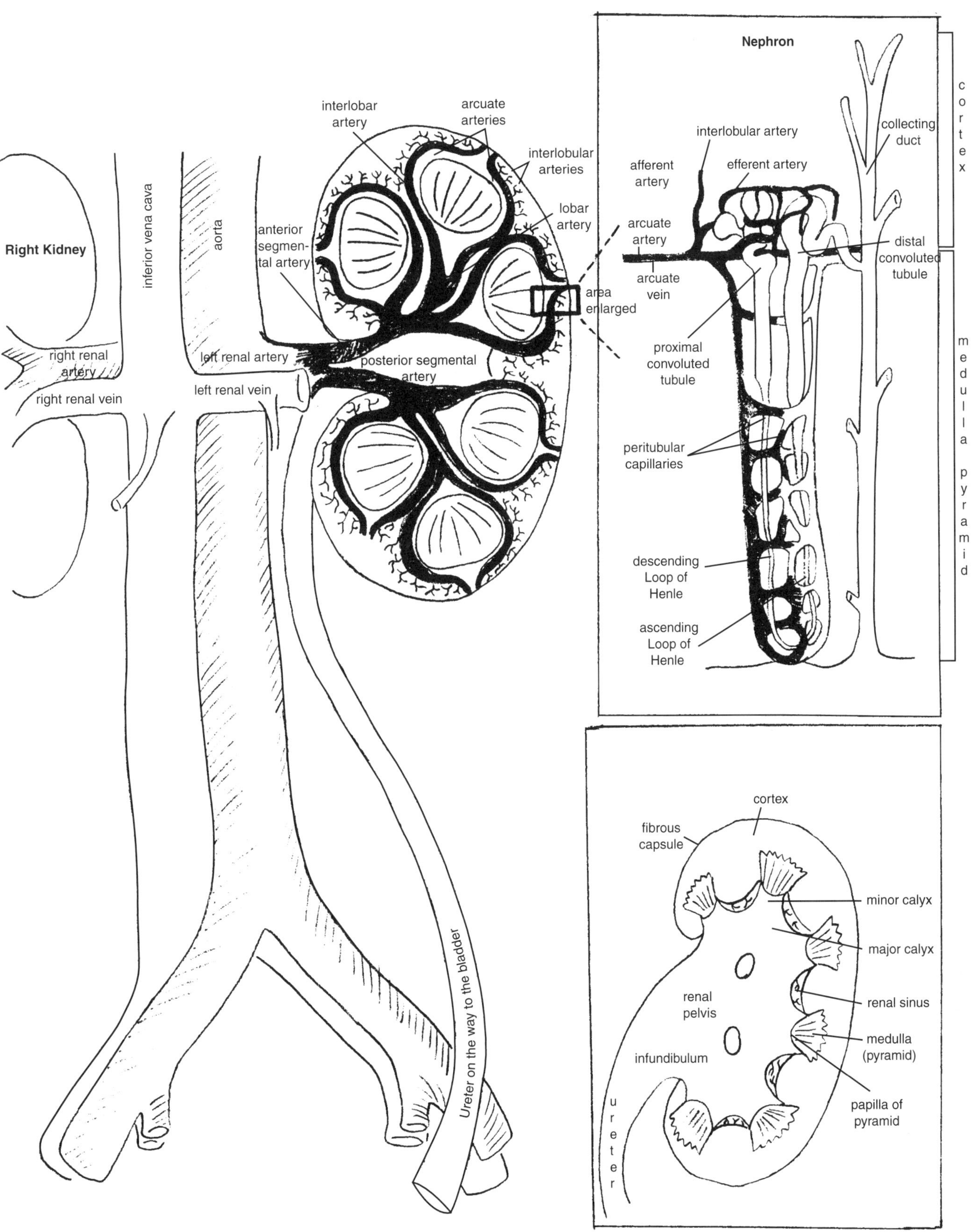
Right Kidney
inferior vena cava
aorta
interlobar artery
arcuate arteries
interlobular arteries
lobar artery
anterior segmental artery
area enlarged
right renal artery
right renal vein
left renal artery
left renal vein
posterior segmental artery
Ureter on the way to the bladder
Nephron
interlobular artery
collecting duct
afferent artery
efferent artery
arcuate artery
arcuate vein
distal convoluted tubule
proximal convoluted tubule
peritubular capillaries
descending Loop of Henle
ascending Loop of Henle
cortex
medulla pyramid
cortex
fibrous capsule
minor calyx
major calyx
renal sinus
renal pelvis
medulla (pyramid)
infundibulum
papilla of pyramid
ureter

NOTES

FILTRATION, REABSORPTION, AND SECRETION

- Filtered plasma must pass through three layers to get to the Bowman's capsule in the glomerulus
  - capillary fenestrated endothelial lining
  - negatively charged basement membrane (charge barrier)
  - podocytes of Bowman's capsule (size barrier)
- Substances easily filtered: isotonic plasma, positively charged particles, glucose, amino acids, water, Na^+, K^+, Ca^{2+}, and small proteins (<7000 Daltons)
- Substances NOT filtered under normal circumstances: large proteins (>70,000 Daltons) such as albumin, and negatively charged proteins

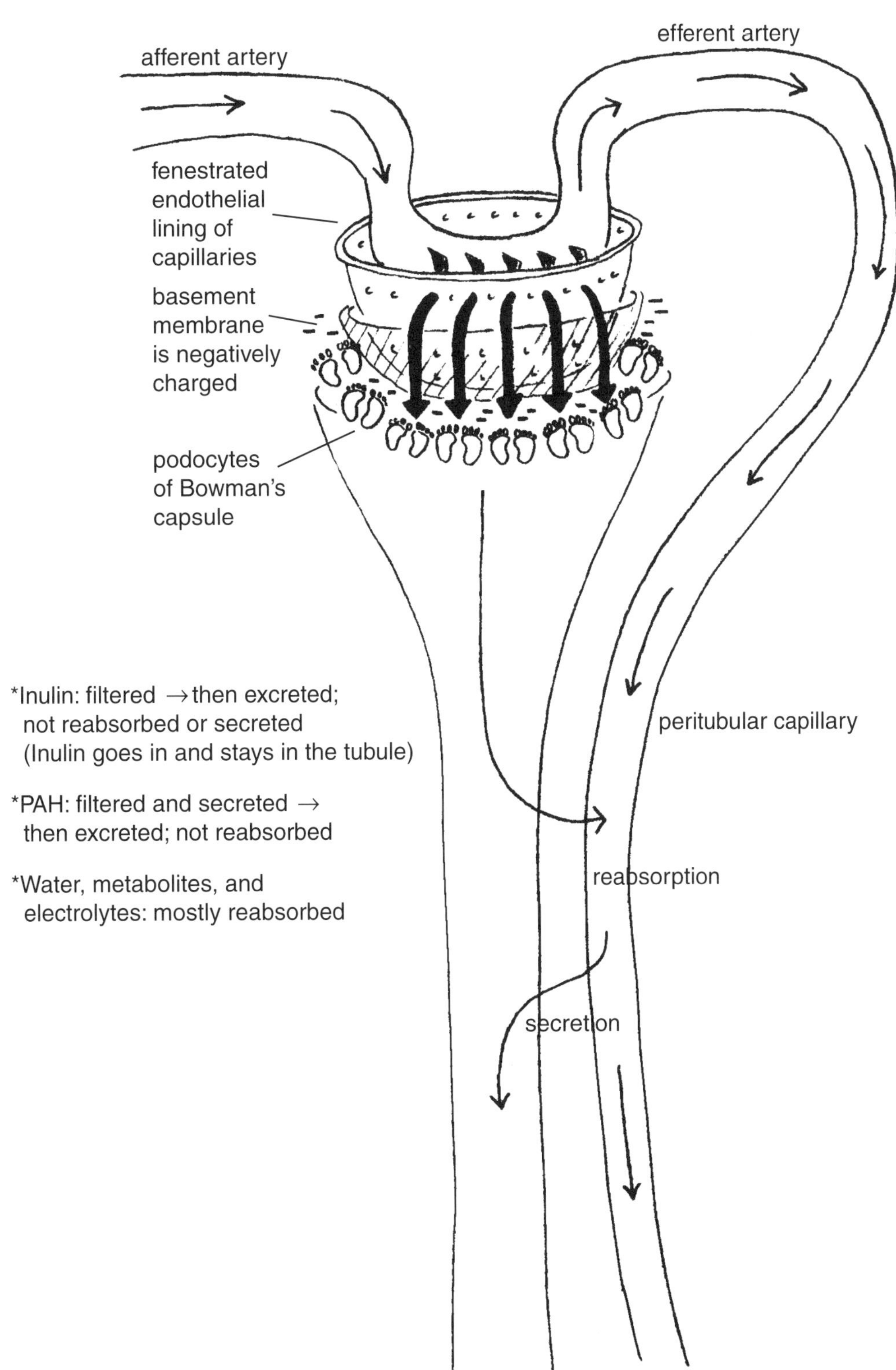
afferent artery
efferent artery
fenestrated endothelial lining of capillaries
basement membrane is negatively charged
podocytes of Bowman's capsule
*Inulin: filtered → then excreted; not reabsorbed or secreted (Inulin goes in and stays in the tubule)
*PAH: filtered and secreted → then excreted; not reabsorbed
*Water, metabolites, and electrolytes: mostly reabsorbed
peritubular capillary
reabsorption
secretion

NOTES

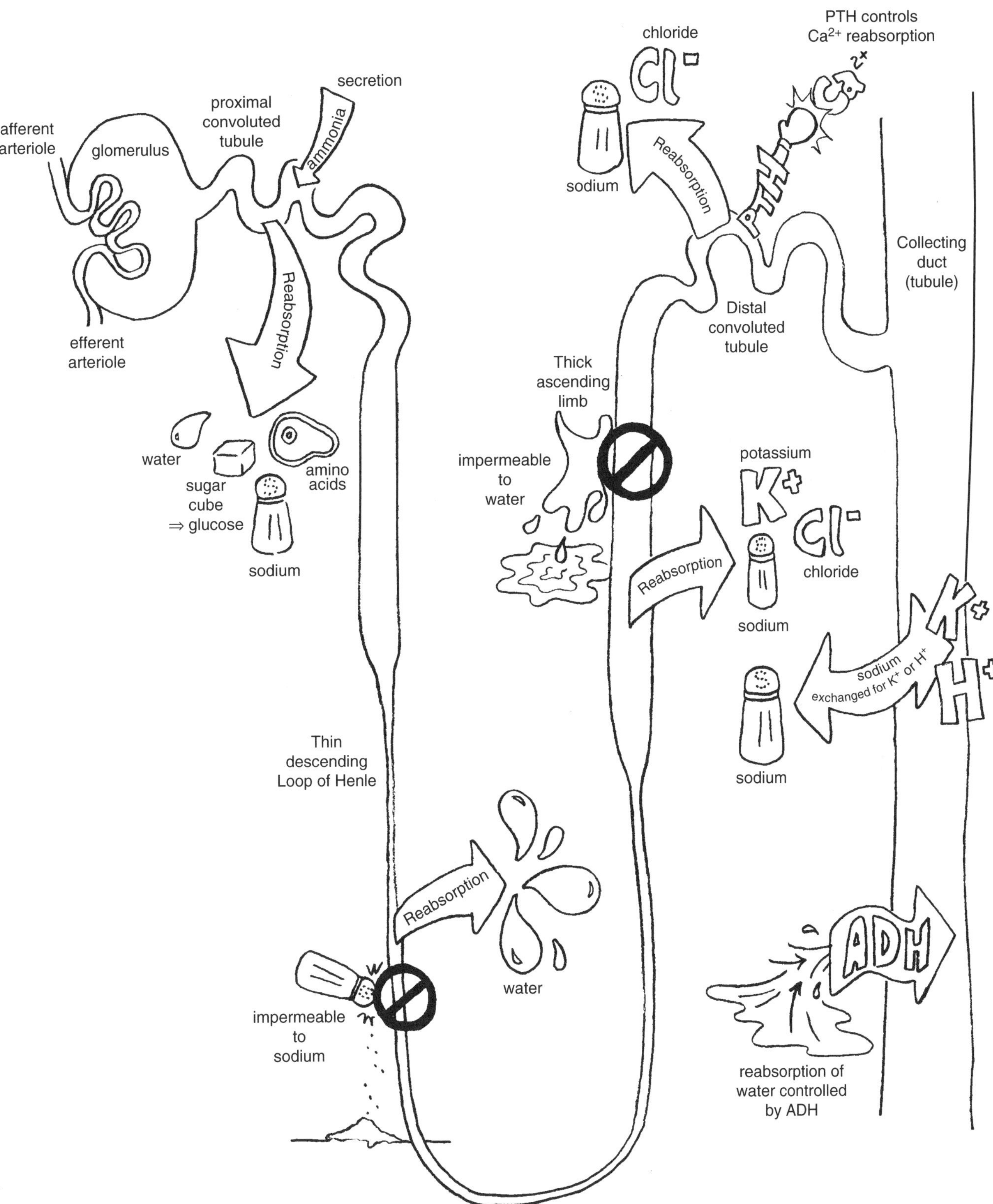
afferent arteriole
glomerulus
proximal convoluted tubule
secretion
ammonia
Reabsorption
efferent arteriole
water
sugar cube ⇒ glucose
amino acids
sodium
Thin descending Loop of Henle
Reabsorption
water
impermeable to sodium
chloride
Cl⁻
sodium
Reabsorption
PTH controls Ca2+ reabsorption
PTH
Ca2+
Collecting duct (tubule)
Distal convoluted tubule
Thick ascending limb
impermeable to water
potassium
K+
Cl⁻
Reabsorption
sodium
chloride
K+
sodium exchanged for K+ or H+
H+
sodium
ADH
reabsorption of water controlled by ADH

NOTES

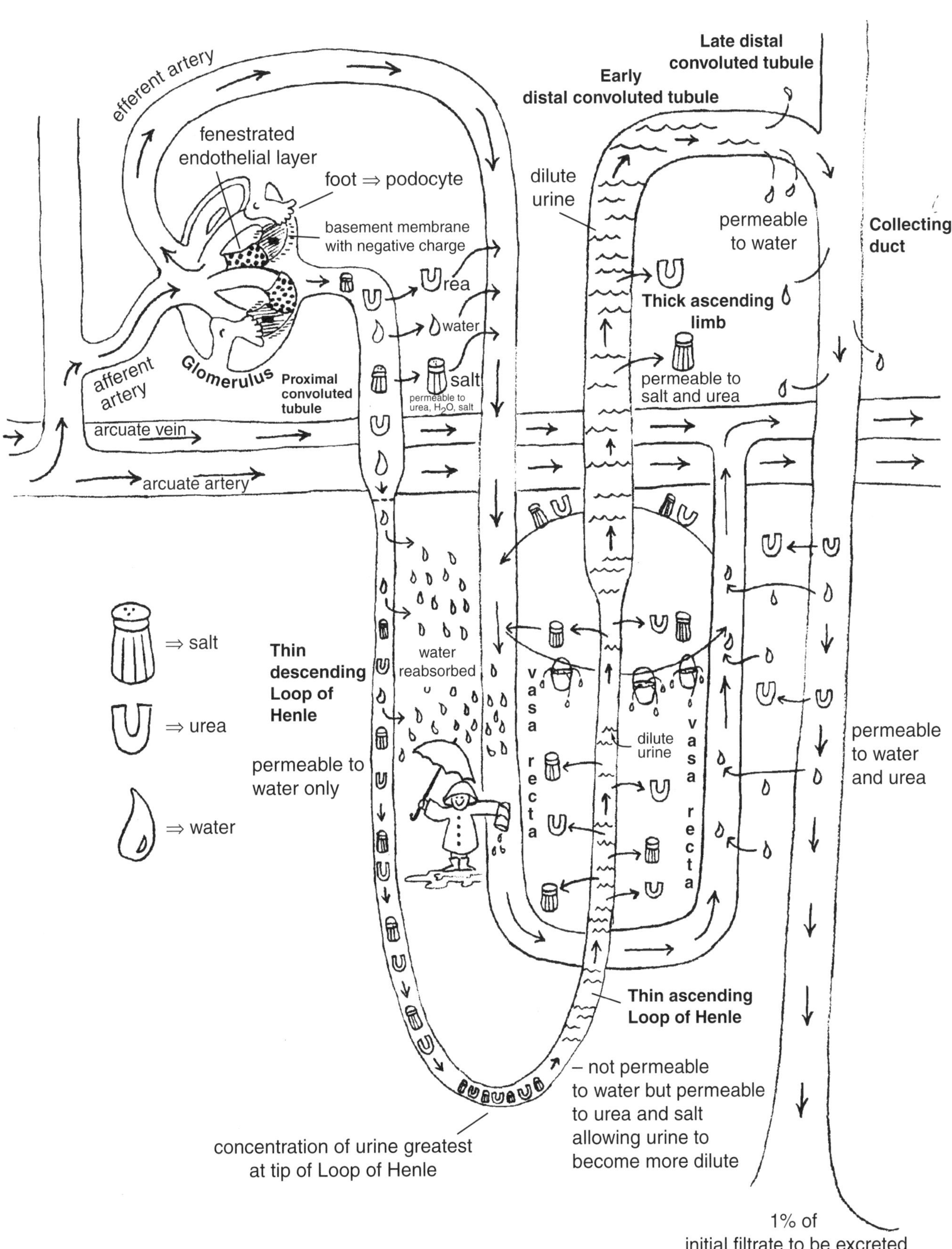
Late distal convoluted tubule
Early distal convoluted tubule
efferent artery
fenestrated endothelial layer
foot ⇒ podocyte
basement membrane with negative charge
dilute urine
permeable to water
Collecting duct
Urea
water
Thick ascending limb
salt
permeable to urea, H_2O, salt
permeable to salt and urea
afferent artery
Glomerulus
Proximal convoluted tubule
arcuate vein
arcuate artery
⇒ salt
⇒ urea
⇒ water
Thin descending Loop of Henle
permeable to water only
water reabsorbed
vasa recta
dilute urine
vasa recta
permeable to water and urea
Thin ascending Loop of Henle
– not permeable to water but permeable to urea and salt allowing urine to become more dilute
concentration of urine greatest at tip of Loop of Henle
1% of initial filtrate to be excreted

NOTES

Glomerular Capillary Pressures

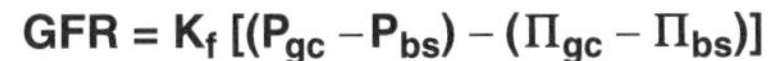

$$GFR = K_f [(P_{gc} - P_{bs}) - (\Pi_{gc} - \Pi_{bs})]$$

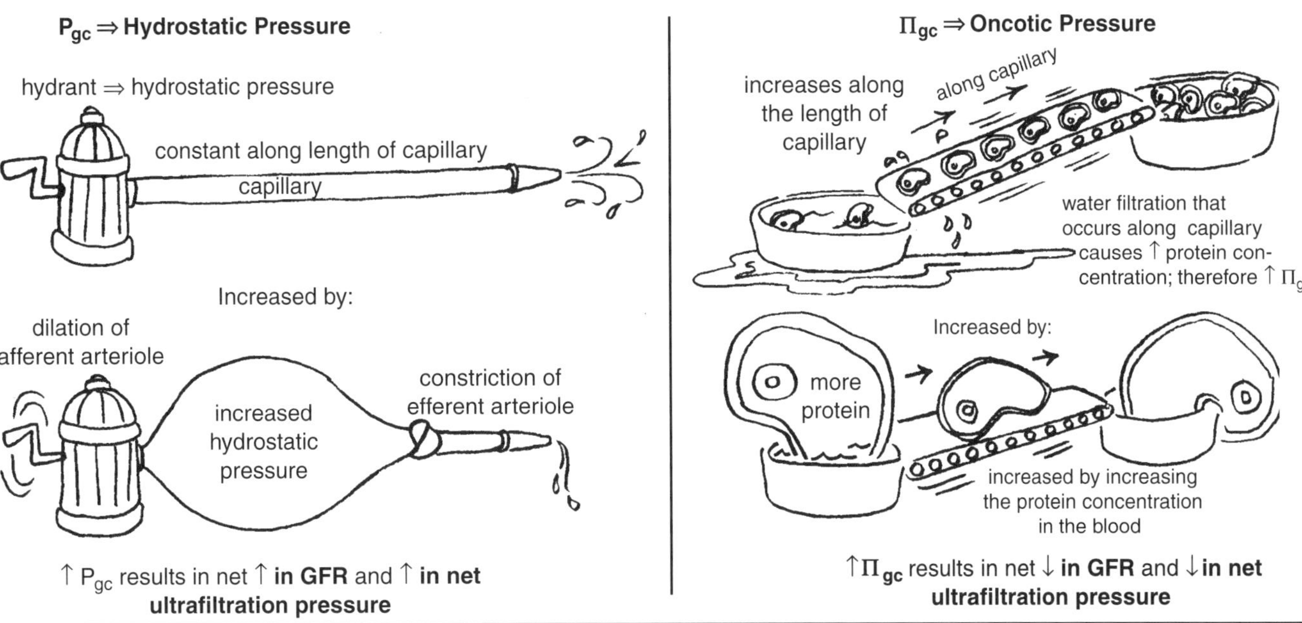
P_{gc} ⇒ Hydrostatic Pressure
hydrant ⇒ hydrostatic pressure
constant along length of capillary
capillary
Increased by:
dilation of afferent arteriole
increased hydrostatic pressure
constriction of efferent arteriole
↑ P_{gc} results in net ↑ in GFR and ↑ in net ultrafiltration pressure
Π_{gc} ⇒ Oncotic Pressure
increases along the length of capillary
along capillary
water filtration that occurs along capillary causes ↑ protein concentration; therefore ↑ Π_{gc}
Increased by:
more protein
increased by increasing the protein concentration in the blood
↑Π_{gc} results in net ↓ in GFR and ↓ in net ultrafiltration pressure

Bowman's Space Pressures

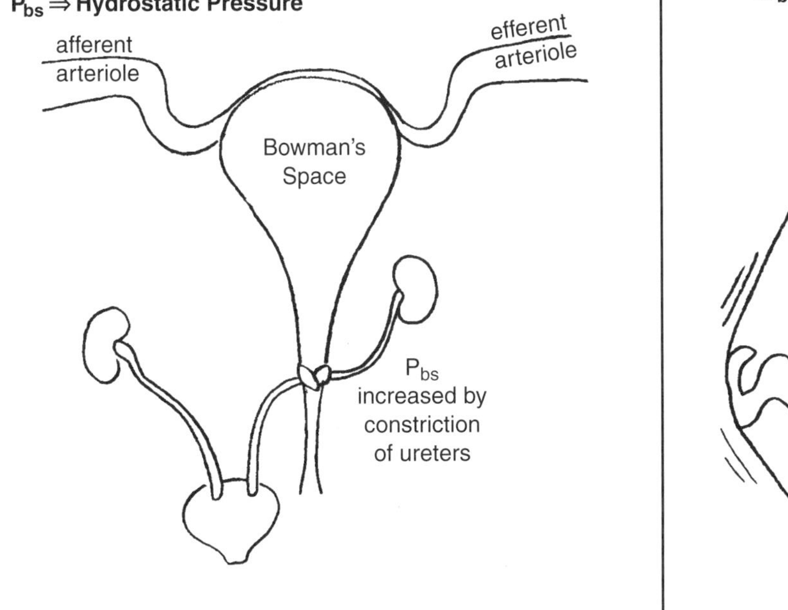
P_{bs} ⇒ Hydrostatic Pressure
afferent arteriole
efferent arteriole
Bowman's Space
P_{bs} increased by constriction of ureters

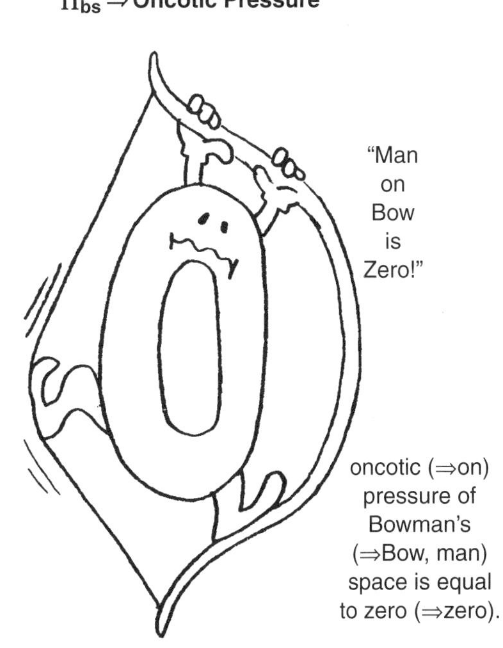
Π_{bs} ⇒ Oncotic Pressure
"Man on Bow is Zero!"
oncotic (⇒on) pressure of Bowman's (⇒Bow, man) space is equal to zero (⇒zero).

NOTES

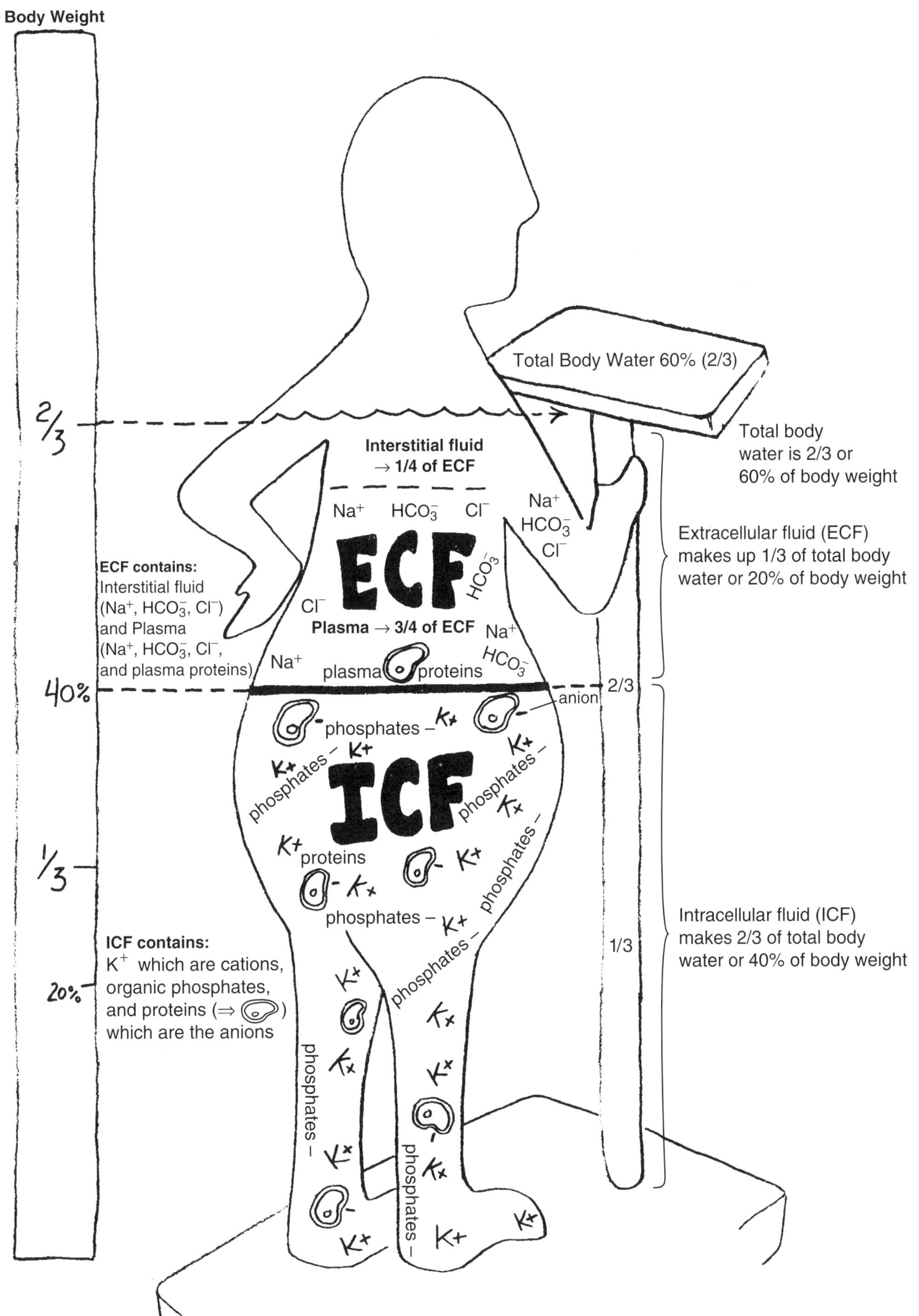
Body Weight
2/3
40%
1/3
20%
Total Body Water 60% (2/3)
Total body water is 2/3 or 60% of body weight
Interstitial fluid → 1/4 of ECF
Na+ HCO3− Cl−
ECF
Cl−
HCO3−
Plasma → 3/4 of ECF
Na+
plasma proteins
ECF contains:
Interstitial fluid (Na+, HCO3−, Cl−) and Plasma (Na+, HCO3−, Cl−, and plasma proteins)
Extracellular fluid (ECF) makes up 1/3 of total body water or 20% of body weight
anion
2/3
phosphates –
K+
ICF
proteins
1/3
ICF contains:
K+ which are cations, organic phosphates, and proteins (⇒) which are the anions
Intracellular fluid (ICF) makes 2/3 of total body water or 40% of body weight

NOTES

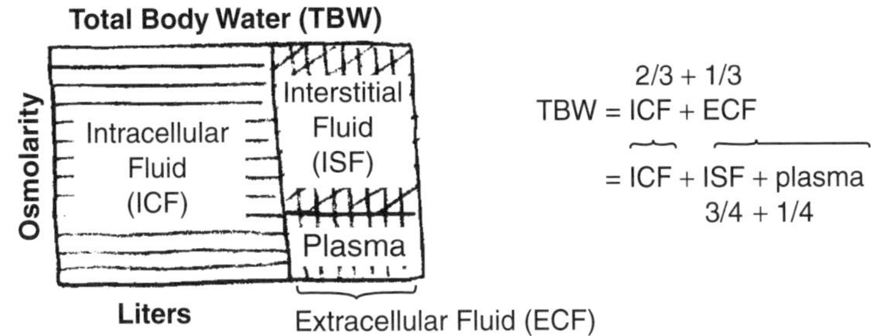
Total Body Water (TBW)
Osmolarity
Intracellular Fluid (ICF)
Interstitial Fluid (ISF)
Plasma
Liters
Extracellular Fluid (ECF)
2/3 + 1/3
TBW = ICF + ECF
= ICF + ISF + plasma
3/4 + 1/4

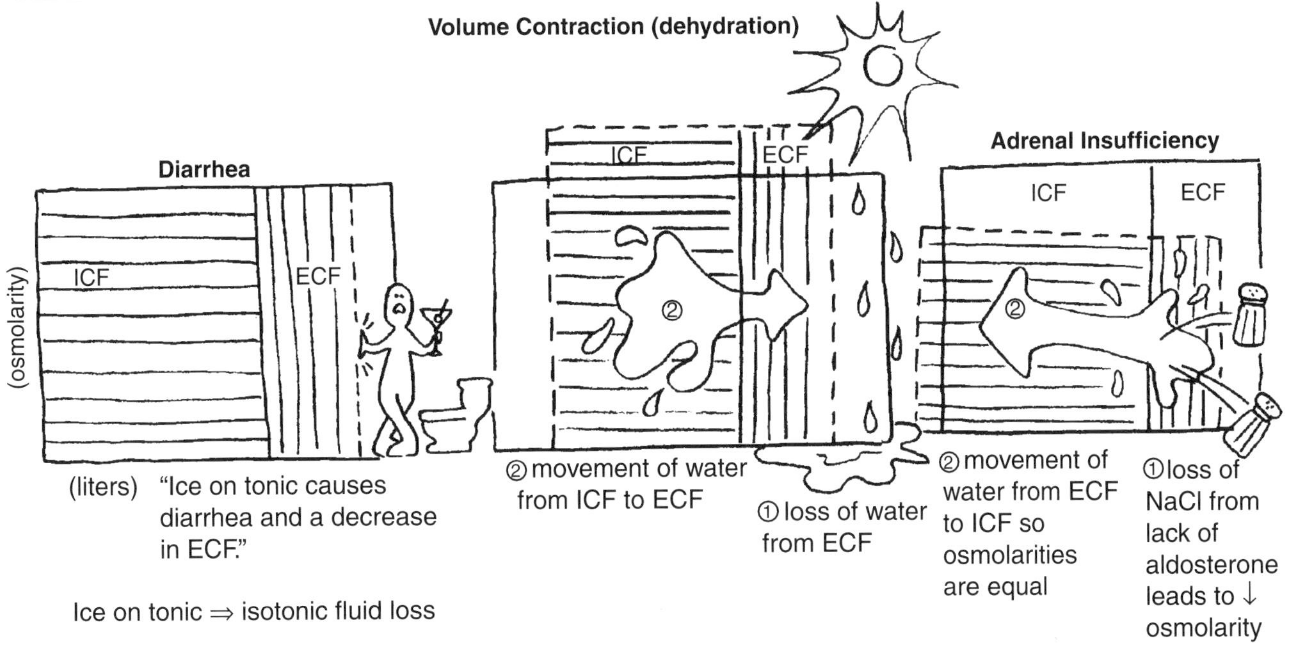
Volume Contraction (dehydration)
Diarrhea
(osmolarity)
ICF
ECF
(liters)
"Ice on tonic causes diarrhea and a decrease in ECF."
Ice on tonic ⇒ isotonic fluid loss
ICF
ECF
② movement of water from ICF to ECF
① loss of water from ECF
Adrenal Insufficiency
ICF
ECF
② movement of water from ECF to ICF so osmolarities are equal
① loss of NaCl from lack of aldosterone leads to ↓ osmolarity

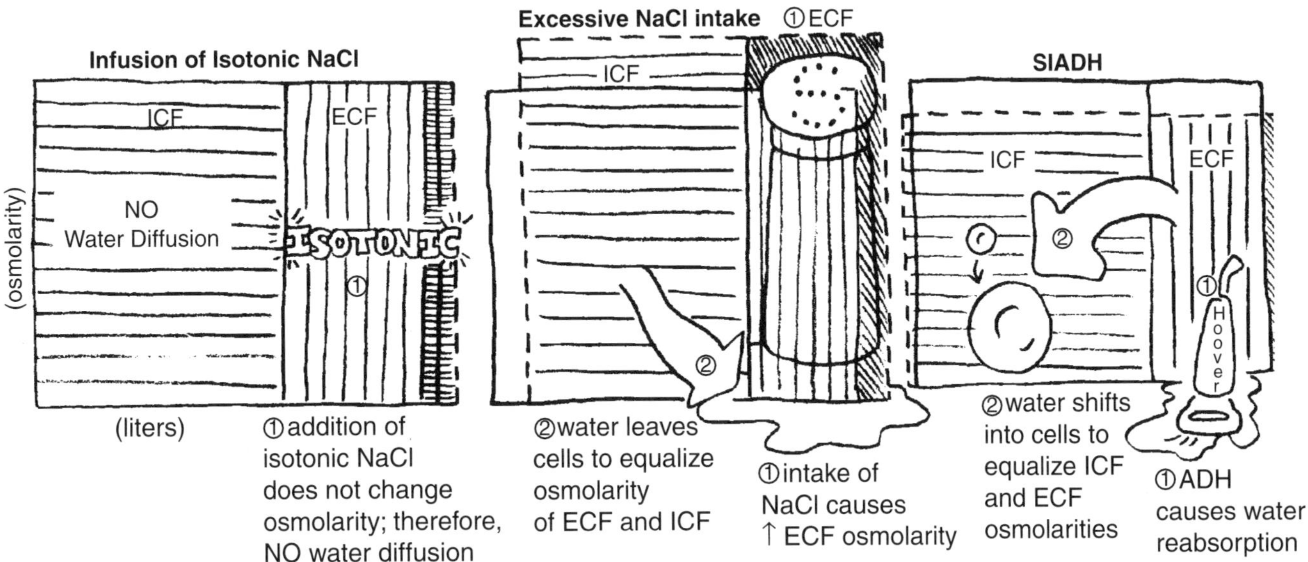
Volume Expansion (overhydration)
Infusion of Isotonic NaCl
ICF
ECF
(osmolarity)
NO Water Diffusion
ISOTONIC
①
(liters)
① addition of isotonic NaCl does not change osmolarity; therefore, NO water diffusion
Excessive NaCl intake
① ECF
ICF
② water leaves cells to equalize osmolarity of ECF and ICF
① intake of NaCl causes ↑ ECF osmolarity
SIADH
ICF
ECF
Hoover
② water shifts into cells to equalize ICF and ECF osmolarities
① ADH causes water reabsorption

NOTES

RENIN-ANGIOTENSIN SYSTEM

- Decrease in arterial pressure → JG cells secrete renin → renin cleaves angiotensinogen to angiotensin I → angiotensin I cleaves to angiotensin II by angiotensin-converting enzyme → angiotensin II causes increased thirst, vasoconstriction, ↑ aldosterone, and ↑ ADH production → collectively lead to increase in blood pressure and intravascular volume

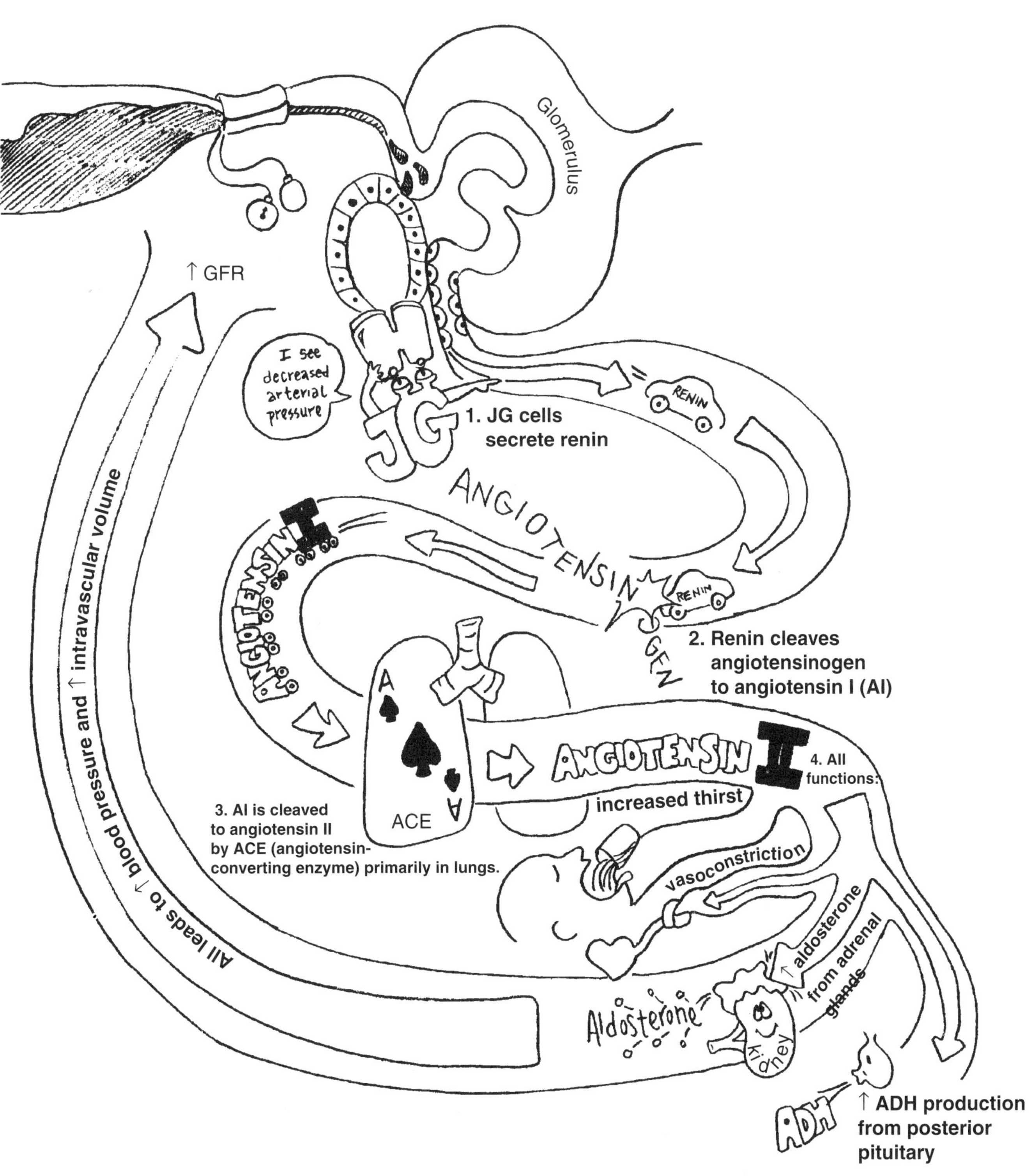
Glomerulus
↑ GFR
I see decreased arterial pressure
JG
1. JG cells secrete renin
RENIN
ANGIOTENSINOGEN
RENIN
2. Renin cleaves angiotensinogen to angiotensin I (AI)
ANGIOTENSIN I
ACE
3. AI is cleaved to angiotensin II by ACE (angiotensin-converting enzyme) primarily in lungs.
ANGIOTENSIN II
4. All functions:
increased thirst
vasoconstriction
↑ aldosterone from adrenal glands
Aldosterone
kidney
ADH
↑ ADH production from posterior pituitary
All leads to ↓ blood pressure and ↑ intravascular volume

NOTES

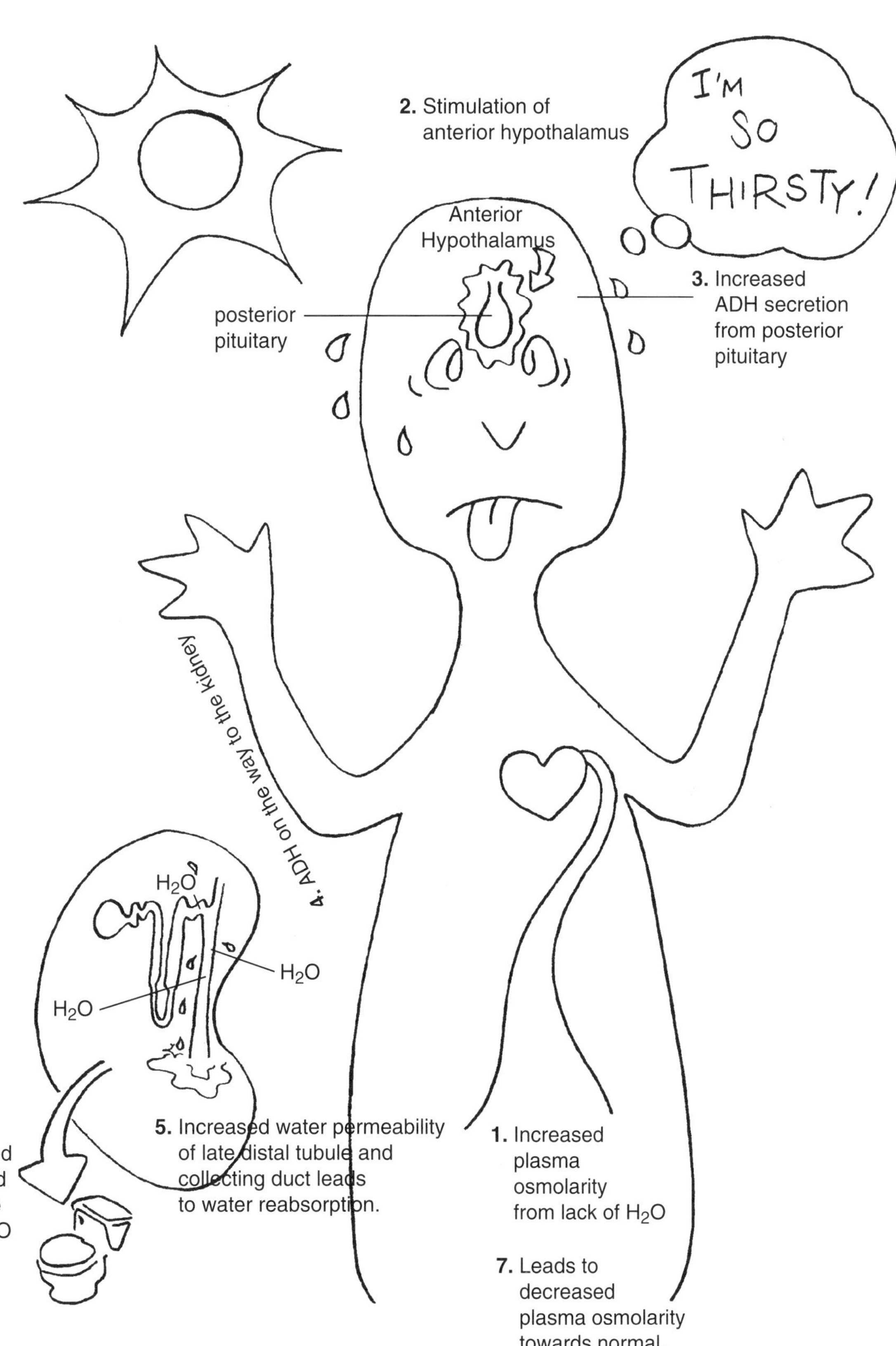
I'M SO THIRSTY!
2. Stimulation of anterior hypothalamus
Anterior Hypothalamus
posterior pituitary
3. Increased ADH secretion from posterior pituitary
4. ADH on the way to the kidney
H_2O
H_2O
H_2O
1. Increased plasma osmolarity from lack of H_2O
5. Increased water permeability of late distal tubule and collecting duct leads to water reabsorption.
6. Urine becomes more concentrated (↑ osmolarity) and less urine volume (secondary to H_2O reabsorption)
7. Leads to decreased plasma osmolarity towards normal.

NOTES

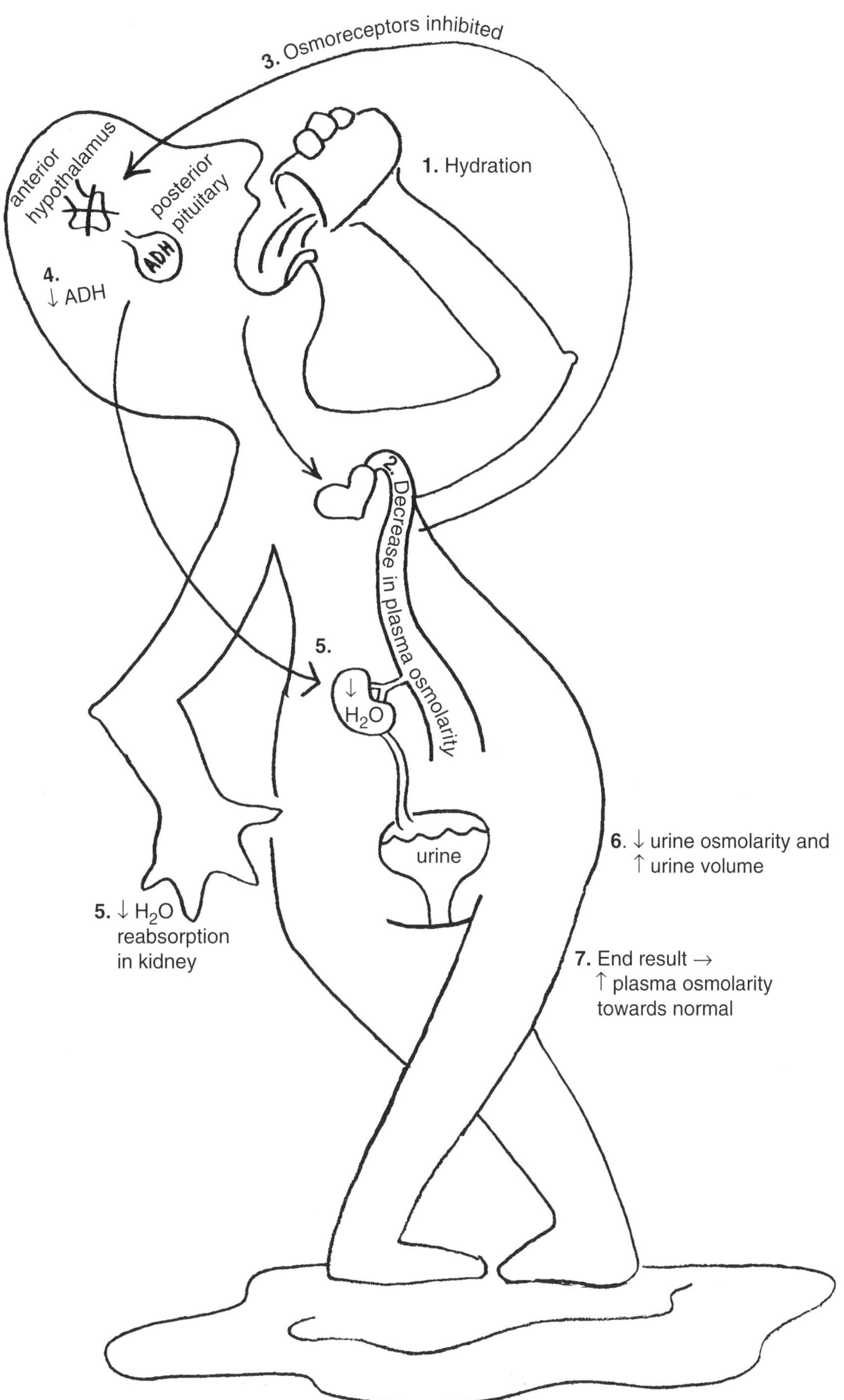
3. Osmoreceptors inhibited
anterior hypothalamus
posterior pituitary
ADH
1. Hydration
4. ↓ ADH
2. Decrease in plasma osmolarity
5.
↓ H_2O
urine
6. ↓ urine osmolarity and ↑ urine volume
5. ↓ H_2O reabsorption in kidney
7. End result → ↑ plasma osmolarity towards normal

NOTES

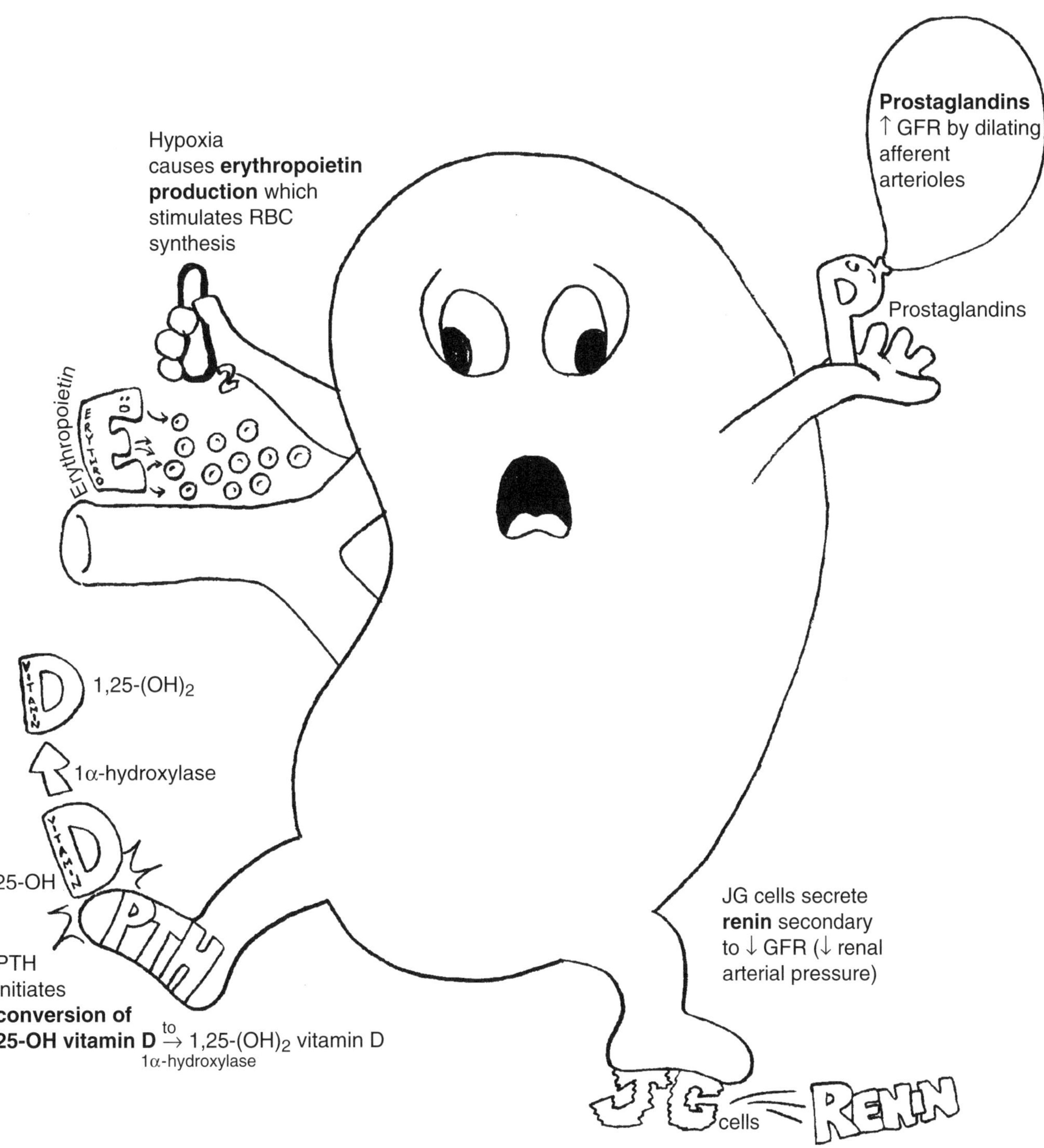
Hypoxia
causes **erythropoietin production** which stimulates RBC synthesis
Erythropoietin
ERYTHRO
Prostaglandins
↑ GFR by dilating afferent arterioles
Prostaglandins
1,25-$(OH)_2$
VITAMIN
1α-hydroxylase
25-OH
PTH
PTH initiates **conversion of 25-OH vitamin D** $\xrightarrow[\text{1}\alpha\text{-hydroxylase}]{\text{to}}$ 1,25-$(OH)_2$ vitamin D
JG cells secrete **renin** secondary to ↓ GFR (↓ renal arterial pressure)
JG cells
RENIN

NOTES

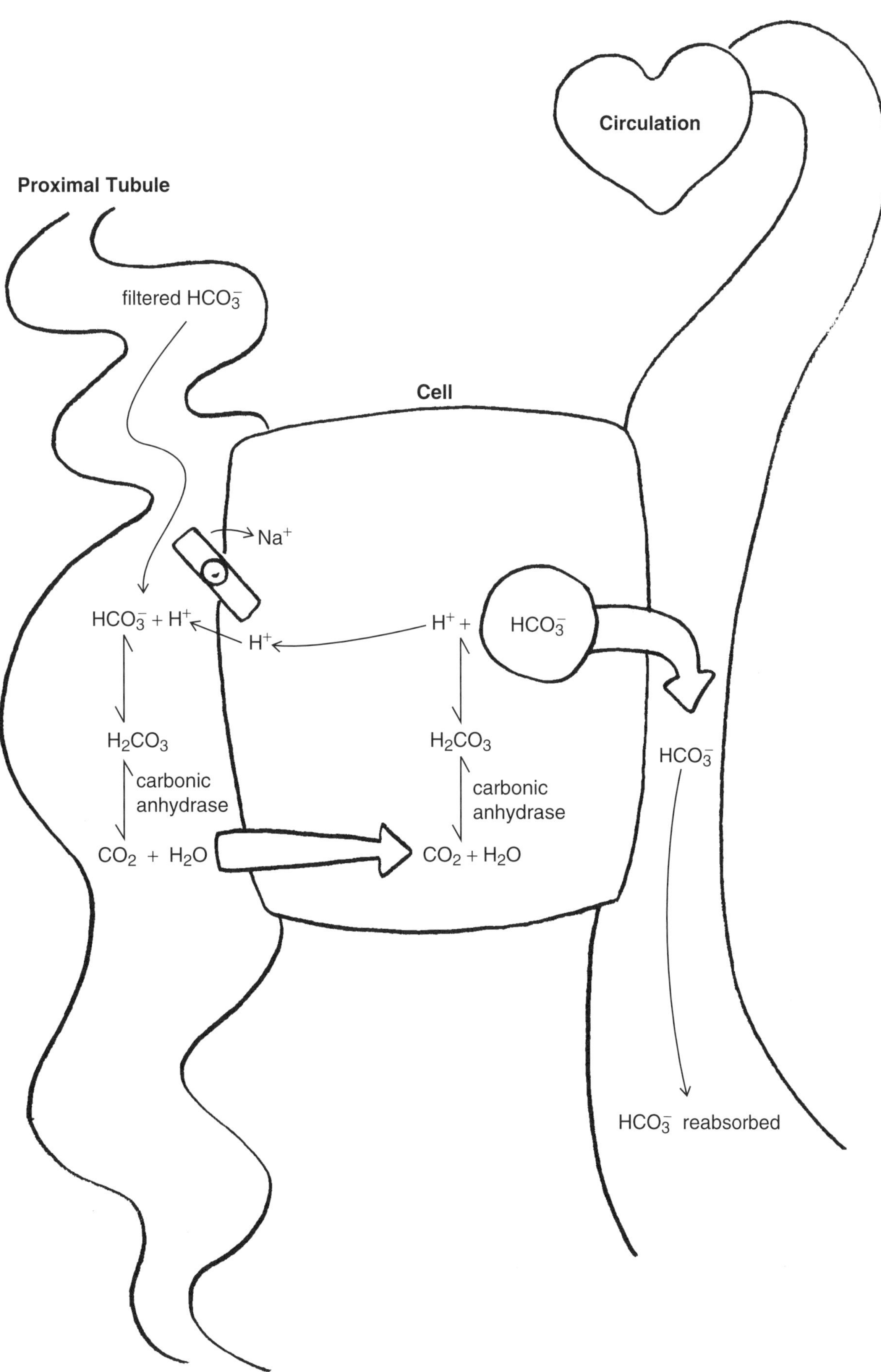
Circulation
Proximal Tubule
filtered HCO_3^-
Cell
Na^+
$HCO_3^- + H^+$
H^+
$H^+ +$
HCO_3^-
H_2CO_3
carbonic anhydrase
$CO_2 + H_2O$
H_2CO_3
carbonic anhydrase
$CO_2 + H_2O$
HCO_3^-
HCO_3^- reabsorbed

NOTES

METABOLIC ACIDOSIS

- Increase in acid causes decrease in HCO_3^-
- HCO_3^- consumed by acid (HA)
  - $HCO_3^- + HA \rightarrow A^- + CO_2 + H_2O$
- In order to conserve HCO_3^- kidneys reabsorb and regenerate HCO_3^-
- Ammonium ion (NH_4^+) production increased, which provides a mechanism for H^+ excretion in urine
- Normal gap metabolic acidosis: **D**iarrhea, **U**reteral diversion, **R**TA, **H**yperalimentation, **A**mmonium chloride, **M**isc.
- Elevated gap metabolic acidosis: **M**ethanol, **U**remia, **D**KA, **P**araldehyde ingestion, **I**schemia, **L**actic acidosis, **E**thylene glycol, **S**alicylates
- Respiratory compensation occurs in the form of increased ventilation releasing CO_2 and increasing pH
- To calculate pCO_2:
  - $pCO_2 = 1.5\ [HCO_3^-] + 8\ (\pm 2)$
  - Then compare to actual measured pCO_2 on ABG
  - If pCO_2 actual < pCO_2 calculated, then respiratory alkalosis coexists with metabolic acidosis
  - If pCO_2 actual > pCO_2 calculated, then respiratory acidosis coexists with metabolic acidosis
  - If pCO_2 actual = pCO_2 calculated, then metabolic acidosis exists alone

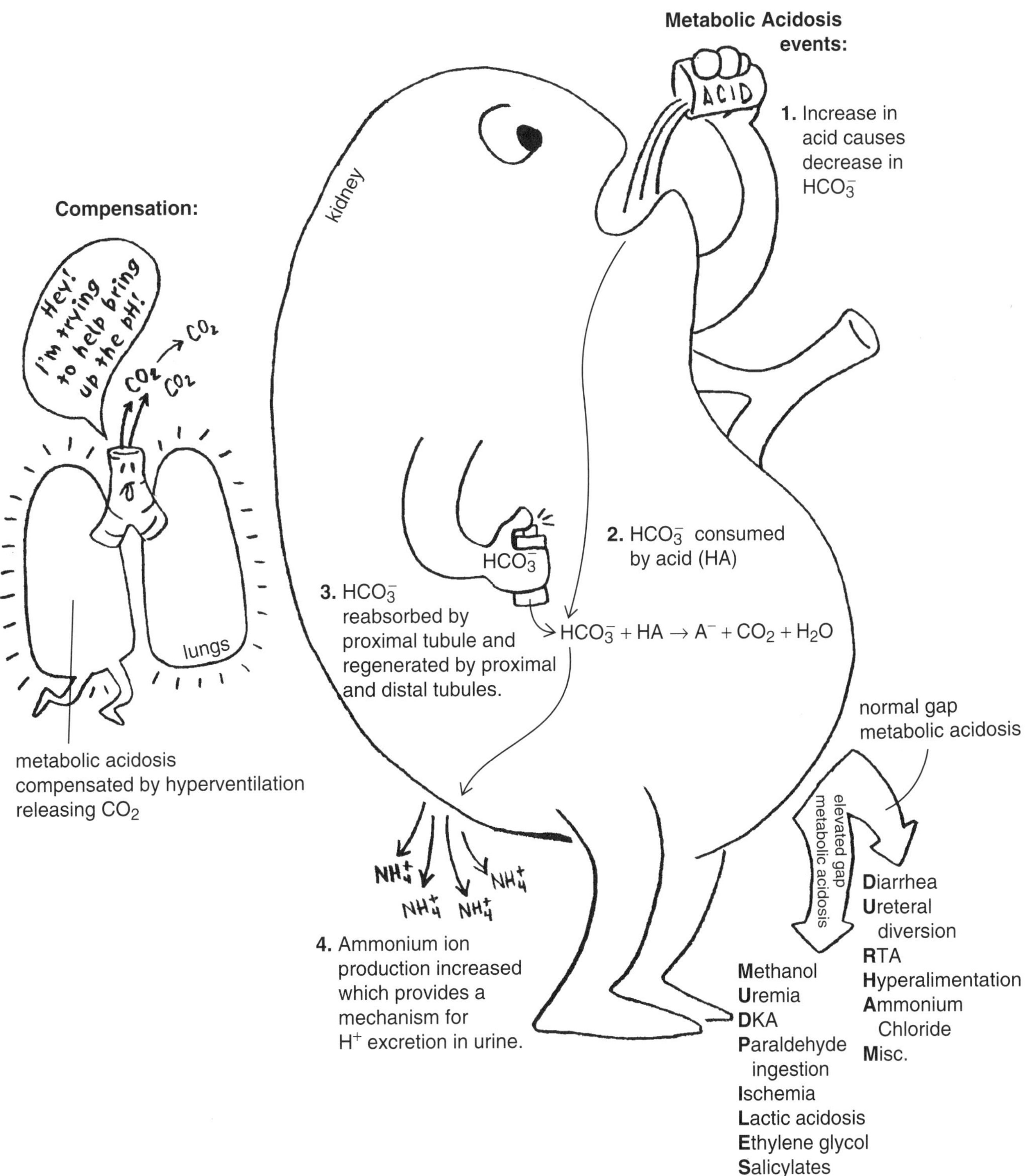
Metabolic Acidosis events:
ACID
1. Increase in acid causes decrease in HCO_3^-
kidney
Compensation:
Hey! I'm trying to help bring up the pH!
CO_2
CO_2
CO_2
lungs
metabolic acidosis compensated by hyperventilation releasing CO_2
HCO_3^-
2. HCO_3^- consumed by acid (HA)
3. HCO_3^- reabsorbed by proximal tubule and regenerated by proximal and distal tubules.
$HCO_3^- + HA \rightarrow A^- + CO_2 + H_2O$
normal gap metabolic acidosis
elevated gap metabolic acidosis
NH_4^+
NH_4^+
NH_4^+
NH_4^+
4. Ammonium ion production increased which provides a mechanism for H^+ excretion in urine.
Methanol
Uremia
DKA
Paraldehyde ingestion
Ischemia
Lactic acidosis
Ethylene glycol
Salicylates
Diarrhea
Ureteral diversion
RTA
Hyperalimentation
Ammonium Chloride
Misc.

NOTES

METABOLIC ALKALOSIS

SALINE RESPONSIVE METABOLIC ALKALOSIS

1. Extracellular volume depletion
2. Loss of Na^+, Cl^-, H_2O, and ↓ GFR (↓ HCO_3^- filtered; therefore ↑ pH)
3. ↑ angiotensin II production
4. Angiotensin II causes ↑ renal avidity for Na^+
5. Because Cl^- is low HCO_3^- is reabsorbed with Na^+ as $NaHCO_3^-$; therefore ↑HCO_3^- concentrations further ↑ pH
6. Treatment includes normal saline that ↑ Cl^- and ↑ Na^+; therefore stopping HCO_3^- reabsorption

SALINE NONRESPONSIVE METABOLIC ALKALOSIS

1. Causes of ↑ aldosterone include Cushing syndrome, primary hyperaldosteronism, and ACTH-secreting tumors
2. Aldosterone causes Na^+ reabsorption and H^+ secretion secondary to Na^+/H^+ exchange
3. Aldosterone causes ↑ HCO_3^- generation
4. Metabolic alkalosis with ↑ intravascular volume results

RESPIRATORY COMPENSATION

Metabolic alkalosis ↓ ventilation, which ↑ pCO_2 and ↓ pH

- To calculate pCO_2:
  - $pCO_2 = 0.9\,[HCO_3^-] + 16$
  - Compare to actual pCO_2 measured from ABG
  - If pCO_2 actual $<$ pCO_2 calculated, then respiratory alkalosis coexists with metabolic alkalosis
  - If pCO_2 actual $>$ pCO_2 calculated, then respiratory acidosis coexists with metabolic alkalosis
  - If pCO_2 actual $=$ pCO_2 calculated, then only metabolic alkalosis exists

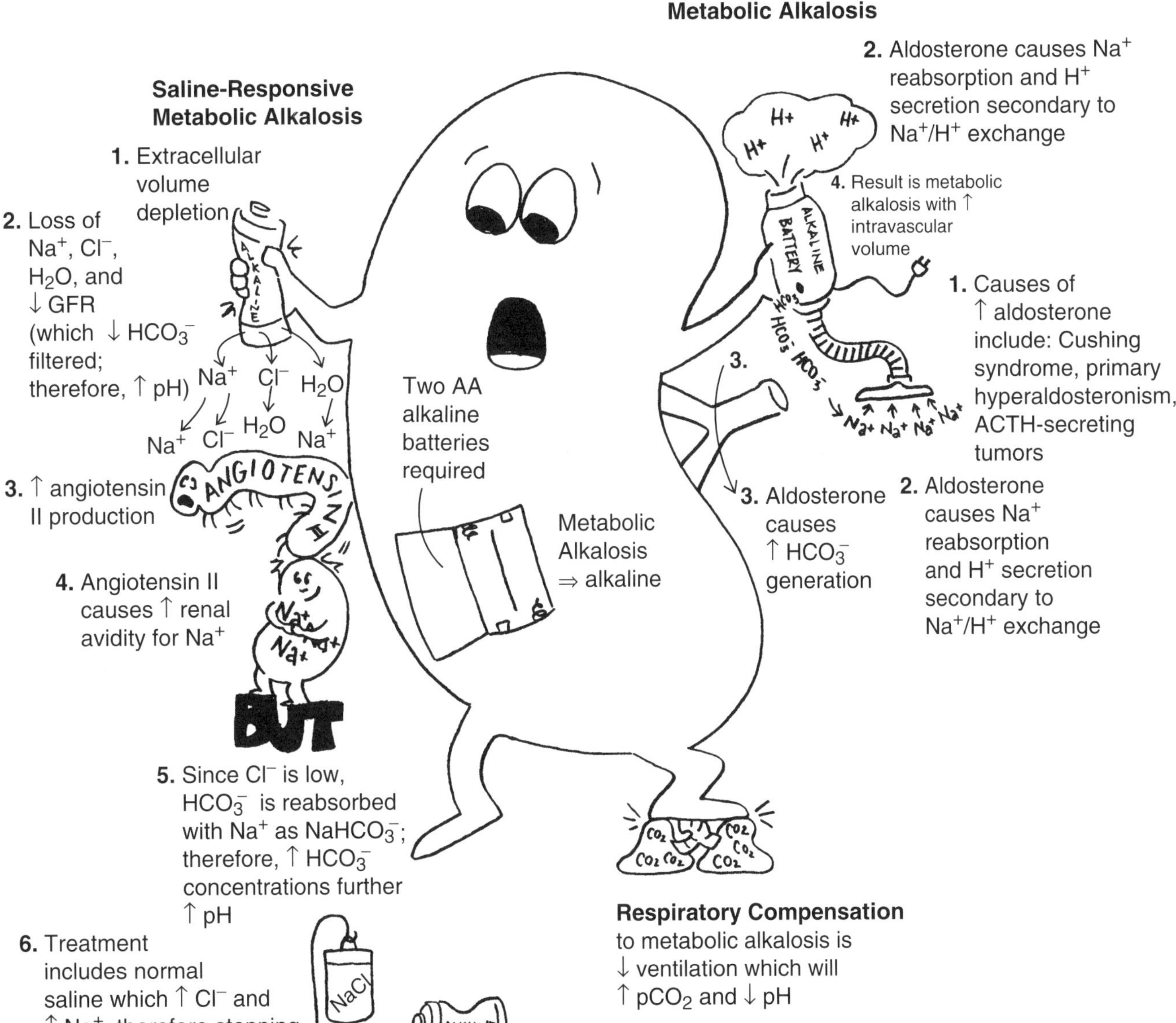
Saline-Responsive Metabolic Alkalosis
1. Extracellular volume depletion
2. Loss of Na^+, Cl^-, H_2O, and ↓ GFR (which ↓ HCO_3^- filtered; therefore, ↑ pH)
ALKALINE
Na^+ Cl^- H_2O
Na^+ Cl^- H_2O Na^+
3. ↑ angiotensin II production
ANGIOTENSIN II
4. Angiotensin II causes ↑ renal avidity for Na^+
Na^+
BUT
5. Since Cl^- is low, HCO_3^- is reabsorbed with Na^+ as $NaHCO_3^-$; therefore, ↑ HCO_3^- concentrations further ↑ pH
6. Treatment includes normal saline which ↑ Cl^- and ↑ Na^+, therefore stopping HCO_3^- reabsorption
NaCl
ALKALINE
Two AA alkaline batteries required
Metabolic Alkalosis ⇒ alkaline
Saline Nonresponsive Metabolic Alkalosis
2. Aldosterone causes Na^+ reabsorption and H^+ secretion secondary to Na^+/H^+ exchange
H^+ H^+ H^+ H^+
4. Result is metabolic alkalosis with ↑ intravascular volume
ALKALINE BATTERY
1. Causes of ↑ aldosterone include: Cushing syndrome, primary hyperaldosteronism, ACTH-secreting tumors
HCO_3^- HCO_3^- HCO_3^-
Na^+ Na^+ Na^+ Na^+
3.
3. Aldosterone causes ↑ HCO_3^- generation
2. Aldosterone causes Na^+ reabsorption and H^+ secretion secondary to Na^+/H^+ exchange
CO_2 CO_2 CO_2 CO_2 CO_2 CO_2
Respiratory Compensation to metabolic alkalosis is ↓ ventilation which will ↑ pCO_2 and ↓ pH

NOTES

RESPIRATORY ACIDOSIS

- Causes include COPD, asthma, foreign body aspiration, pneumothorax, emphysema, bronchiectasis, and pulmonary edema
- Pathological process causes primary increase in pCO_2 concentration in lungs (secondary to decreased ventilation rate)
- Increase in CO_2 causes a shift to the right, which results in increased H^+ and HCO_3^- concentrations ($CO_2 + H_2O \rightarrow H^+ + HCO_3^-$)
- Relatively larger increase in H^+ than in HCO_3^- causes ↓ pH; H^+ is measured in nanoequivalents/L and HCO_3^- in milliequivalents/L; any increase in H^+ concentration is therefore relatively larger than in the same increase in HCO_3^- concentration.
- Renal compensation consists of HCO_3^- reabsorption
- For every 10 mm Hg increase in pCO_2:
  - pH will ↓ by 0.08 (acute) and ↓ by 0.03 (chronic)
  - HCO_3^- will ↓ by 1 mEq/L (acute) and ↓ by 4 mEq/L (chronic)
  - If pH or HCO_3^- measured < calculated, then metabolic acidosis coexists with respiratory acidosis
  - If pH or HCO_3^- measured > calculated, then metabolic alkalosis coexists with respiratory acidosis
  - If pH or HCO_3^- = calculated, then only respiratory acidosis exists

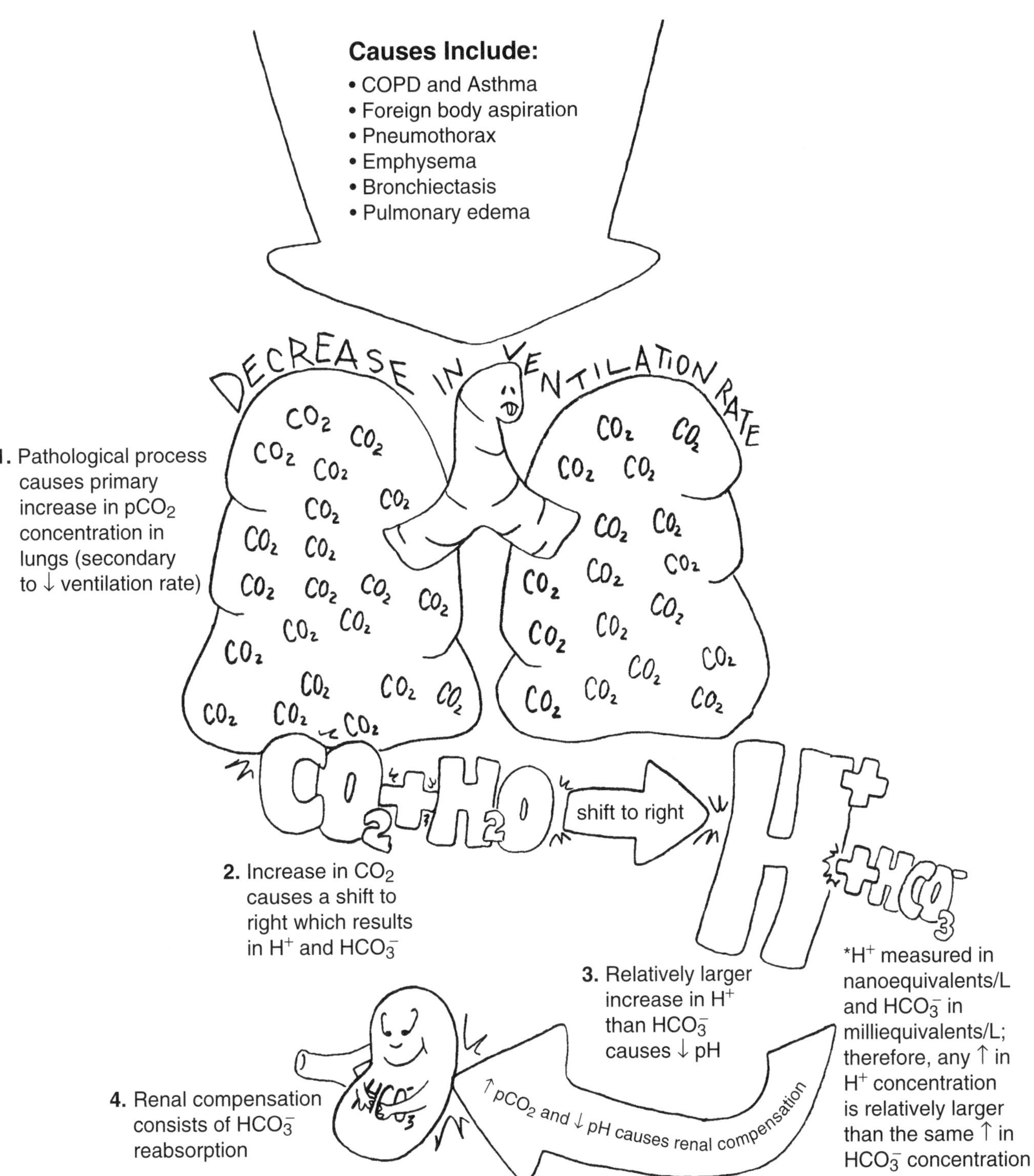
Causes Include:
• COPD and Asthma
• Foreign body aspiration
• Pneumothorax
• Emphysema
• Bronchiectasis
• Pulmonary edema
DECREASE IN VENTILATION RATE
1. Pathological process causes primary increase in pCO2 concentration in lungs (secondary to ↓ ventilation rate)
CO2 + H2O
shift to right
H+ + HCO3-
2. Increase in CO2 causes a shift to right which results in H+ and HCO3-
3. Relatively larger increase in H+ than HCO3- causes ↓ pH
*H+ measured in nanoequivalents/L and HCO3- in milliequivalents/L; therefore, any ↑ in H+ concentration is relatively larger than the same ↑ in HCO3- concentration
↑ pCO2 and ↓ pH causes renal compensation
4. Renal compensation consists of HCO3- reabsorption

NOTES

RESPIRATORY ALKALOSIS

- Causes include pneumonia, pulmonary embolism (PE), congestive heart failure (CHF), interstitial fibrosis, cerebral vascular accident (CVA), salicylates, fever, hyperthyroidism, and hepatic failure
- Pathological process causes ↓ in pCO_2 secondary to increased ventilation rate
- Decrease in pCO_2 causes shift to left that results in ↓ H^+ and ↓ HCO_3^- (but relatively more of ↓ in H^+ than ↓ in HCO_3^-; therefore, ↑ pH)
  - $CO_2 + H_2O \leftarrow H^+ + HCO_3^-$
- Renal compensation is ↑ excretion of HCO_3^- and inhibition of HCO_3^- regeneration
- For every 10 mm Hg ↓ in pCO_2:
  - pH will ↑ by 0.08 (acute) and ↑ 0.03 (chronic)
  - HCO_3^- ↓ by 2 mEq/L (acute) and ↓ by 5 mEq/L (chronic)
  - If pH or HCO_3^- measured < calculated, then metabolic acidosis coexists with respiratory alkalosis.
  - If pH or HCO_3^- measured > calculated, then metabolic alkalosis coexists with respiratory alkalosis.
  - If measured pH or HCO_3^- = calculated, then respiratory alkalosis exists alone.

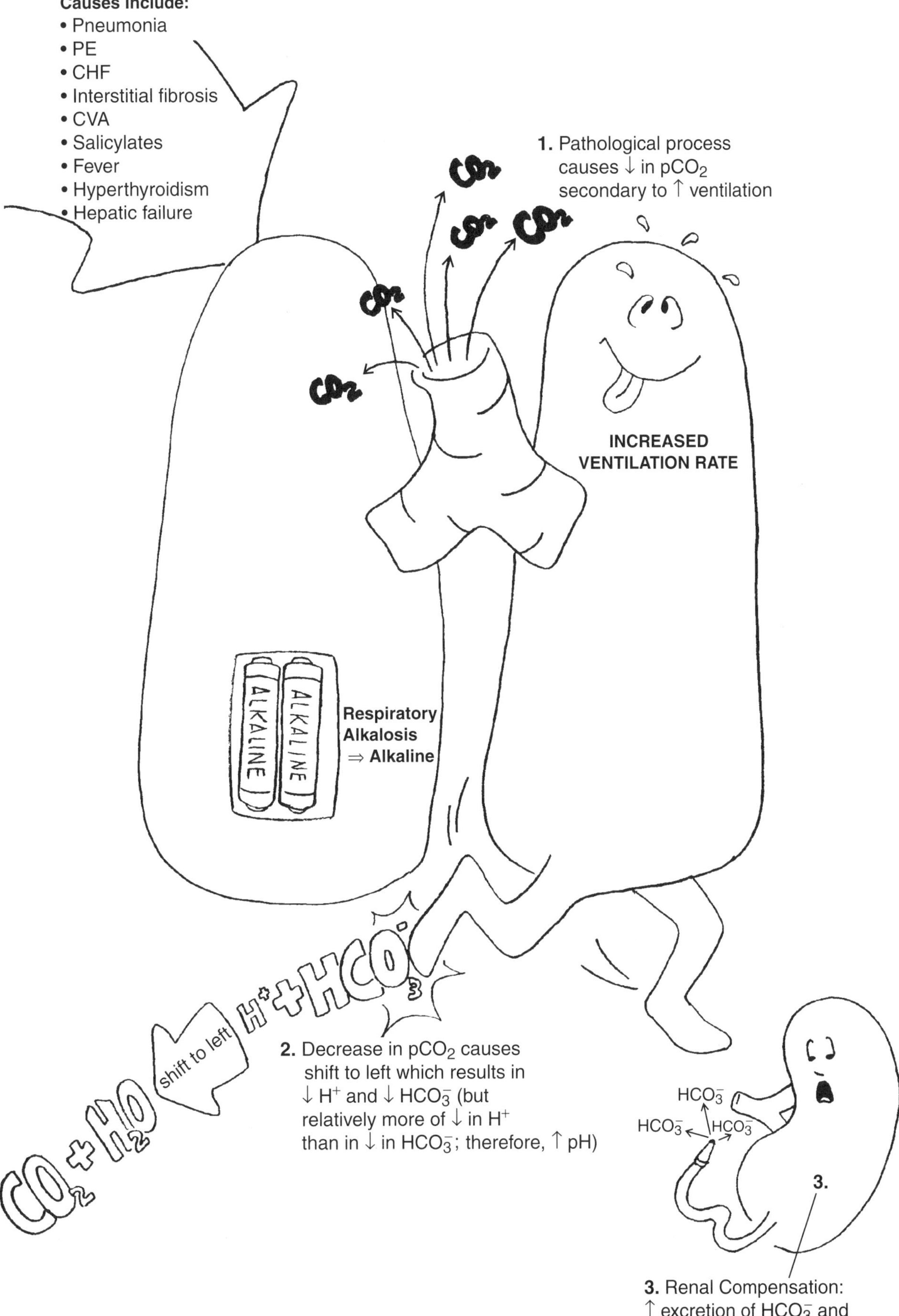
Causes Include:
• Pneumonia
• PE
• CHF
• Interstitial fibrosis
• CVA
• Salicylates
• Fever
• Hyperthyroidism
• Hepatic failure
1. Pathological process causes ↓ in pCO_2 secondary to ↑ ventilation
CO_2
CO_2
CO_2
CO_2
CO_2
INCREASED VENTILATION RATE
ALKALINE
ALKALINE
Respiratory Alkalosis ⇒ Alkaline
$CO_2 + H_2O$
shift to left
$H^+ + HCO_3^-$
2. Decrease in pCO_2 causes shift to left which results in ↓ H^+ and ↓ HCO_3^- (but relatively more of ↓ in H^+ than in ↓ in HCO_3^-; therefore, ↑ pH)
HCO_3^-
HCO_3^-
HCO_3^-
3.
3. Renal Compensation: ↑ excretion of HCO_3^- and inhibited generation of HCO_3^-

NOTES

BLADDER

- Storage sac for urine
- Four layers
    - mucosa → innermost layer; transitional epithelium allows distention of bladder as it fills
    - submucosa
    - muscularis
    - serosa (adventitia)
- Rugae → folds of mucosa that allow bladder distention
- Detrusor muscle is smooth muscle
- Blood supply to bladder
    - superior and inferior vesicular arteries that arise from internal iliac arteries
- Urethra
    - internal sphincter → involuntary; smooth muscle
    - external spincter → voluntary; skeletal muscle

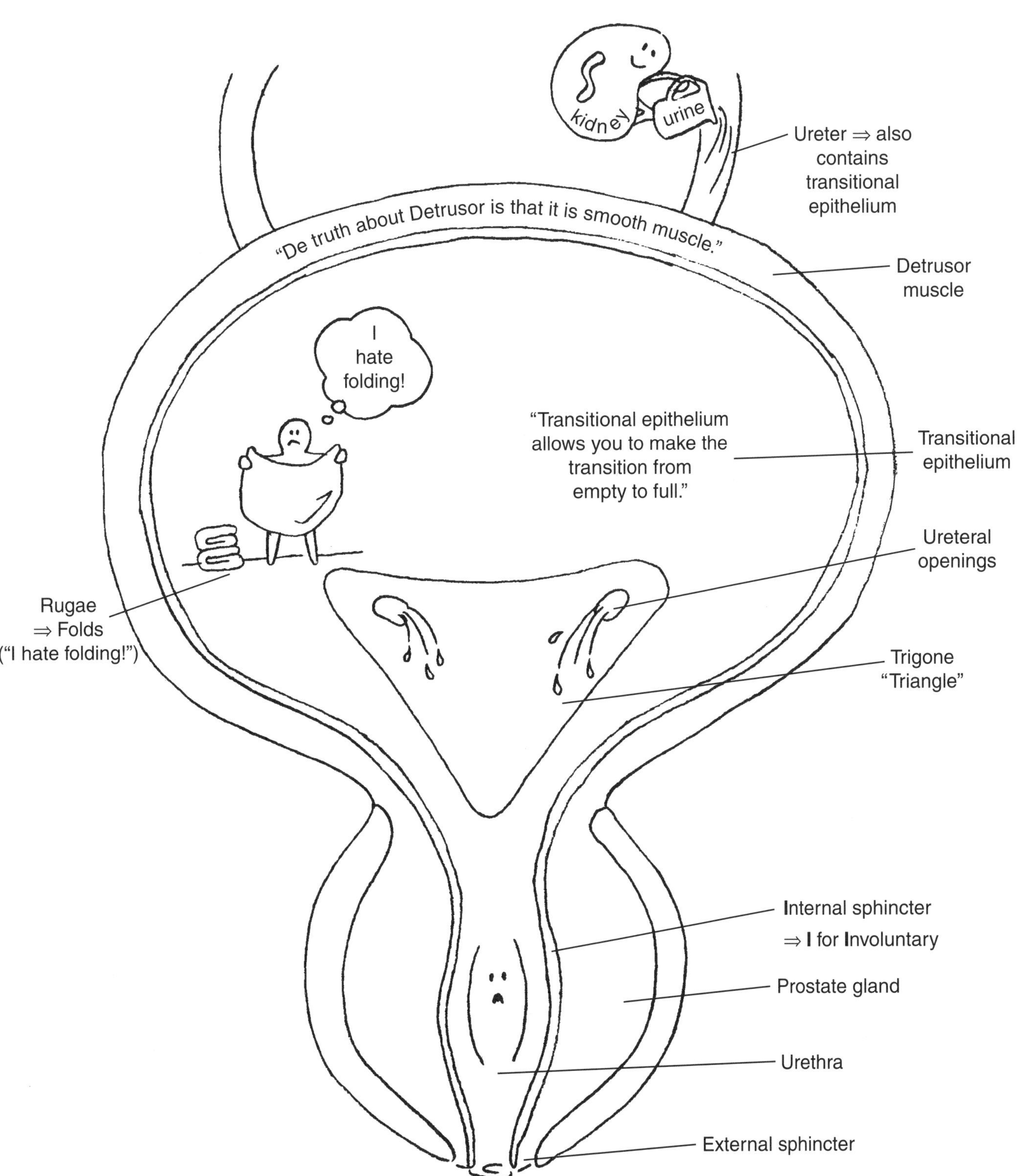
kidney
urine
Ureter ⇒ also contains transitional epithelium
"De truth about Detrusor is that it is smooth muscle."
Detrusor muscle
I hate folding!
"Transitional epithelium allows you to make the transition from empty to full."
Transitional epithelium
Ureteral openings
Rugae ⇒ Folds ("I hate folding!")
Trigone "Triangle"
Internal sphincter ⇒ I for Involuntary
Prostate gland
Urethra
External sphincter

NOTES

FEMALE REPRODUCTIVE ANATOMY

Uterus

- Endometrium → innermost layer
- Myometrium → middle, smooth muscle layer
- Serosa → outermost layer
- Fundus – top of the uterus
- Isthmus – area above the cervical canal

Cervix

- Joins vagina
- External os, opening to the vagina
- Cervix exposed to the vagina covered with stratified squamous epithelium and farther up the cervix through the external os, toward the cervical canal, the epithelium changes to simple columnar (transition zone); area important due to association with neoplastic transformation

Fallopian Tubes

- Isthmus joins fallopian tubes to the uterus
- Ampulla is the central portion
- Infundibulum is the portion joined to the fimbria
- Fimbria gathers oocyte from ovary at ovulation

Ovary

- 3–5 cm long, 2–3 cm wide, and 1–3 cm thick
- Shrinks at menopause

Ligaments

- Broad
    - double layer of peritoneum
    - extends from uterine sides to lateral walls of pelvis and to pelvis floor
- Uterosacral
    - extends from sides of cervix to sacrum
- Round
    - extends from uterine fundus inferolaterally to labia majora → eventually joins inguinal ligament
    - contains Samson's artery (branch of ovarian artery)
- Cardinal
    - lateral support to cervix
    - contains uterine artery

Blood Supply

- Arteries
    - uterine artery branches off hypogastric (anterior branch of internal iliac) artery; anastomoses with ovarian artery; passes over ureters anteriorly (water [ureters] under the bridge [uterine artery])
    - ovarian artery directly branches from abdominal aorta
    - vaginal artery is a branch of hypogastric artery
- Veins
    - right ovarian vein drains into inferior vena cava
    - left ovarian vein drains into left renal vein

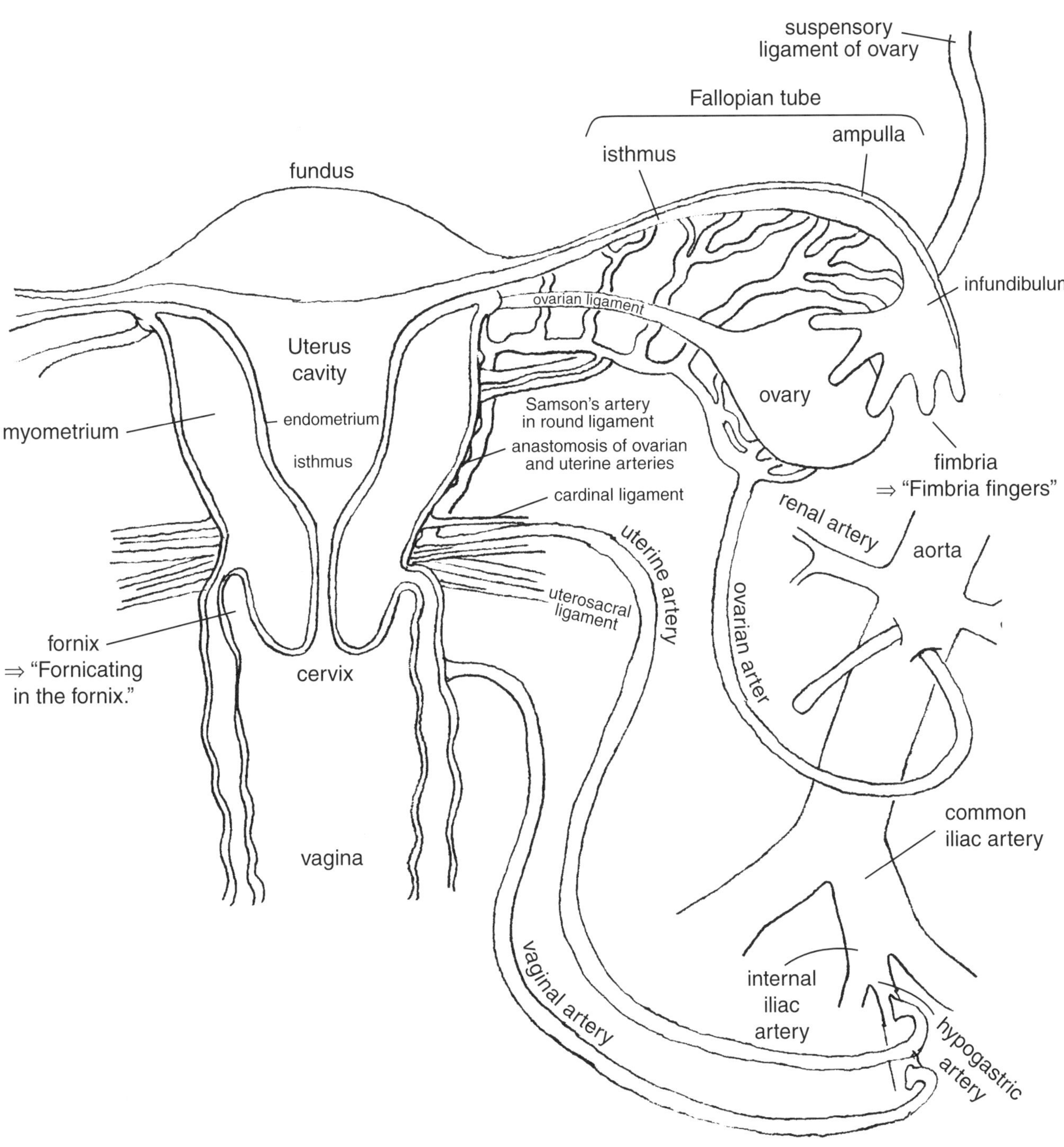
suspensory
ligament of ovary
Fallopian tube
isthmus
ampulla
fundus
infundibulum
ovarian ligament
Uterus
cavity
ovary
myometrium
endometrium
isthmus
Samson's artery
in round ligament
anastomosis of ovarian
and uterine arteries
fimbria
⇒ "Fimbria fingers"
cardinal ligament
renal artery
aorta
uterine artery
uterosacral
ligament
ovarian arter
fornix
⇒ "Fornicating
in the fornix."
cervix
common
iliac artery
vagina
internal
iliac
artery
vaginal artery
hypogastric
artery

NOTES

REPRODUCTIVE CYCLE

- GnRH secreted in pulsatile manner by hypothalamic arcuate nucleus
  - causes anterior pituitary to secrete FSH and LH in pulsatile manner
- Menstruation—beginning of follicular phase of the cycle
  - lowest concentrations of estradiol, progesterone, and LH
  - FSH increases in beginning of menstruation
- FSH involved with selection and maturation of follicles for next cycle
  - binds granulosa cell receptors on primary oocyte
    - causes granulosa cells to reproduce thereby increasing their number
  - FSH causes granulosa cells to secrete estradiol
- Estradiol
  - upregulates LH receptors on theca cells
    - theca cells eventually secrete androgen precursors of estradiol
  - prepares granulosa and theca cells to produce progesterone after ovulation
  - negative feedback on pituitary to ↓ FSH; positive feedback to ↑ LH
- Dominant follicle chosen
  - secretes increasing amounts of estradiol
  - positive estradiol feedback to pituitary to ↑ LH secretion; causes endometrium to thicken
  - at day 11–13, LH surge occurs, causing ovulation
  - FSH also increases but reason and effects unknown
- After ovulation follicle converts to corpus luteum
  - corpus luteum produces progesterone
    - mittelschmerz—pain experienced at ovulation by some women
- Luteal phase
  - progesterone dominates hormone
  - during LH surge → LH binds to receptors in granulosa and theca cells of follicle → after ovulation (as follicle is converted to corpus luteum) these cells then produce progesterone
  - progesterone production lasts approximately 11 days
  - if no fertilization occurs → progesterone decreases and a new cycle begins with endometrial sloughing
  - if fertilization does occur → corpus luteum is rescued by hCG produced by placenta
  - progesterone needed for implantation and to sustain pregnancy for early first trimester
  - progesterone has negative pituitary feedback to ↓ FSH and LH; if no implantation, the progesterone will begin to decrease → FSH will then ↑, stimulating beginning of another cycle

Phases of Endometrium

- Proliferative phase
  - occurs during ovary follicular phase
  - ↑ estrogen stimulates endometrial spiral arteries to form and progesterone receptors to develop
- Secretory phase
  - occurs during luteal phase
  - progesterone causes mucous glands to form
  - endometrium thickens in preparation for implantation
- Menstrual phase
  - ↓ estradiol and progesterone cause endometrial sloughing; bleeding from spiral artery constriction

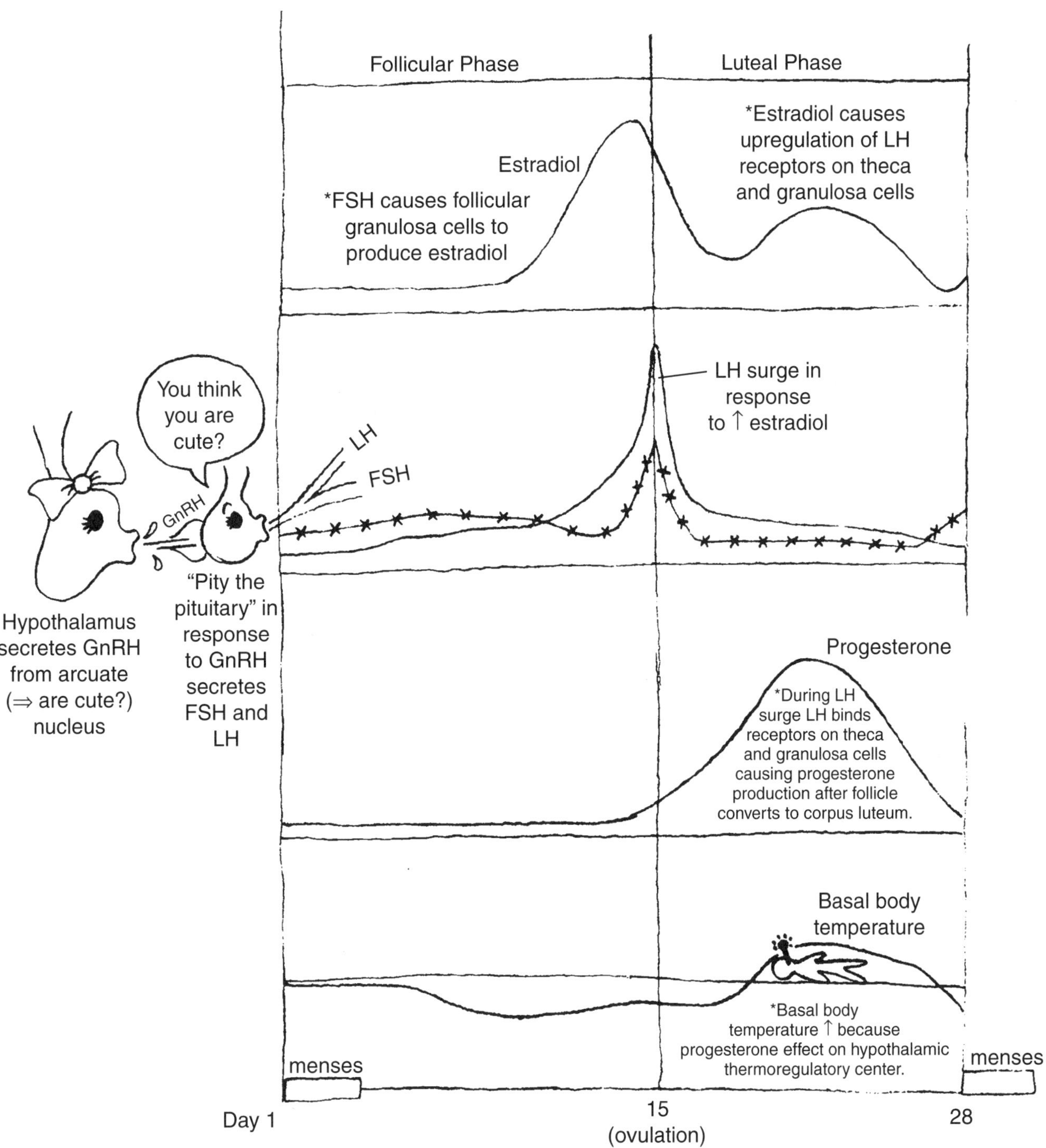
Follicular Phase
Luteal Phase
Estradiol
*FSH causes follicular granulosa cells to produce estradiol
*Estradiol causes upregulation of LH receptors on theca and granulosa cells
You think you are cute?
GnRH
LH
FSH
LH surge in response to ↑ estradiol
"Pity the pituitary" in response to GnRH secretes FSH and LH
Hypothalamus secretes GnRH from arcuate (⇒ are cute?) nucleus
Progesterone
*During LH surge LH binds receptors on theca and granulosa cells causing progesterone production after follicle converts to corpus luteum.
Basal body temperature
*Basal body temperature ↑ because progesterone effect on hypothalamic thermoregulatory center.
menses
menses
Day 1
15 (ovulation)
28

NOTES

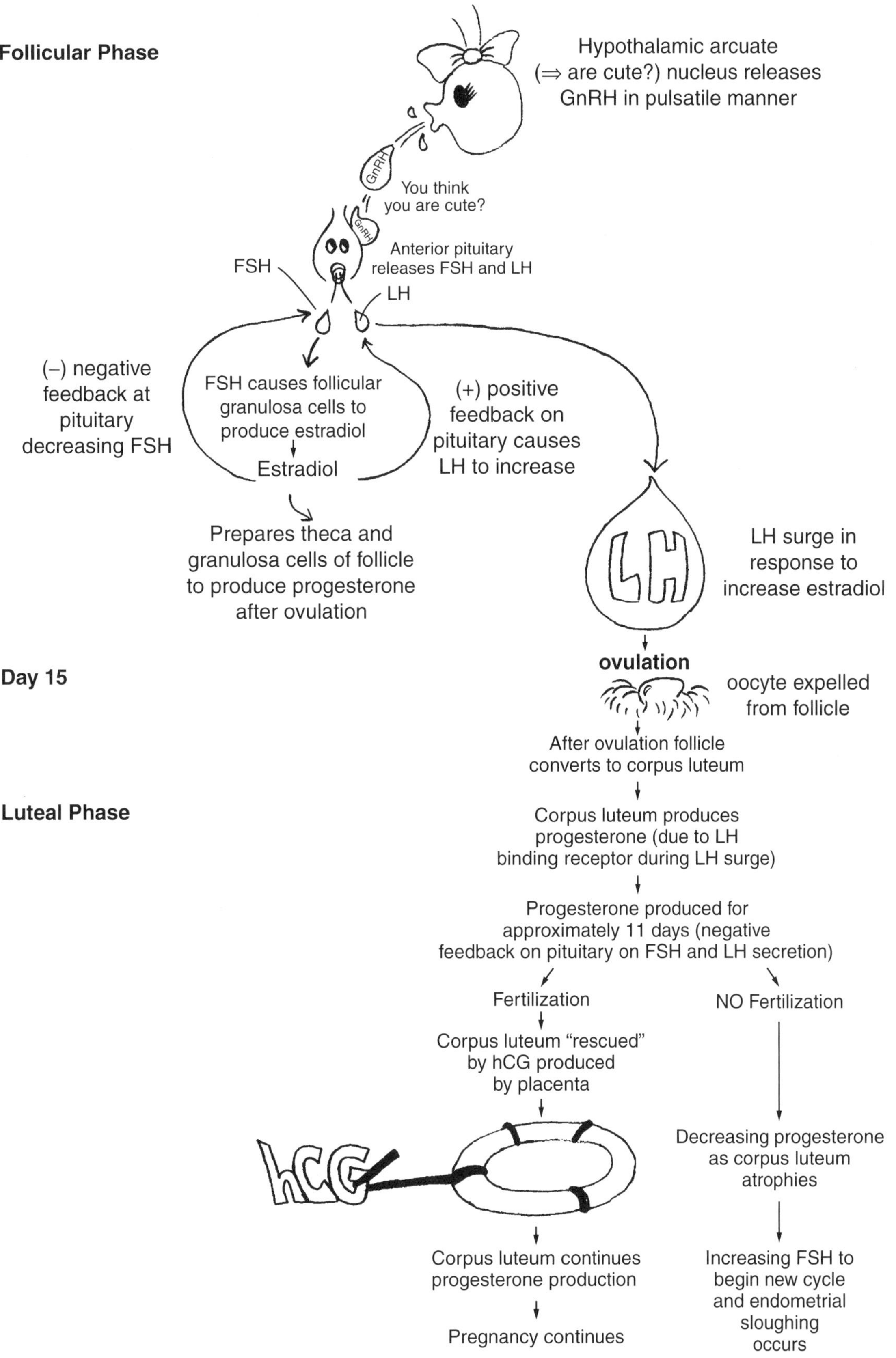
Follicular Phase
Hypothalamic arcuate (⇒ are cute?) nucleus releases GnRH in pulsatile manner
GnRH
You think you are cute?
GnRH
Anterior pituitary releases FSH and LH
FSH
LH
(–) negative feedback at pituitary decreasing FSH
FSH causes follicular granulosa cells to produce estradiol
Estradiol
(+) positive feedback on pituitary causes LH to increase
Prepares theca and granulosa cells of follicle to produce progesterone after ovulation
LH
LH surge in response to increase estradiol
Day 15
ovulation
oocyte expelled from follicle
After ovulation follicle converts to corpus luteum
Luteal Phase
Corpus luteum produces progesterone (due to LH binding receptor during LH surge)
Progesterone produced for approximately 11 days (negative feedback on pituitary on FSH and LH secretion)
Fertilization
Corpus luteum "rescued" by hCG produced by placenta
hCG
Corpus luteum continues progesterone production
Pregnancy continues
NO Fertilization
Decreasing progesterone as corpus luteum atrophies
Increasing FSH to begin new cycle and endometrial sloughing occurs

NOTES

MALE REPRODUCTIVE ANATOMY AND EJACULATION PATHWAY

Testes

- Paired ovoid organs where spermatogenesis takes place
- Each testis divided into lobules (250–300) containing 3–4 tightly convoluted seminiferous tubules where spermatogenesis actually takes place
- Contains interstitial cells that produce and secrete male sex hormones
- Sperm removed from testes via efferent ductules to the epididymis
- Testicular arteries arise from abdominal aorta below the renal arteries
- Right testicular vein drains to inferior vena cava; left testicular vein drains into left renal vein

Epididymis

- Located posterior to testis; contains a head, body, and tail
- Stores spermatozoa and transports these from seminiferous tubules to ductus deferens

Ductus Deferens

- Transports sperm from epididymis to ejaculatory duct
- Originates at tail of epididymis → exits scrotum → penetrates inguinal canal → enters pelvic cavity → travels along the medial side of the ureter and passes bladder → teminal portion of ductus deferens is ampulla that joins the ejaculatory duct
- contained primarily within spermatic cord (consists of ductus deferens, spermatic vessels, nerves, cremaster muscle, lymph vessels, and connective tissue); spermatic cord extends from testis to inguinal ring

Ejaculatory Ducts

- Formed by ductus deferens ampulla and seminal vesicle duct
- Pierces prostate gland and then ejects sperm along with additives into the prostatic urethra

Seminal Vesicles

- Secretes fluid that enhances sperm longevity and movement; 60% of semen volume is seminal vesicle secretion

Prostate Gland

- Surrounds beginning of urethra below the bladder
- Divided into five lobules formed by urethra and ejaculatory ducts
- Secretes liquid that assists sperm with motility (provides liquid to travel within); alkalinity of liquid protects sperm from acidic environment in the female vagina

Bulbourethral Glands

- Located inferior to prostate gland (also known as Cowper's glands)
- Stimulated glands secrete a mucoid substance prior to ejaculation, which neutralizes urine residue in urethra

Urethra

- Common tube for urinary and reproductive systems
- Consists of prostatic, membranous, and penile urethra

Penis

- Composed of erectile tissue that becomes erect when engorged with blood during stimulation
- Shaft of penis composed of three columns of erectile tissue: two corpus cavernosum; one corpus spongiosum

Male Reproductive Anatomy and Ejaculation Pathway

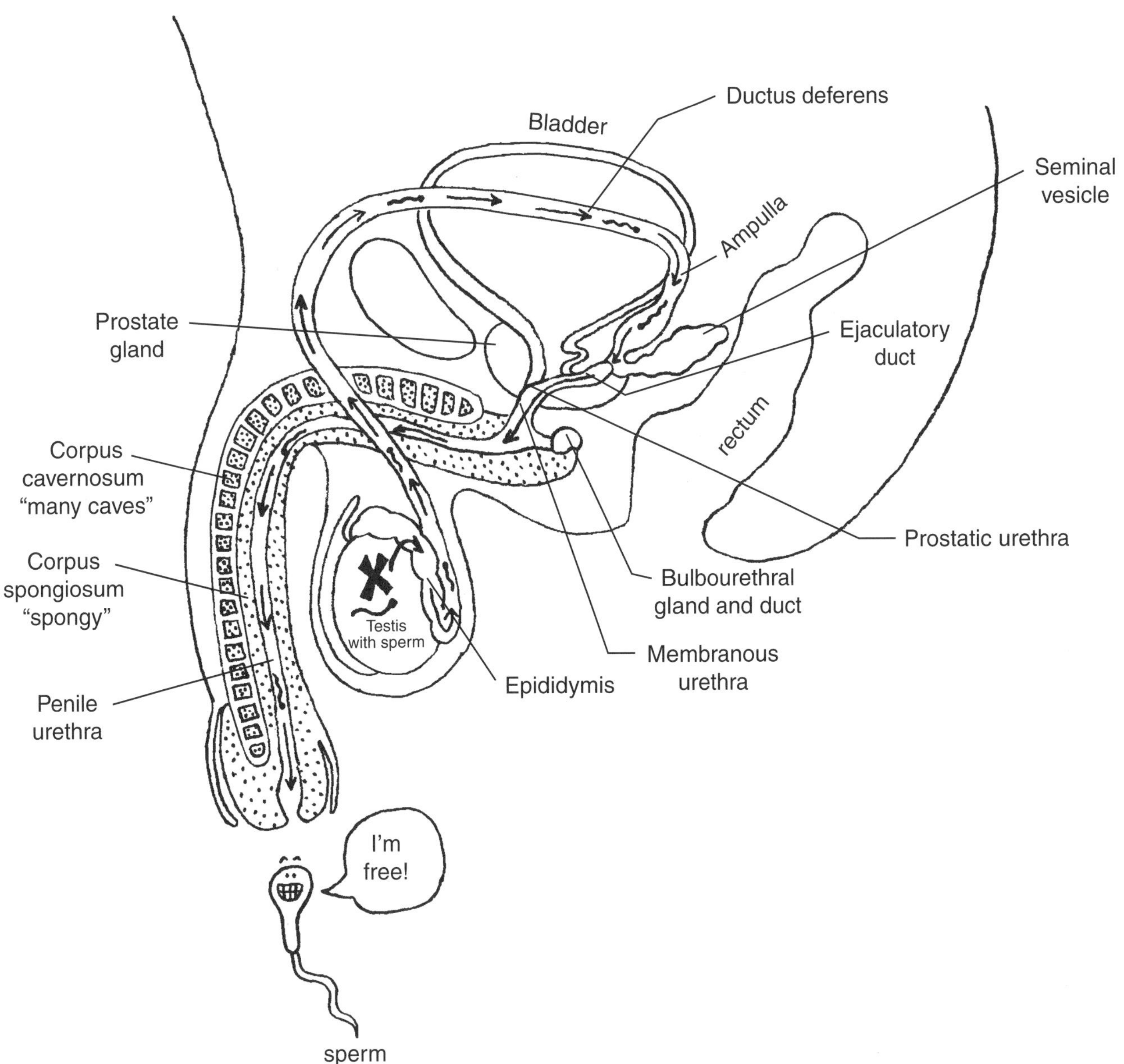

NOTES

HORMONAL REGULATION

- GnRh released in pulsatile manner from hypothalamic arcuate nucleus that stimulates the anterior pituitary to release FSH and LH
- FSH stimulates the Sertoli or nurse cells to maintain spermatogenesis in the testis (S for FSH and Sertoli)
- LH stimulates the Leydig cells to release testosterone (L for LH and Leydig)
- Sertoli cells release inhibin, which causes a decrease in FSH secretion due to negative feedback at the anterior pituitary
- Testosterone stimulates Sertoli cells (through paracrine effect) to maintain spermatogenesis
- Testosterone has inhibitory effects at anterior pituitary (to decrease LH secretion) and hypothalamus (to decrease GnRH release)
- Testosterone responsible for differentiation of Wolffian ducts, male secondary sex characteristics, libido, maintenance of spermatogenesis, and closure of epiphyseal plates in long bones

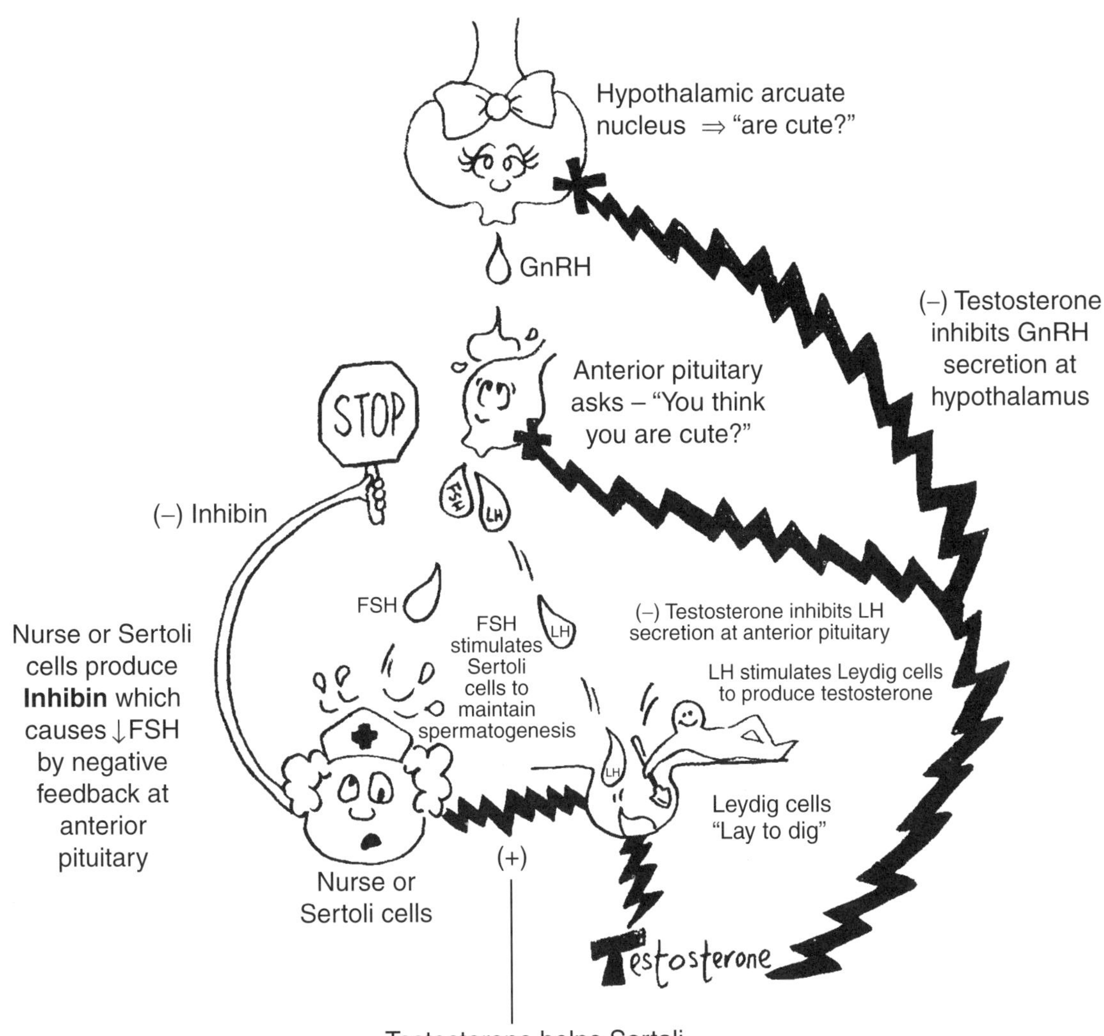
Hypothalamic arcuate nucleus ⇒ "are cute?"
GnRH
(–) Testosterone inhibits GnRH secretion at hypothalamus
STOP
Anterior pituitary asks – "You think you are cute?"
FSH
LH
(–) Inhibin
FSH
LH
FSH stimulates Sertoli cells to maintain spermatogenesis
(–) Testosterone inhibits LH secretion at anterior pituitary
LH stimulates Leydig cells to produce testosterone
Nurse or Sertoli cells produce **Inhibin** which causes ↓FSH by negative feedback at anterior pituitary
LH
Leydig cells "Lay to dig"
(+)
Nurse or Sertoli cells
Testosterone
Testosterone helps Sertoli cells to maintain spermatogenesis

NOTES

SPERMATOGENESIS

- Spermatogonia are stem cells in the outer region of seminferous tubules; diploid cells (46 chromosomes); duplicate themselves by mitosis
- During mitosis only one of spermatogonia remain spermatogonia, whereas the other is a primary spermatocyte that undergoes meiosis
- After first meiotic division of diploid (46 chromosomes) primary spermatocyte → two haploid (23 chromosomes) daughter cells are produced (referred to as secondary spermatocytes)
- These two secondary spermatocytes undergo a second meiotic division and each produces two daughter haploid cells (total: four spermatids)
- One primary spermatocyte therefore produces four spermatids
- Spermatids have interconnected cytoplasm
- Spermiogenesis is the maturation of innerconnected spermatids into separate mature spermatozoa
- Process of spermiogenesis requires the assistance of nurse or Sertoli cells which, among other functions, secrete nutrients
- Nurse cells are linked together by tight junctions forming a blood-testis barrier

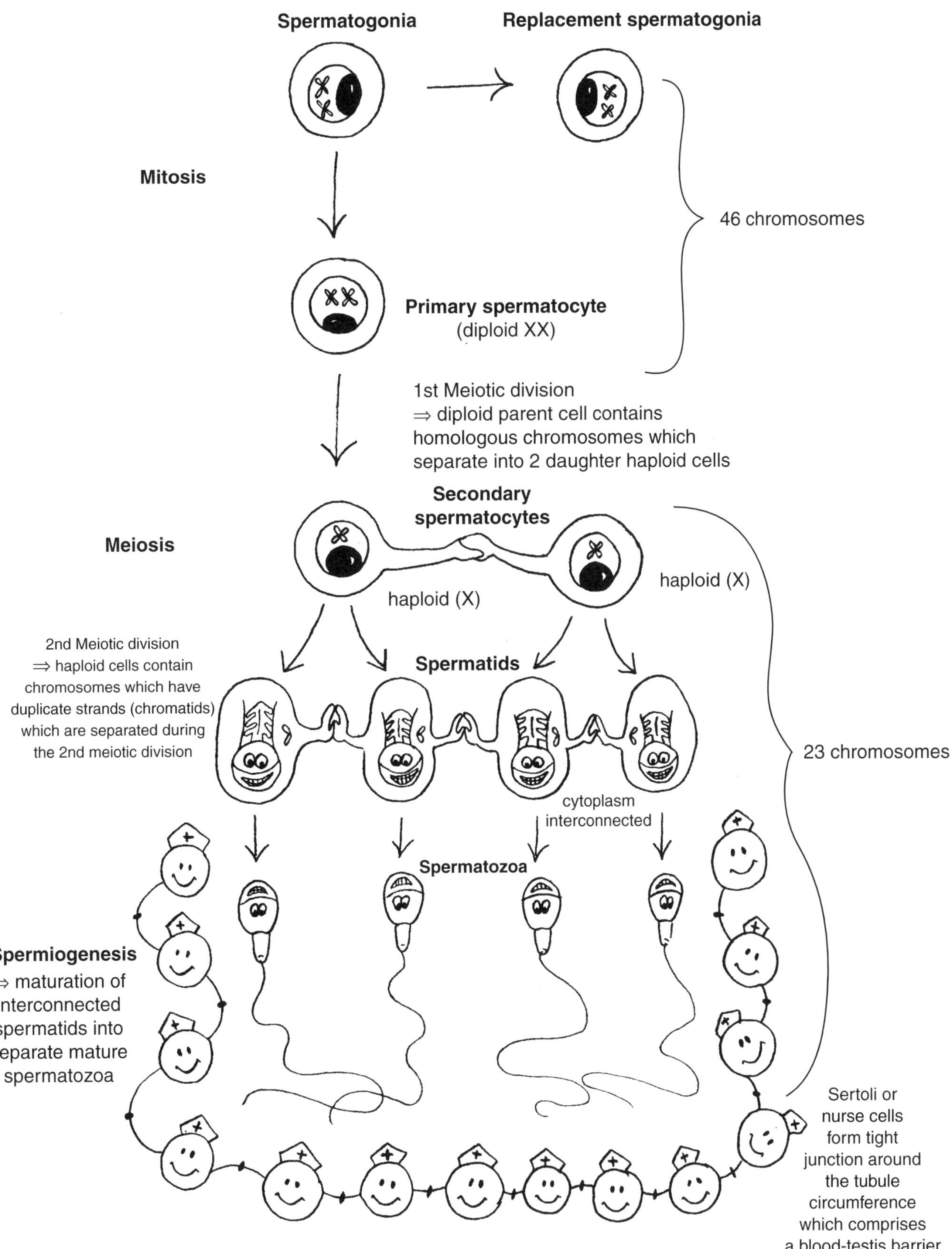
Spermatogonia
Replacement spermatogonia
Mitosis
46 chromosomes
Primary spermatocyte
(diploid XX)
1st Meiotic division
⇒ diploid parent cell contains
homologous chromosomes which
separate into 2 daughter haploid cells
Secondary
spermatocytes
Meiosis
haploid (X)
haploid (X)
2nd Meiotic division
⇒ haploid cells contain
chromosomes which have
duplicate strands (chromatids)
which are separated during
the 2nd meiotic division
Spermatids
23 chromosomes
cytoplasm
interconnected
Spermatozoa
Spermiogenesis
⇒ maturation of
interconnected
spermatids into
separate mature
spermatozoa
Sertoli or
nurse cells
form tight
junction around
the tubule
circumference
which comprises
a blood-testis barrier

NOTES

LAYERS OF TESTIS

- From innermost to outermost
  - tunica albuginea
  - tunica vaginalis (visceral layer, then parietal layer)
  - internal spermatic fascia
  - cremaster muscle
  - cremaster fascia
  - external spermatic fascia
  - dartos fascia
  - skin

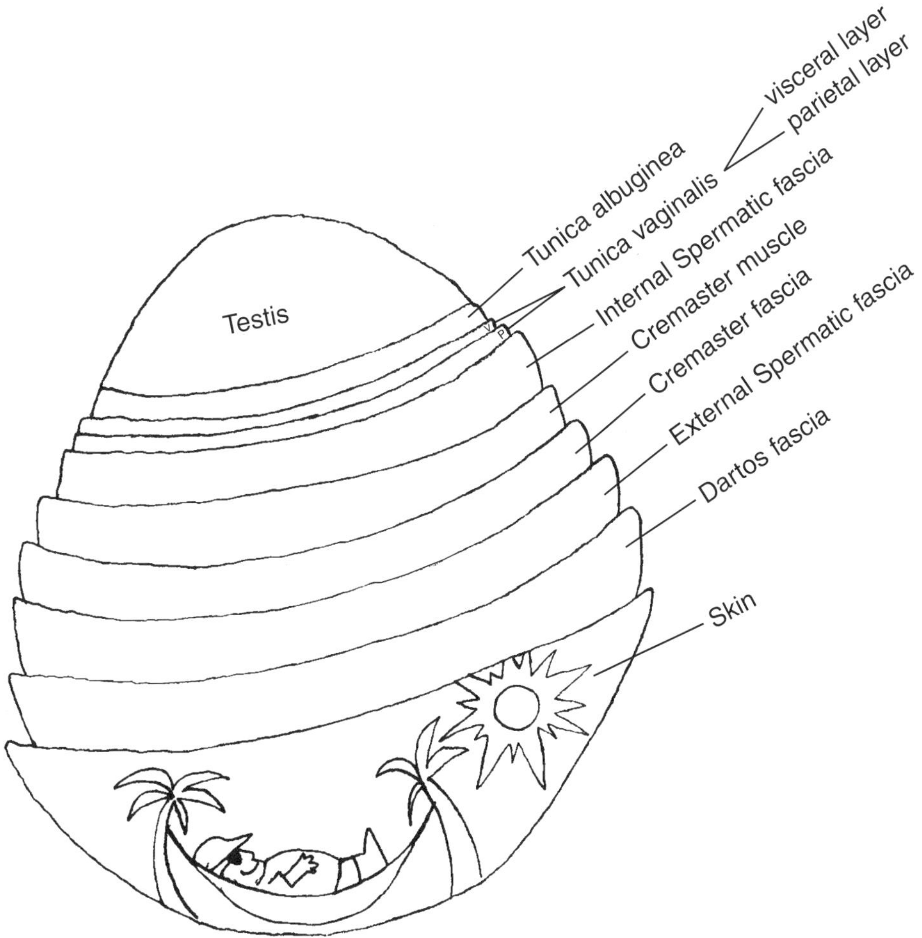

"Total Albinos Totally Veg In Summer, 'Cuz Many Can Form Extra Sun Damage Soon."

Total Albinos ⇒ Tunica Albuginea
Totally Veg ⇒ Tunica Vaginalis
In Summer ⇒ Internal Spermatic fascia
'Cuz Many ⇒ Cremaster Muscle
Can Form ⇒ Cremaster Fascia
Extra Sun ⇒ External Spermatic fascia
Damage ⇒ Dartos fascia
Soon ⇒ Skin

NOTES

NERVOUS SYSTEM ORGANIZATION

- Consists of neurons that are highly integrated in the central nervous system (CNS) and nerves and ganglions in the peripheral nervous system (PNS)
- CNS consists of brain and spinal cord
- PNS divided into somatic nervous system that is voluntary and affects the skeletal system and the autonomic system that controls the viscera and involuntary actions
- The autonomic nervous system is further divided into the parasympathetic and sympathetic nervous systems that will be discussed later in this chapter

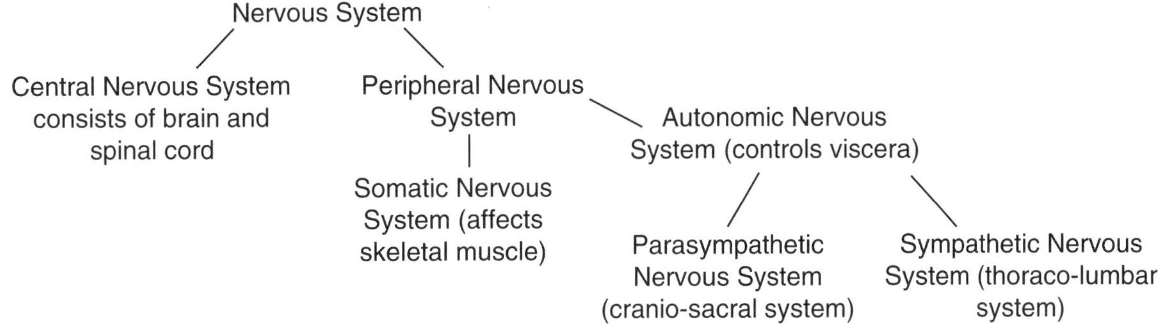
Nervous System
Central Nervous System consists of brain and spinal cord
Peripheral Nervous System
Somatic Nervous System (affects skeletal muscle)
Autonomic Nervous System (controls viscera)
Parasympathetic Nervous System (cranio-sacral system)
Sympathetic Nervous System (thoraco-lumbar system)

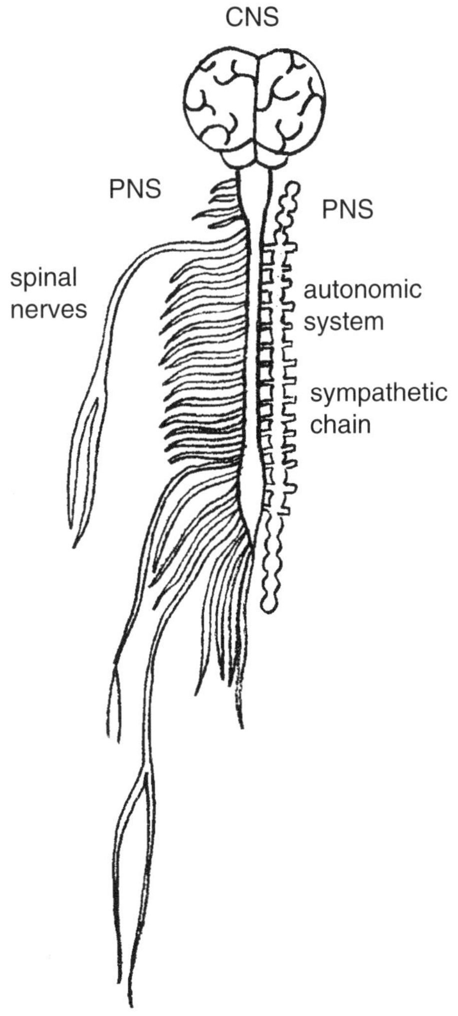
CNS
PNS
PNS
spinal nerves
autonomic system
sympathetic chain

NOTES

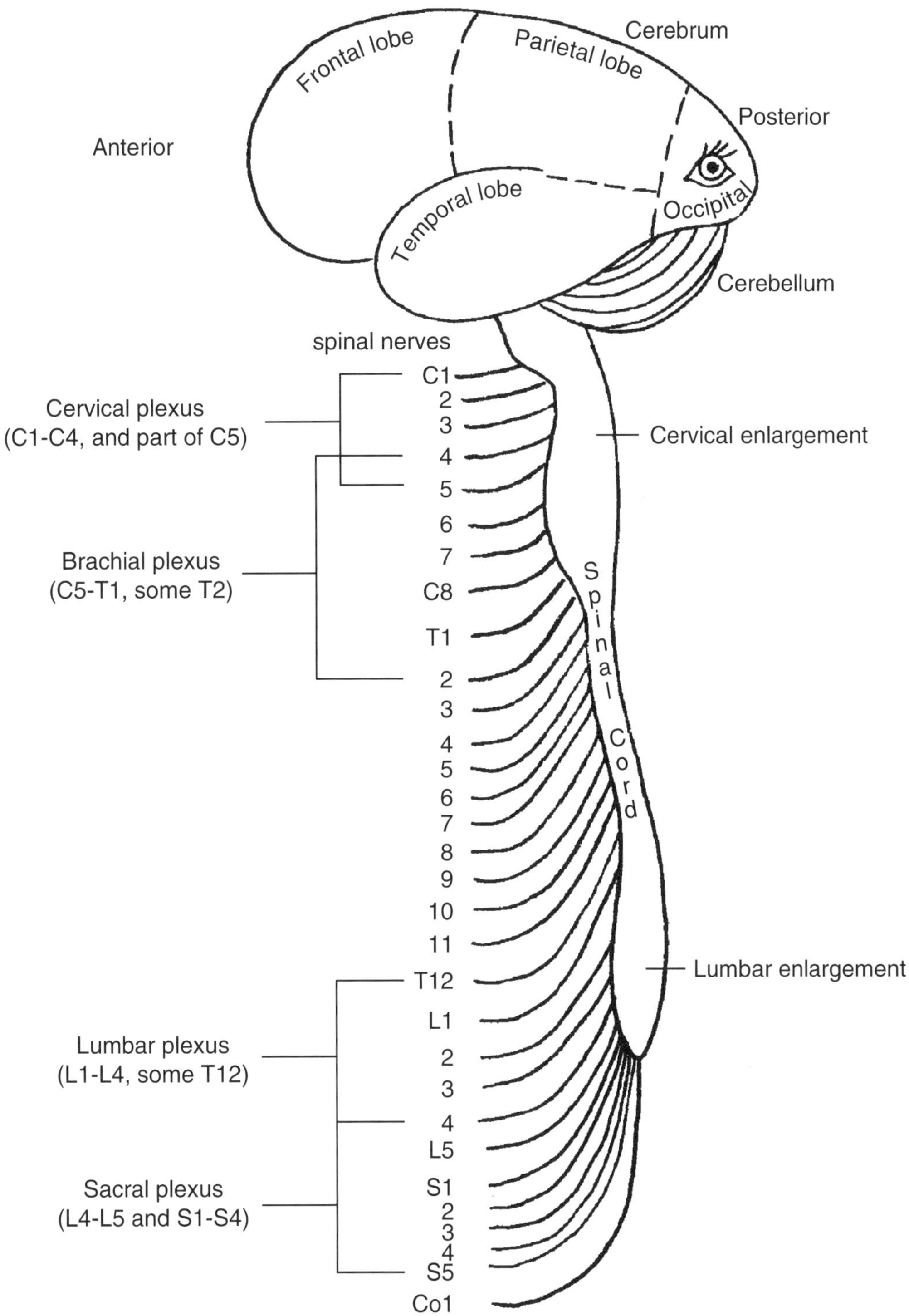
Frontal lobe
Parietal lobe
Cerebrum
Posterior
Anterior
Temporal lobe
Occipital
Cerebellum
spinal nerves
C1
2
3
4
5
6
7
C8
T1
2
3
4
5
6
7
8
9
10
11
T12
L1
2
3
4
L5
S1
2
3
4
S5
Co1
Cervical plexus
(C1-C4, and part of C5)
Brachial plexus
(C5-T1, some T2)
Lumbar plexus
(L1-L4, some T12)
Sacral plexus
(L4-L5 and S1-S4)
Cervical enlargement
Spinal Cord
Lumbar enlargement

NOTES

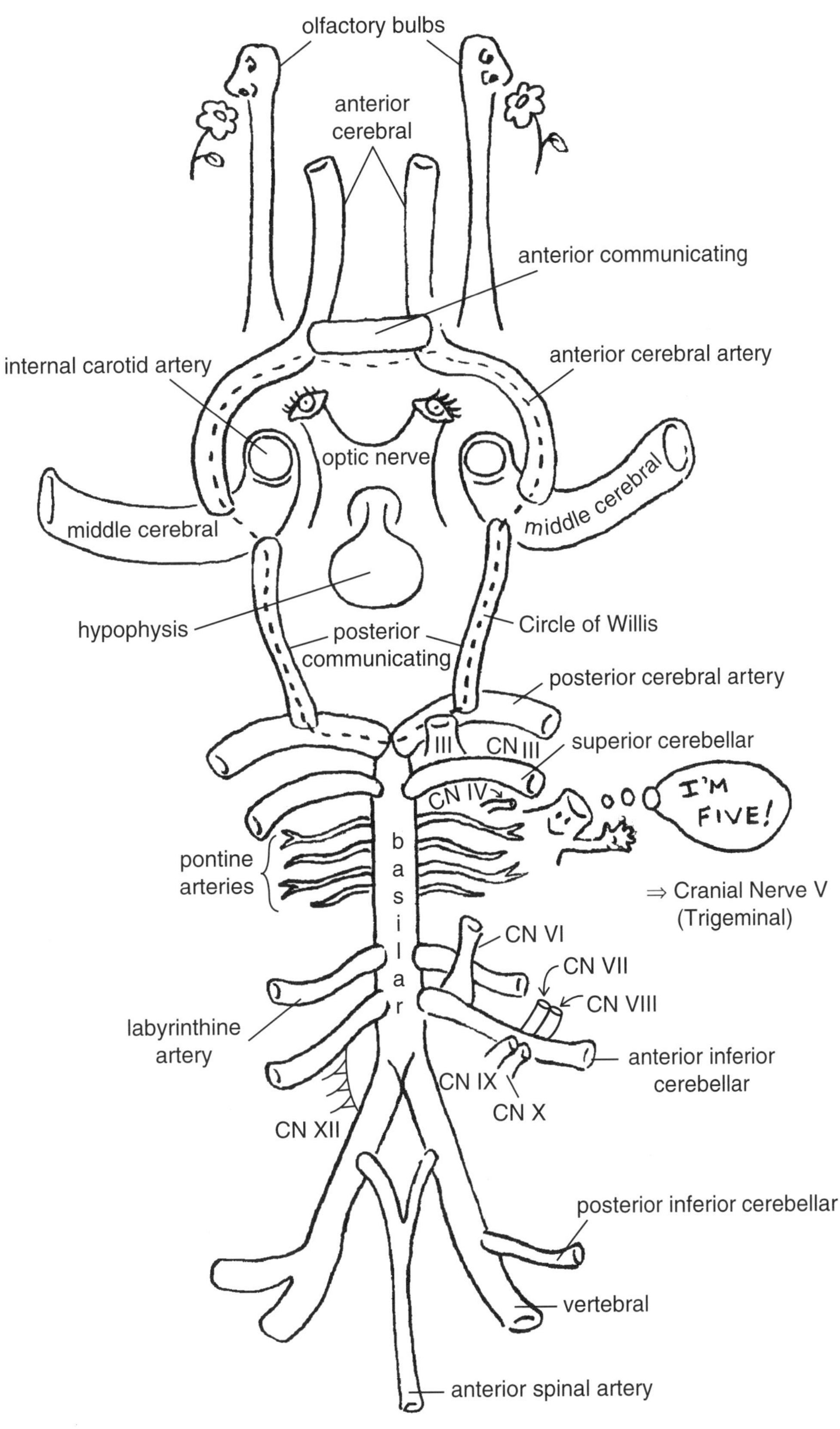
olfactory bulbs
anterior cerebral
anterior communicating
internal carotid artery
anterior cerebral artery
optic nerve
middle cerebral
middle cerebral
hypophysis
posterior communicating
Circle of Willis
posterior cerebral artery
III
CN III
superior cerebellar
CN IV
I'M FIVE!
pontine arteries
basilar
⇒ Cranial Nerve V (Trigeminal)
CN VI
CN VII
CN VIII
labyrinthine artery
anterior inferior cerebellar
CN IX
CN X
CN XII
posterior inferior cerebellar
vertebral
anterior spinal artery

NOTES

CEREBROSPINAL FLUID CIRCULATION (CSF)

- Secreted by the choroids plexus and circulated through subarachnoid space
- CSF is reabsorbed by arachnoid villi projecting into the superior sagittal sinus, one of the veins that drains the brain
- Circulation can be seen in illustration

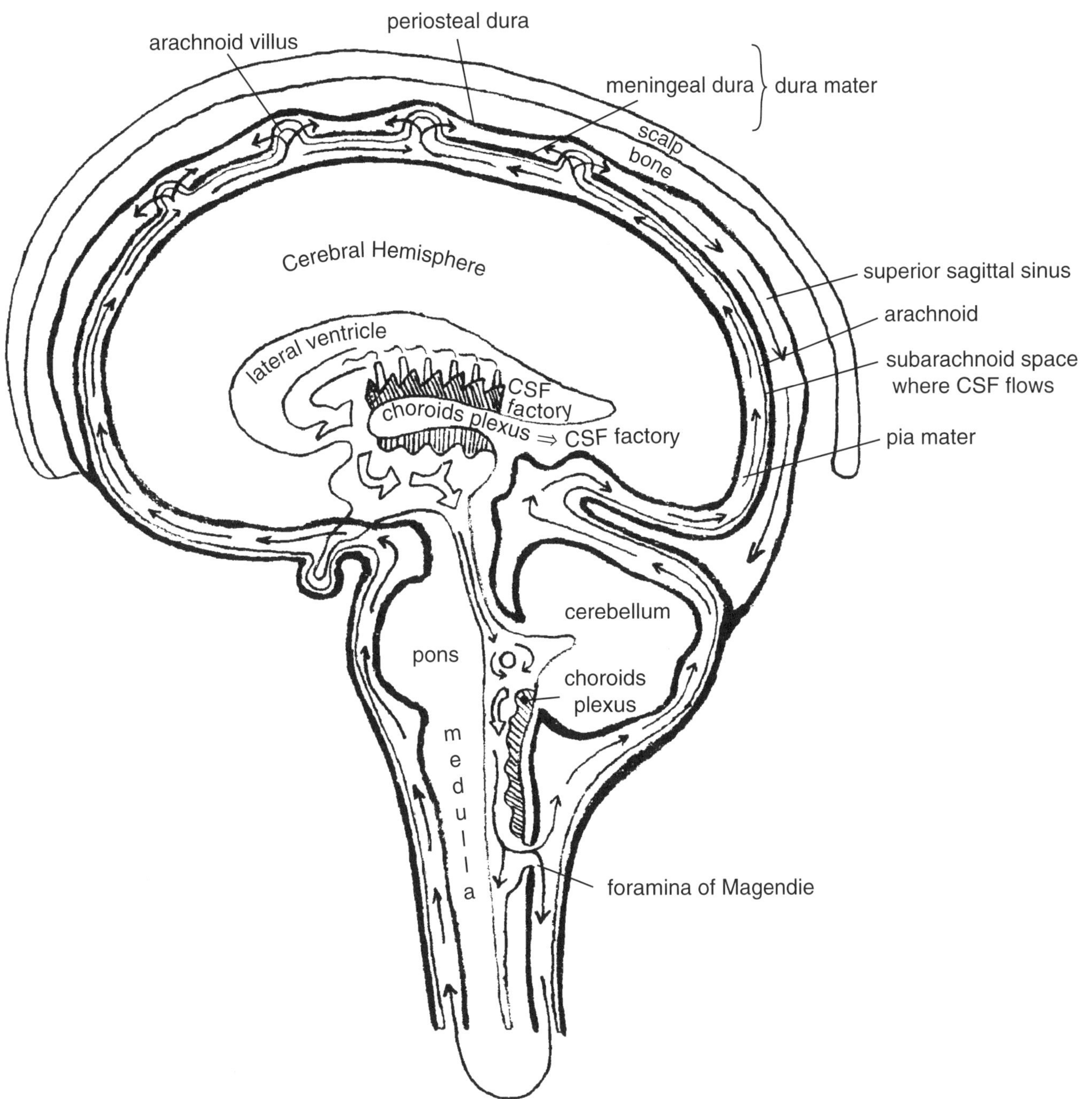
periosteal dura
arachnoid villus
meningeal dura
dura mater
scalp
bone
Cerebral Hemisphere
superior sagittal sinus
arachnoid
subarachnoid space where CSF flows
lateral ventricle
CSF factory
choroids plexus ⇒ CSF factory
pia mater
cerebellum
pons
choroids plexus
medulla
foramina of Magendie

NOTES

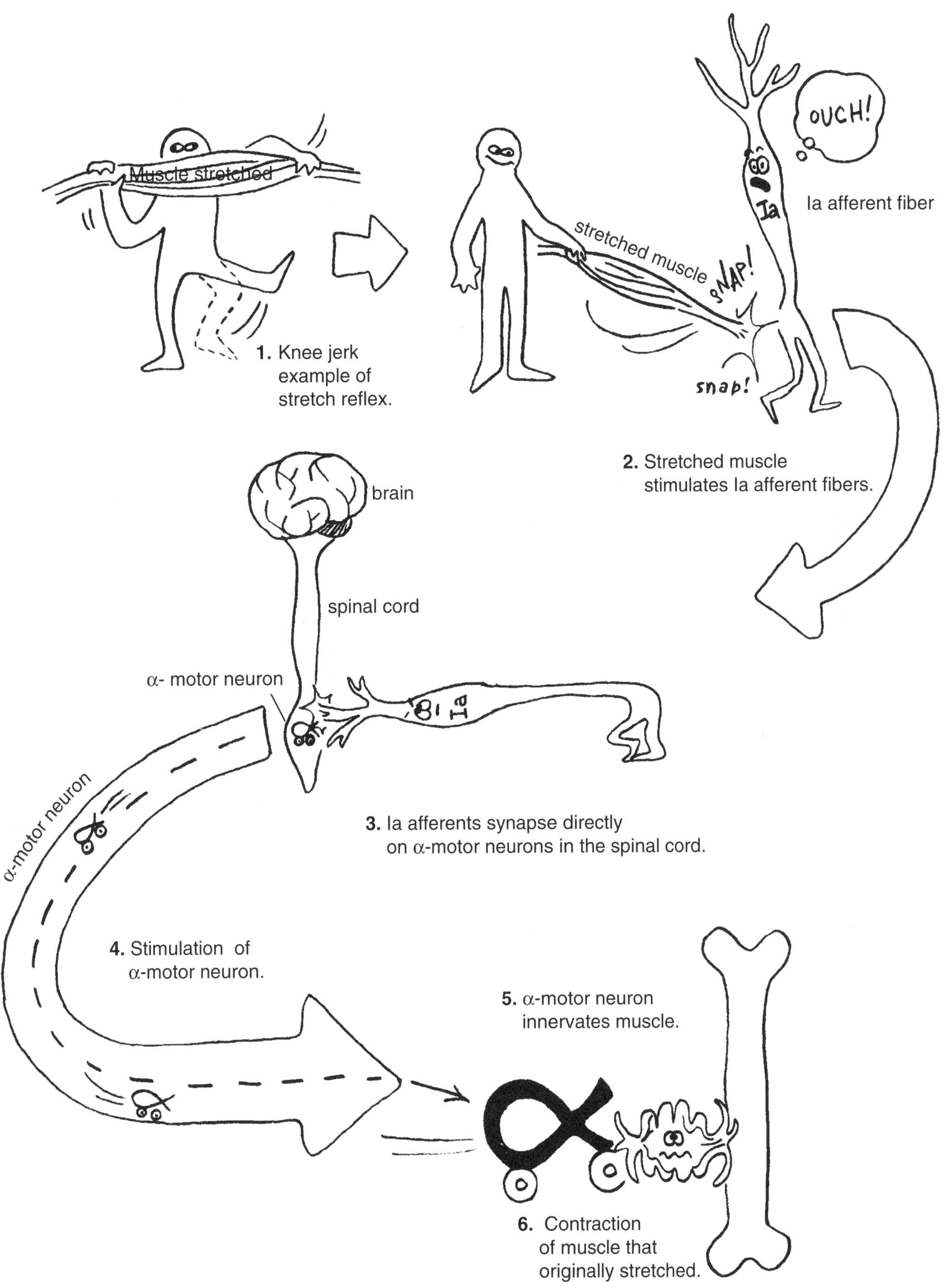
Muscle stretched
1. Knee jerk example of stretch reflex.
OUCH!
Ia
Ia afferent fiber
stretched muscle
SNAP!
snap!
2. Stretched muscle stimulates Ia afferent fibers.
brain
spinal cord
α- motor neuron
Ia
α-motor neuron
3. Ia afferents synapse directly on α-motor neurons in the spinal cord.
4. Stimulation of α-motor neuron.
5. α-motor neuron innervates muscle.
6. Contraction of muscle that originally stretched.

NOTES

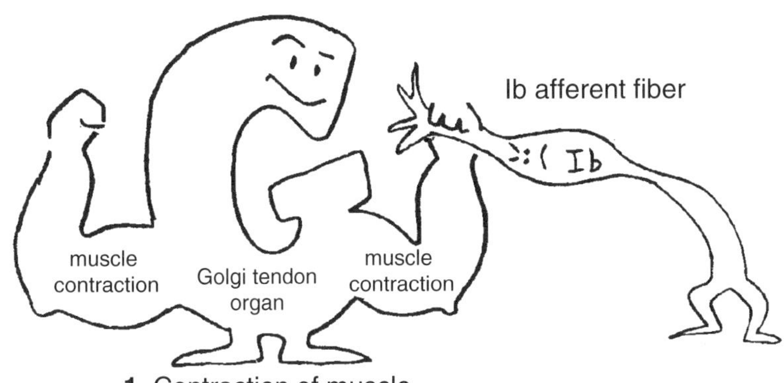

1. Contraction of muscle activates Golgi tendon organs and group Ib afferent fibers.

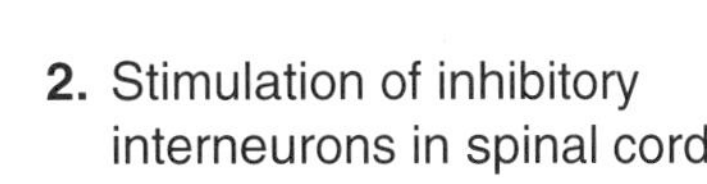

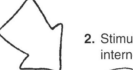

2. Stimulation of inhibitory interneurons in spinal cord.

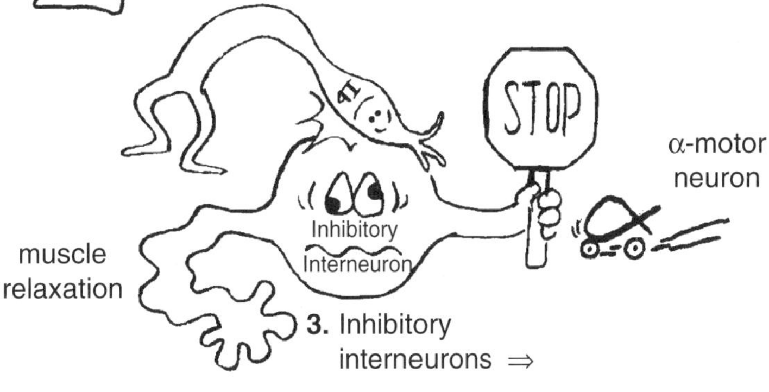

3. Inhibitory interneurons ⇒

4. inhibit α-motor neurons

5. and cause relaxation of muscle that originally contracted

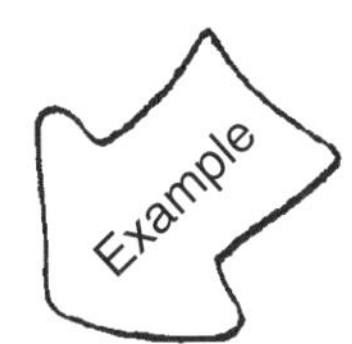

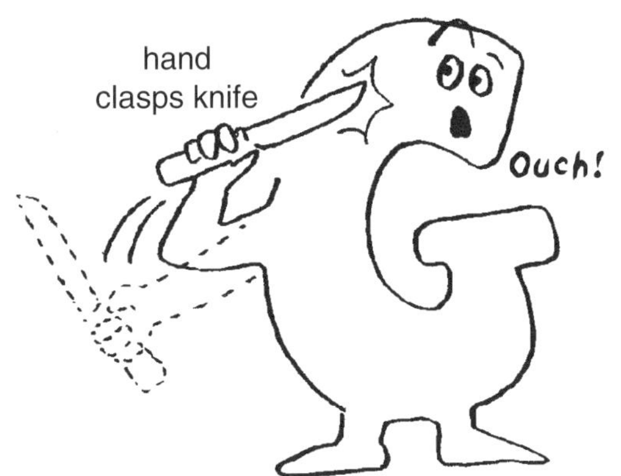

Example of Golgi tendon reflex is clasp-knife reflex (explanation in text)

NOTES

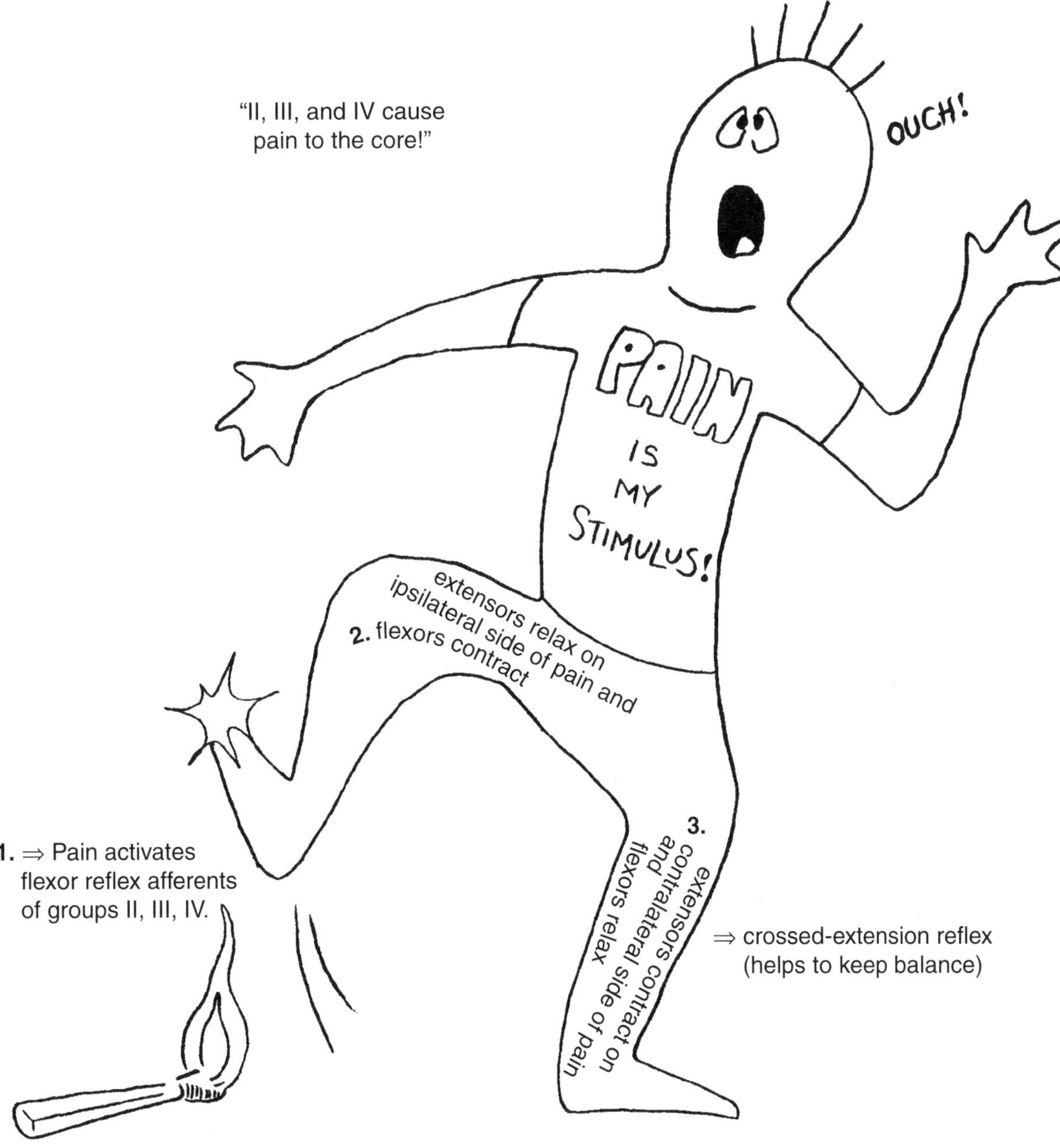
"II, III, and IV cause pain to the core!"
OUCH!
PAIN IS MY STIMULUS!
2. flexors contract
extensors relax on ipsilateral side of pain and
1. ⇒ Pain activates flexor reflex afferents of groups II, III, IV.
3. extensors contract on contralateral side of pain and flexors relax
⇒ crossed-extension reflex (helps to keep balance)

NOTES

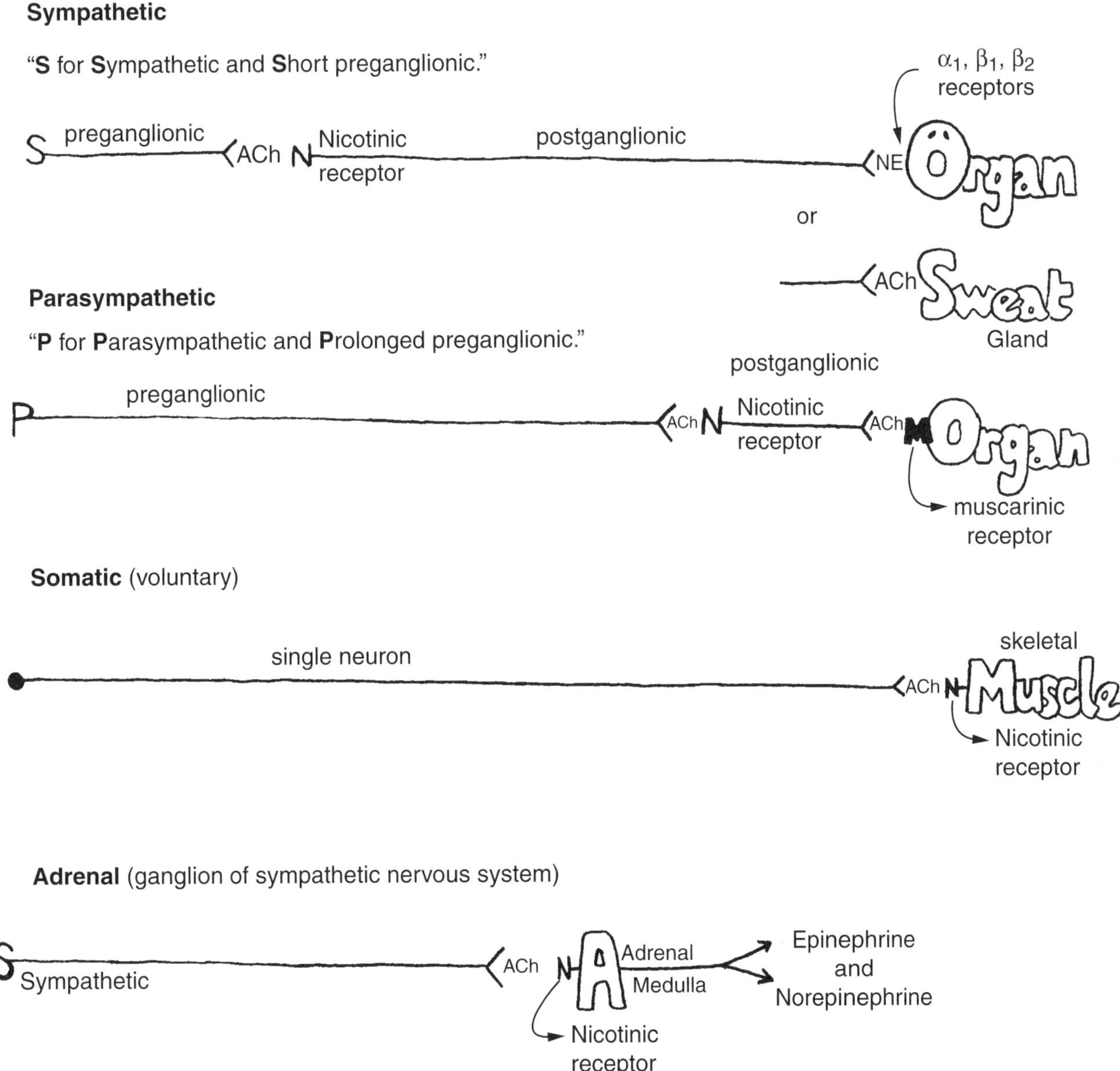
Sympathetic
"S for Sympathetic and Short preganglionic."
α1, β1, β2
receptors
S
preganglionic
ACh
N
Nicotinic
receptor
postganglionic
NE
Organ
or
ACh
Sweat
Gland
Parasympathetic
"P for Parasympathetic and Prolonged preganglionic."
postganglionic
P
preganglionic
ACh
N
Nicotinic
receptor
ACh
M
Organ
muscarinic
receptor
Somatic (voluntary)
skeletal
single neuron
ACh
N
Muscle
Nicotinic
receptor
Adrenal (ganglion of sympathetic nervous system)
S
Sympathetic
ACh
N
A
Adrenal
Medulla
Epinephrine
and
Norepinephrine
Nicotinic
receptor

NOTES

SYMPATHETIC NERVOUS SYSTEM

- Also known as the thoracolumbar nervous system
- Associated with "flight or fight" responses to stimuli such as pupil dilation, increased heart rate, and increased blood flow to muscles and brain
- Preganglionic neuronal cell bodies originate in the lateral horns of T1–L2 → exit spinal cord through anterior roots → join spinal nerves (short distance) → white communicating rami to sympathetic chain → can ascend or descend chain; they synapse with a postganglionic neuron, synapse at level entered, or don't synapse and pass straight through, forming the splanchnic nerves
- Postganglionic neuron exits sympathetic chain via gray communicating rami to join spinal nerves

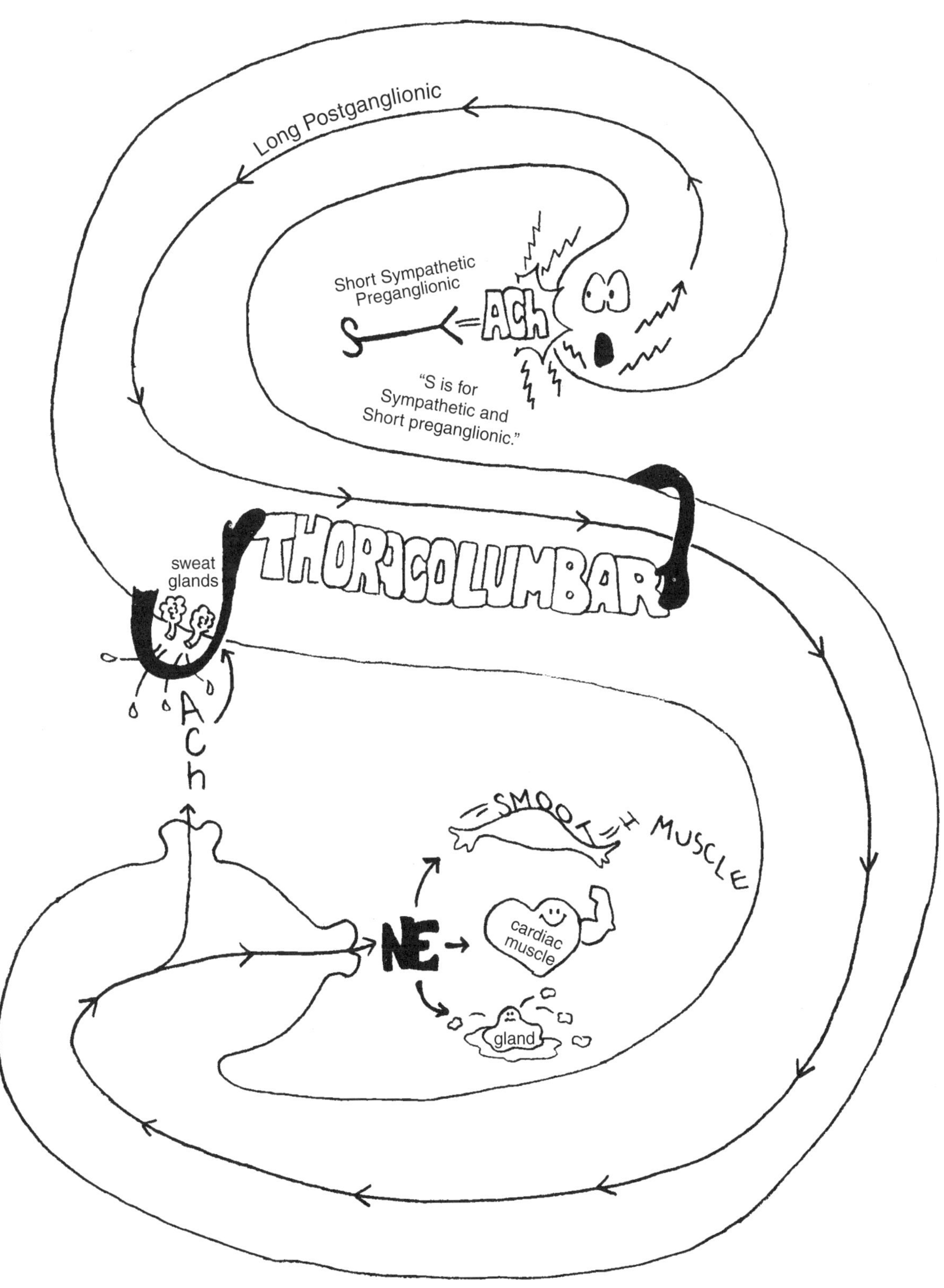
Long Postganglionic
Short Sympathetic Preganglionic
S
ACh
"S is for Sympathetic and Short preganglionic."
THORACOLUMBAR
sweat glands
ACh
SMOOTH MUSCLE
NE
cardiac muscle
gland

NOTES

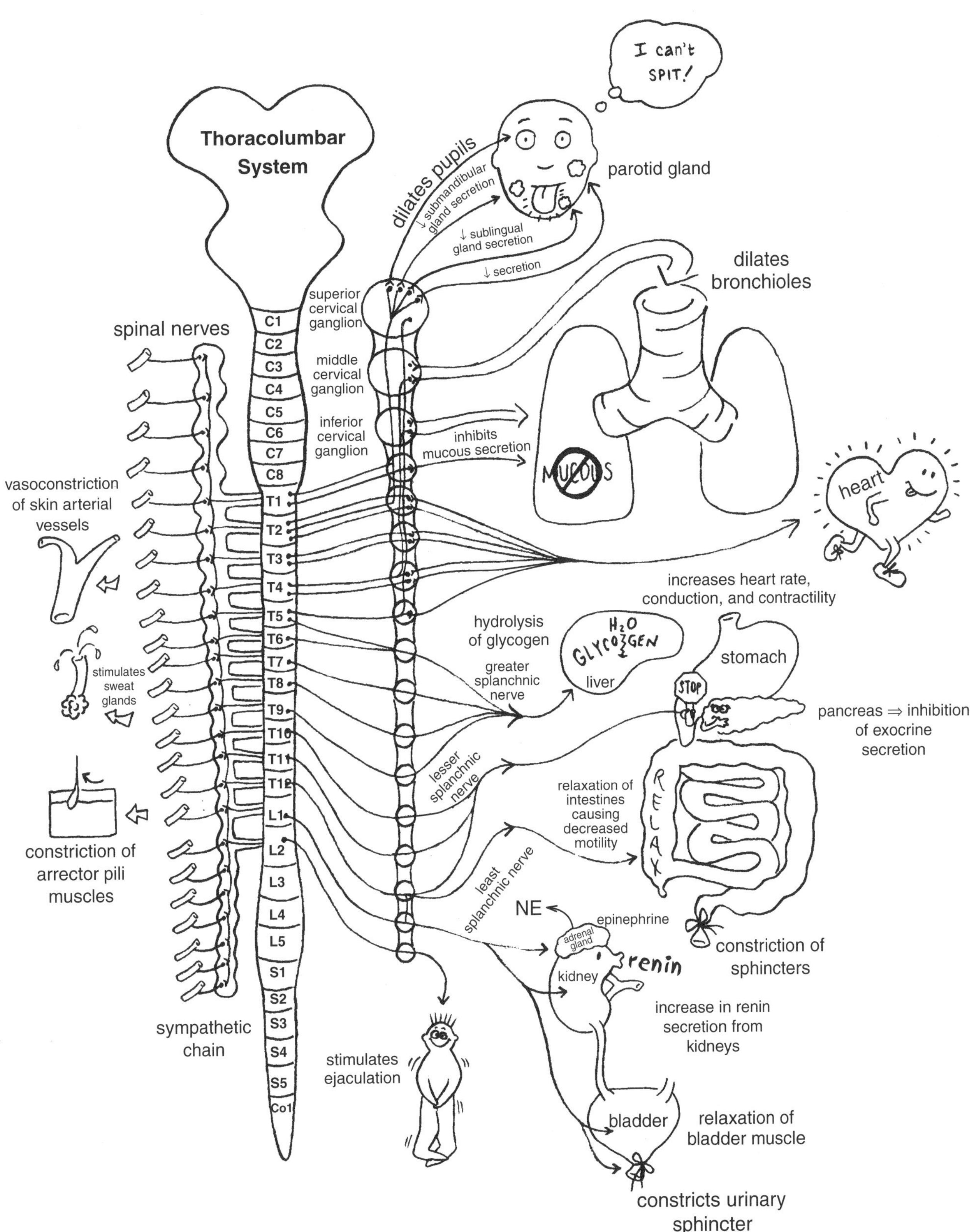
I can't SPIT!
Thoracolumbar System
dilates pupils
↓ submandibular gland secretion
↓ sublingual gland secretion
↓ secretion
parotid gland
dilates bronchioles
superior cervical ganglion
middle cervical ganglion
inferior cervical ganglion
spinal nerves
C1
C2
C3
C4
C5
C6
C7
C8
T1
T2
T3
T4
T5
T6
T7
T8
T9
T10
T11
T12
L1
L2
L3
L4
L5
S1
S2
S3
S4
S5
Co1
inhibits mucous secretion
MUCOUS
heart
increases heart rate, conduction, and contractility
vasoconstriction of skin arterial vessels
hydrolysis of glycogen
H_2O
GLYCOGEN
liver
greater splanchnic nerve
stomach
STOP
pancreas ⇒ inhibition of exocrine secretion
stimulates sweat glands
lesser splanchnic nerve
relaxation of intestines causing decreased motility
RELAX
constriction of arrector pili muscles
least splanchnic nerve
NE
epinephrine
adrenal gland
constriction of sphincters
renin
kidney
increase in renin secretion from kidneys
sympathetic chain
stimulates ejaculation
bladder
relaxation of bladder muscle
constricts urinary sphincter

NOTES

α_1 receptors located on the following:

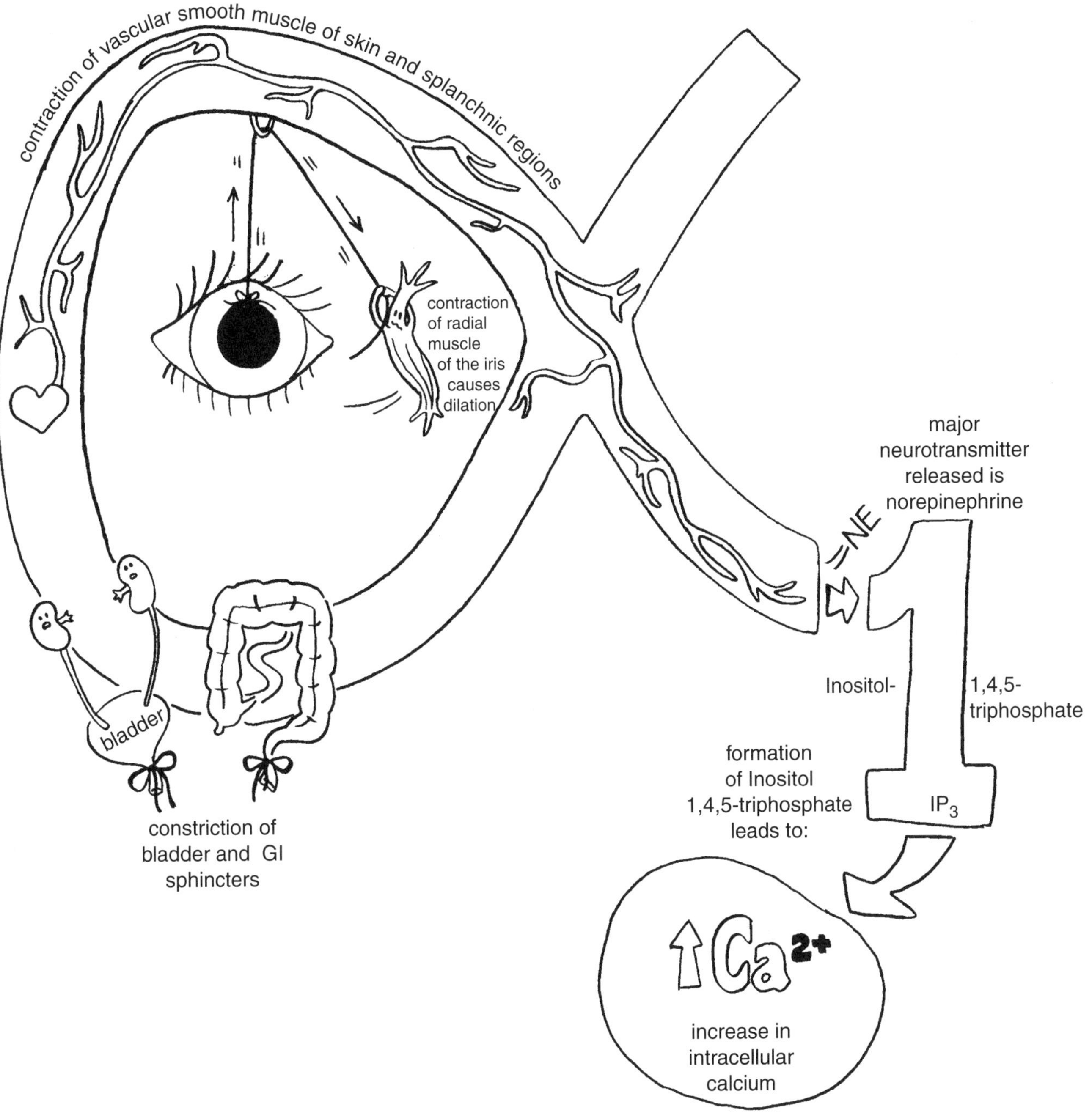
contraction of vascular smooth muscle of skin and splanchnic regions
contraction of radial muscle of the iris causes dilation
bladder
constriction of bladder and GI sphincters
NE
major neurotransmitter released is norepinephrine
Inositol-
1,4,5-triphosphate
formation of Inositol 1,4,5-triphosphate leads to:
IP3
Ca2+
increase in intracellular calcium

NOTES

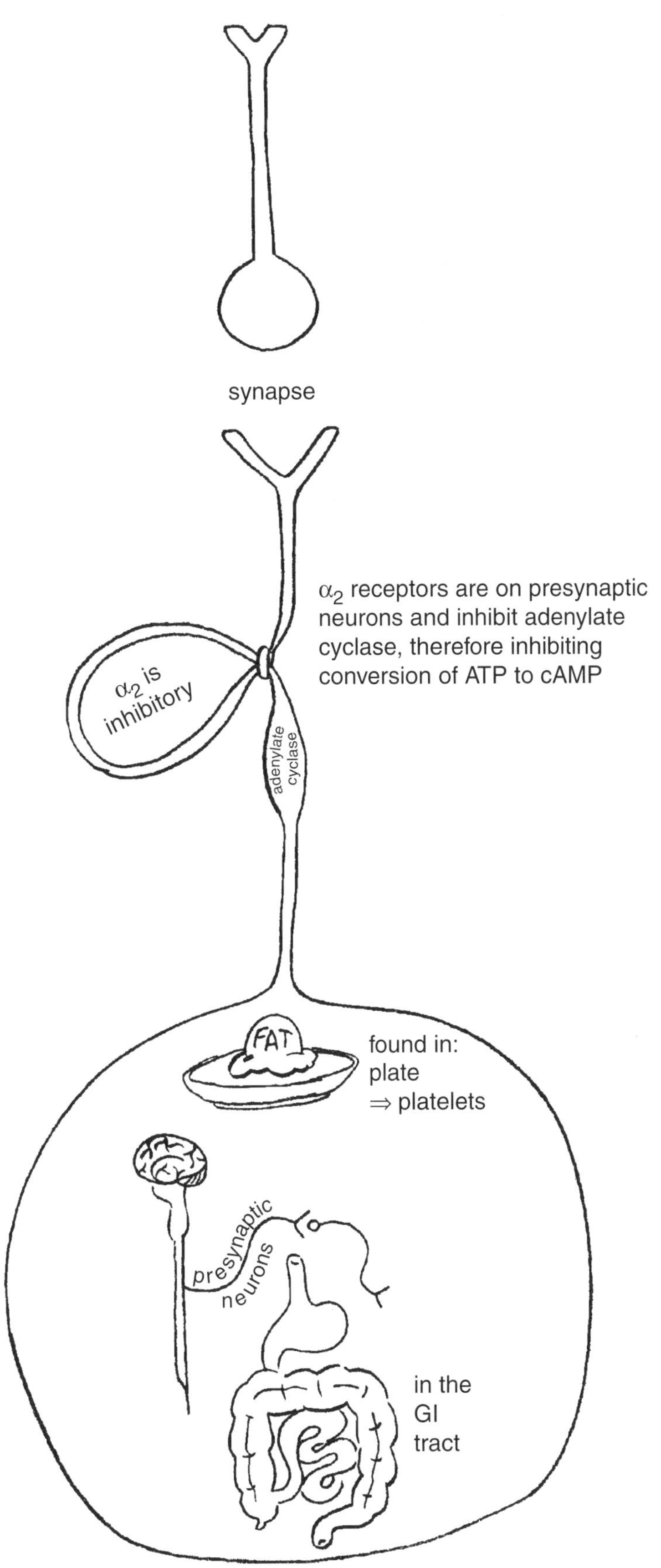
synapse
α_2 receptors are on presynaptic neurons and inhibit adenylate cyclase, therefore inhibiting conversion of ATP to cAMP
α_2 is inhibitory
adenylate cyclase
FAT
found in:
plate
⇒ platelets
presynaptic neurons
in the GI tract

NOTES

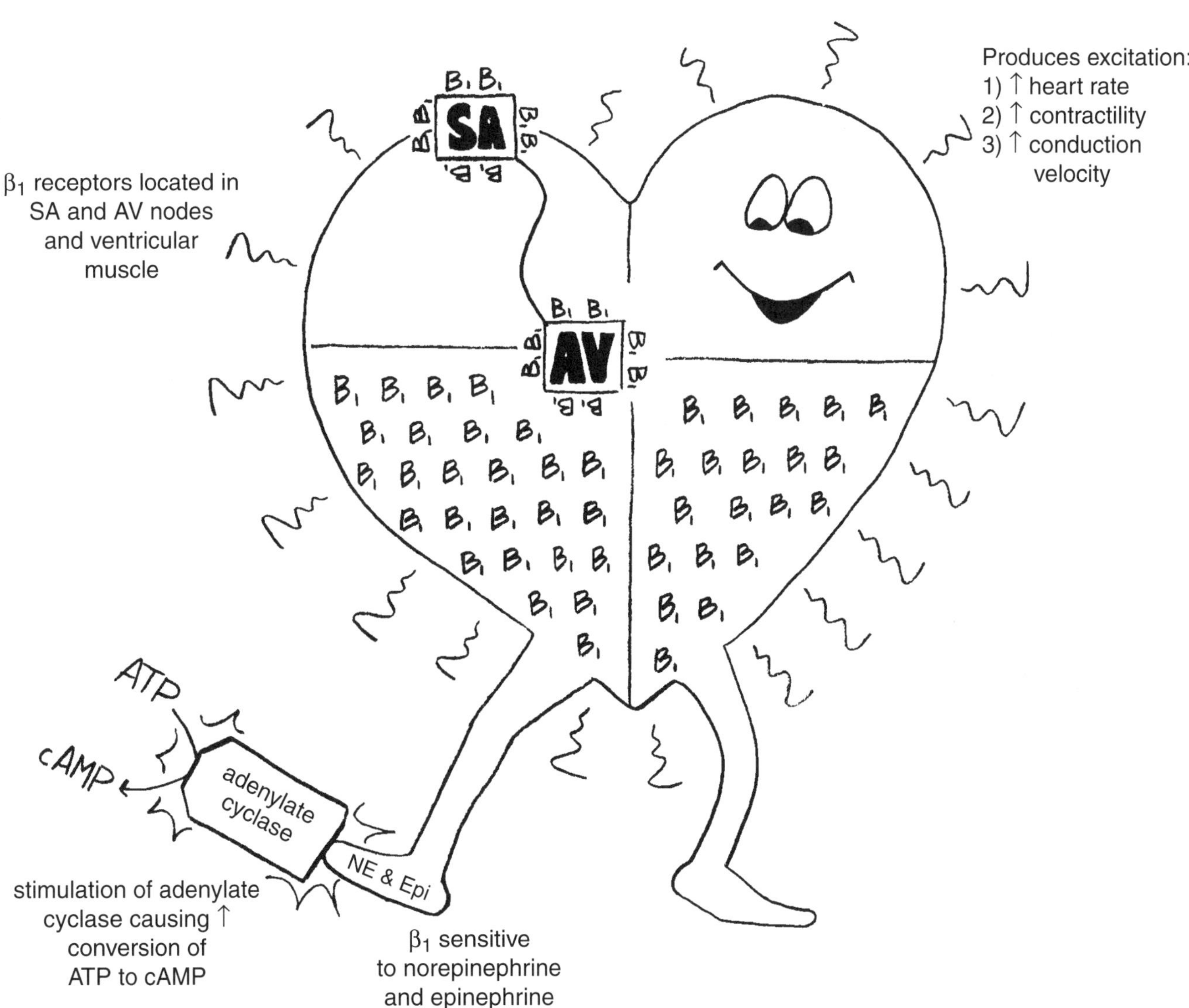
Produces excitation:
1) ↑ heart rate
2) ↑ contractility
3) ↑ conduction velocity
β_1 receptors located in SA and AV nodes and ventricular muscle
SA
AV
ATP
cAMP
adenylate cyclase
NE & Epi
stimulation of adenylate cyclase causing ↑ conversion of ATP to cAMP
β_1 sensitive to norepinephrine and epinephrine

NOTES

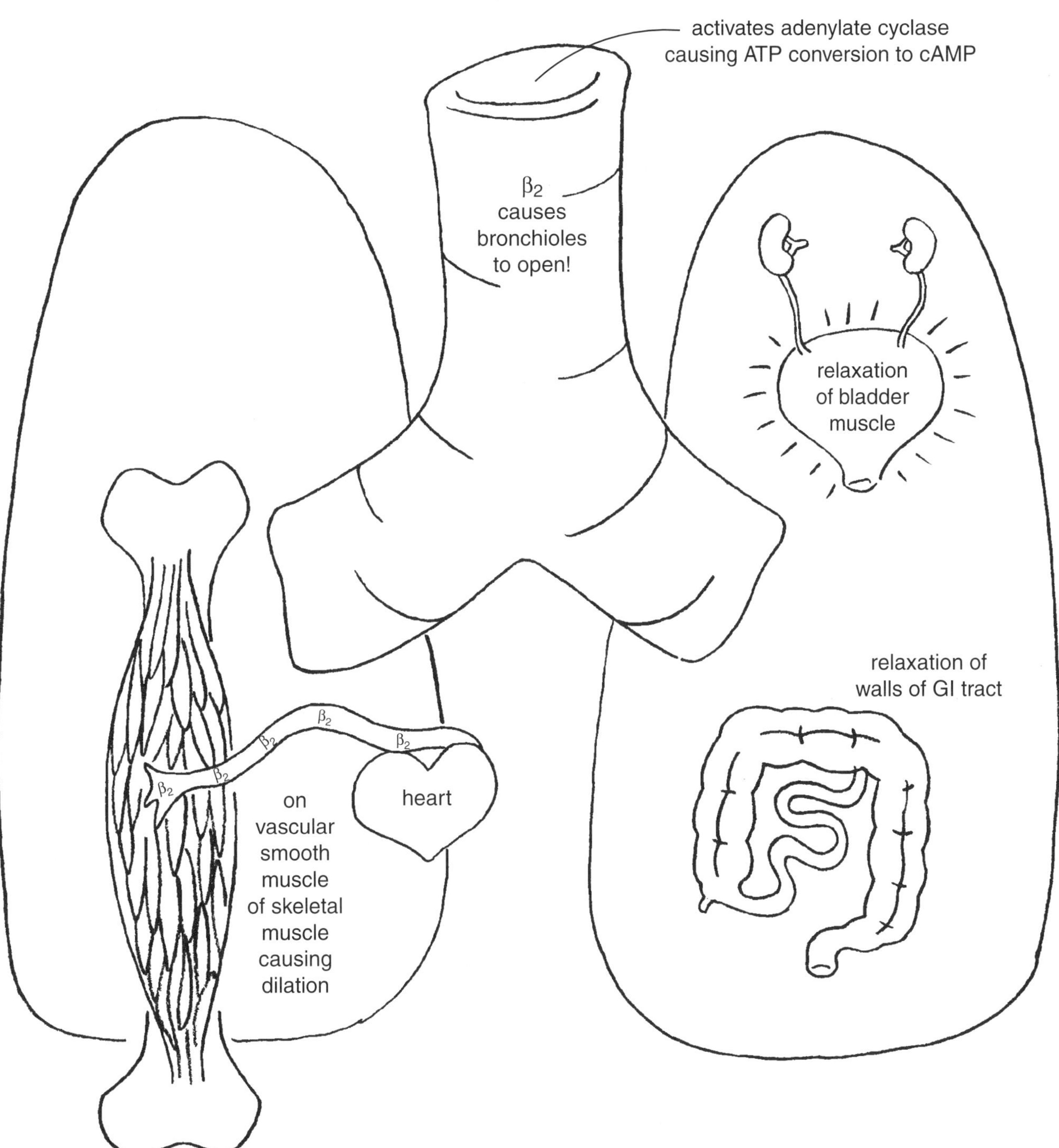
β2 causes relaxation:
activates adenylate cyclase causing ATP conversion to cAMP
β2 causes bronchioles to open!
relaxation of bladder muscle
relaxation of walls of GI tract
β2
β2
β2
β2
β2
heart
on vascular smooth muscle of skeletal muscle causing dilation

NOTES

PARASYMPATHETIC NERVOUS SYSTEM

- Associated with more sedentary activities such as increased gastrointestinal motility, mucous secretions, and bladder constriction
- Also known as the craniosacral system
- Preganglionic cell bodies originate in brain stem and sacral region
- Preganglionic neurons are long, whereas postganglionic neurons tend to be short

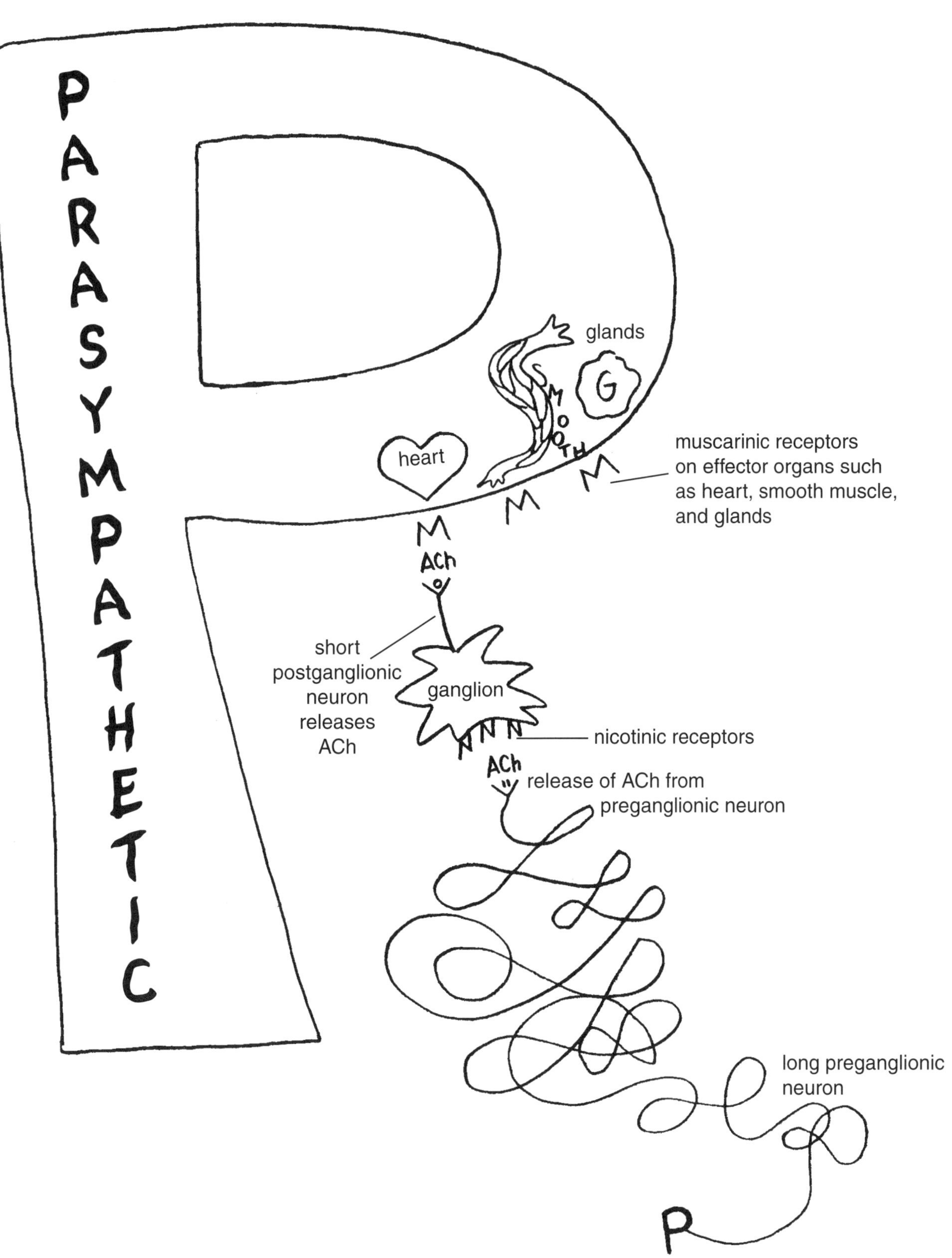
PARASYMPATHETIC
glands
G
SMOOTH
heart
muscarinic receptors on effector organs such as heart, smooth muscle, and glands
M
ACh
short postganglionic neuron releases ACh
ganglion
nicotinic receptors
N
ACh
release of ACh from preganglionic neuron
long preganglionic neuron
P

NOTES

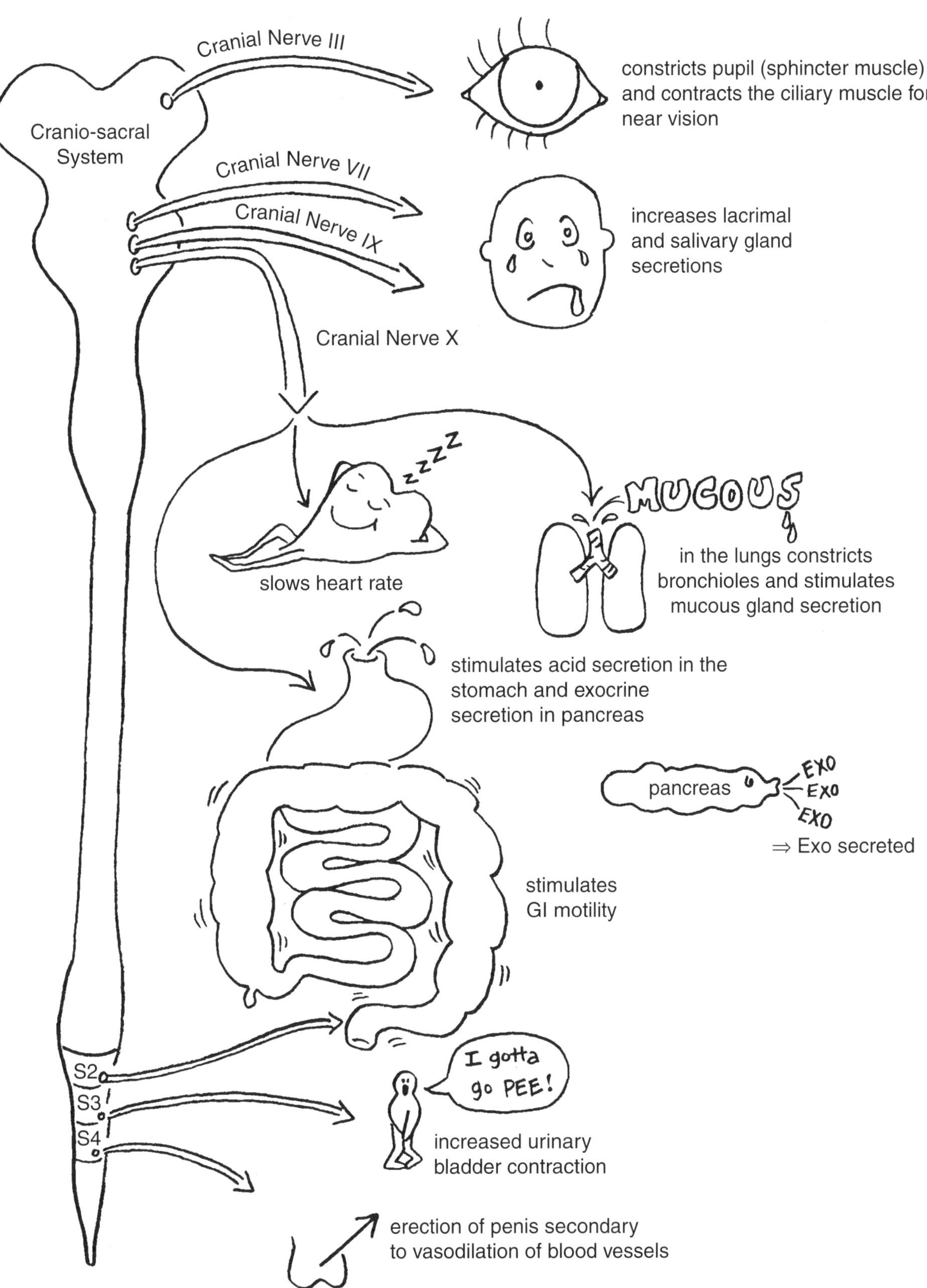
Cranial Nerve III
Cranio-sacral System
constricts pupil (sphincter muscle) and contracts the ciliary muscle for near vision
Cranial Nerve VII
Cranial Nerve IX
increases lacrimal and salivary gland secretions
Cranial Nerve X
MUCOUS
slows heart rate
in the lungs constricts bronchioles and stimulates mucous gland secretion
stimulates acid secretion in the stomach and exocrine secretion in pancreas
pancreas
EXO
EXO
EXO
⇒ Exo secreted
stimulates GI motility
S2
S3
S4
I gotta go PEE!
increased urinary bladder contraction
erection of penis secondary to vasodilation of blood vessels

NOTES

⇒ nicotine cigarette

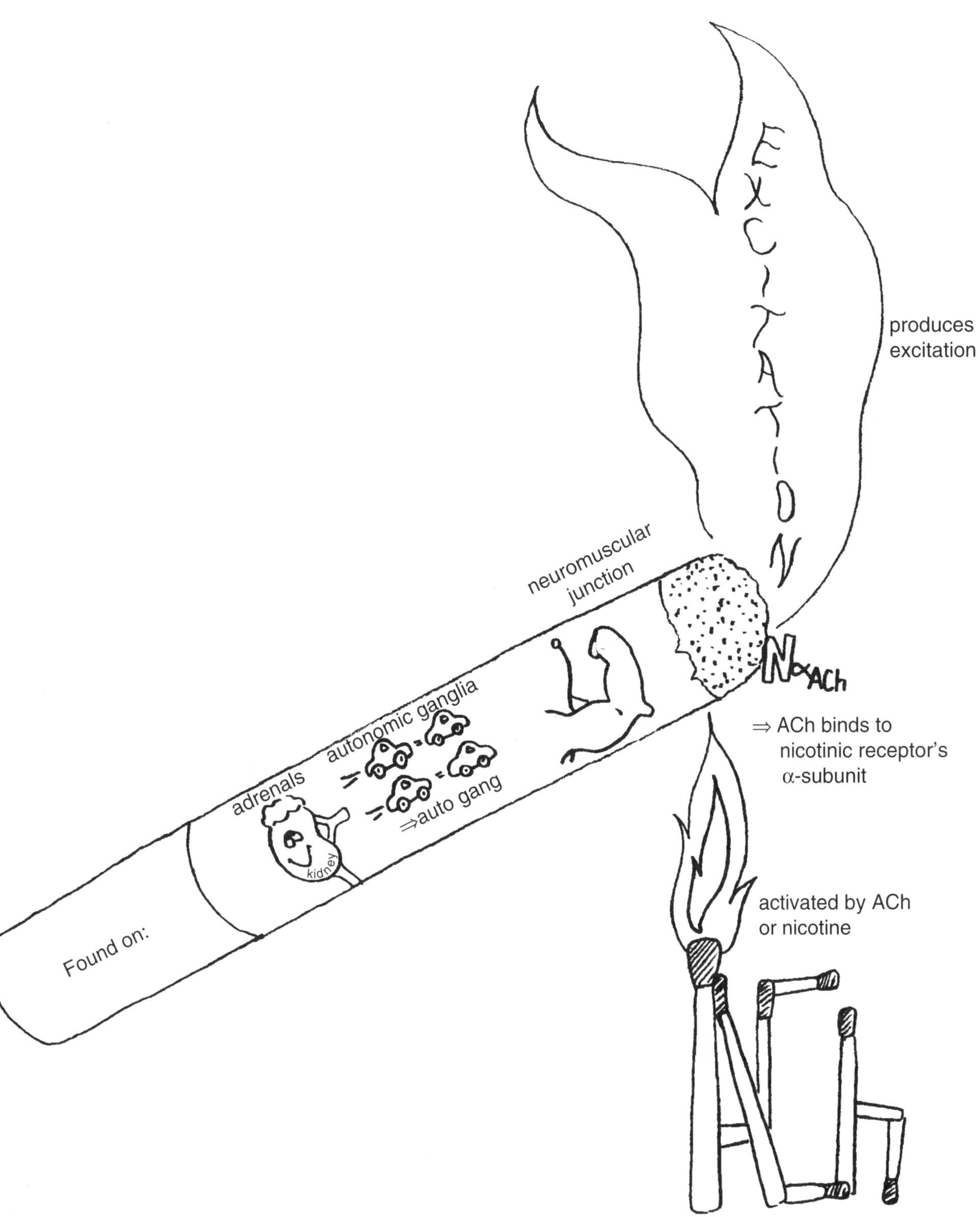
EXCITATION
produces
excitation
neuromuscular
junction
autonomic ganglia
adrenals
kidney
⇒auto gang
Found on:
N α ACh
⇒ ACh binds to
nicotinic receptor's
α-subunit
activated by ACh
or nicotine

NOTES

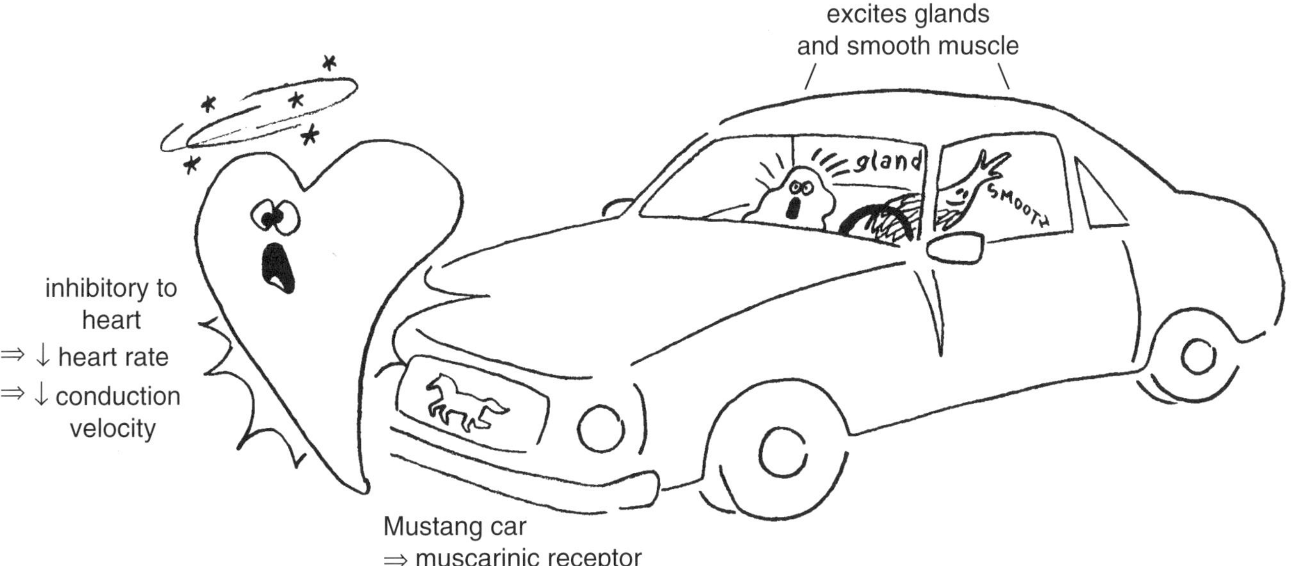
Cholinergic Receptors: Muscarinic Receptor ⇒ Mustang car
excites glands
and smooth muscle
gland
SMOOTH
inhibitory to
heart
⇒ ↓ heart rate
⇒ ↓ conduction
velocity
Mustang car
⇒ muscarinic receptor

NOTES

See Tables 11.1, 11.2, 11.3, and 11.4 in Appendix.

Bones

Anterior

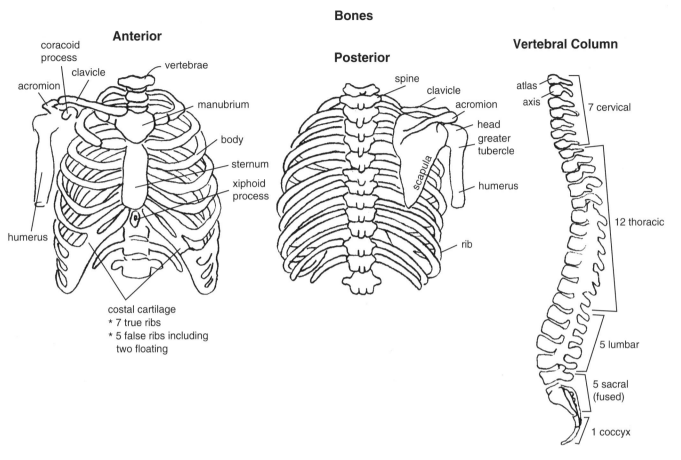

coracoid process
clavicle
acromion
vertebrae
manubrium
body
sternum
xiphoid process
humerus
costal cartilage
* 7 true ribs
* 5 false ribs including two floating

Posterior

spine
clavicle
acromion
head
greater tubercle
scapula
humerus
rib

Vertebral Column

atlas
axis
7 cervical
12 thoracic
5 lumbar
5 sacral (fused)
1 coccyx

Arteries

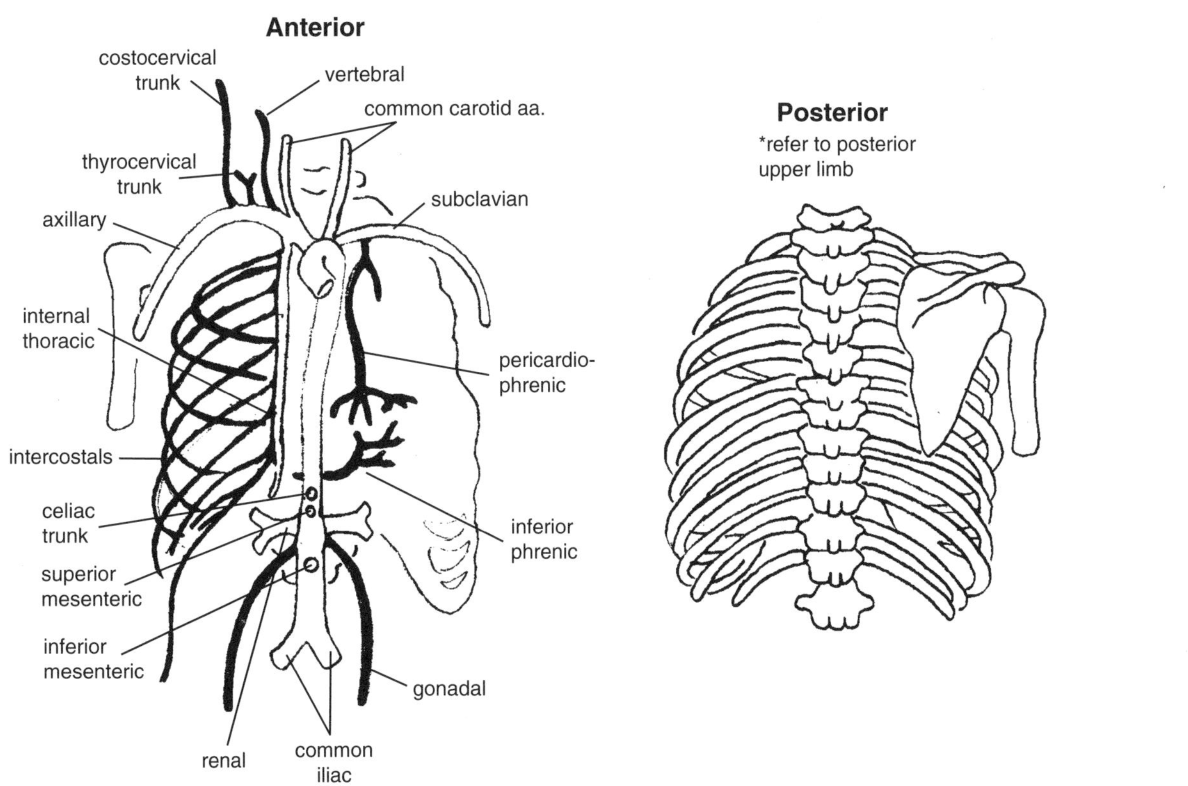

NOTES

See Tables 11.1, 11.2, 11.3, and 11.4 in Appendix.

Nerves

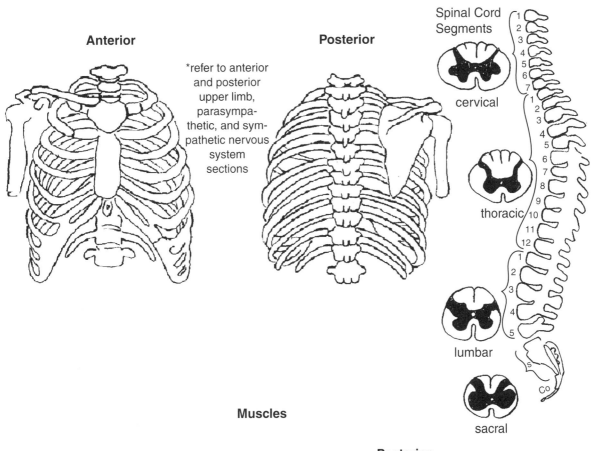

Anterior

Posterior

*refer to anterior and posterior upper limb, parasympathetic, and sympathetic nervous system sections

Vertebral Column

Spinal Cord Segments

cervical

thoracic

lumbar

sacral

Muscles

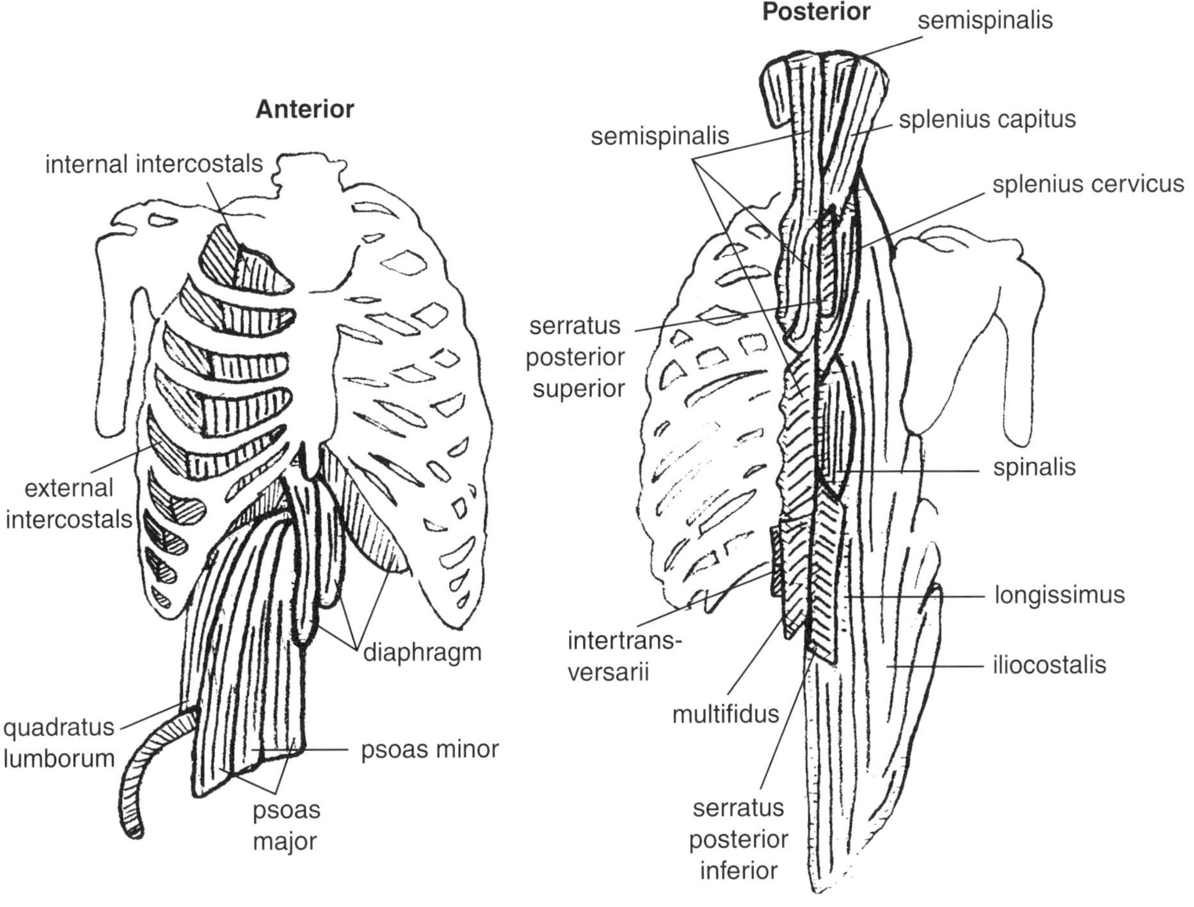

NOTES

See Tables 12.1 and 12.2 in Appendix.

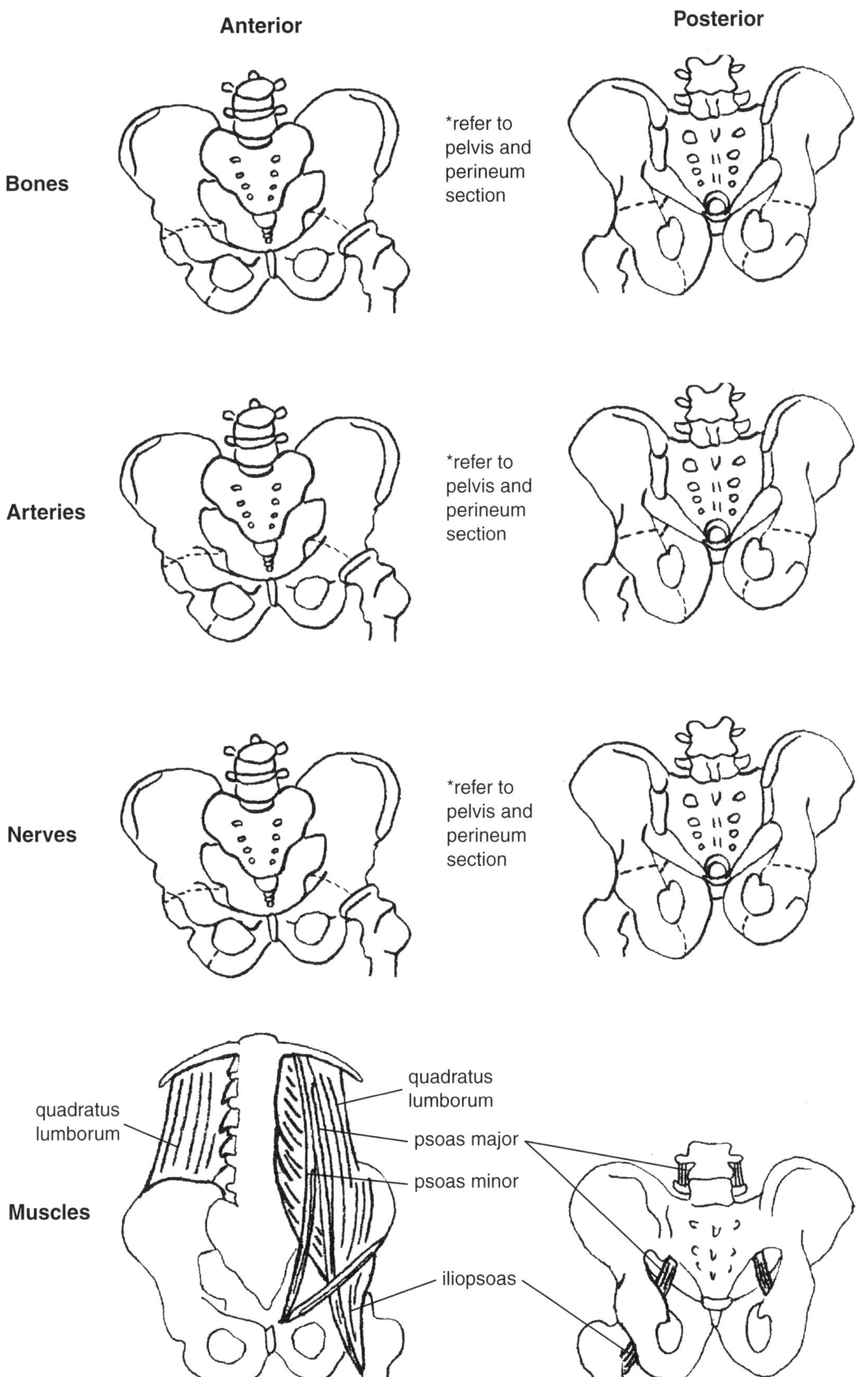
Anterior
Posterior
Bones
*refer to pelvis and perineum section
Arteries
*refer to pelvis and perineum section
Nerves
*refer to pelvis and perineum section
Muscles
quadratus lumborum
quadratus lumborum
psoas major
psoas minor
iliopsoas

NOTES

See Tables 13.1 and 13.2 in Appendix.

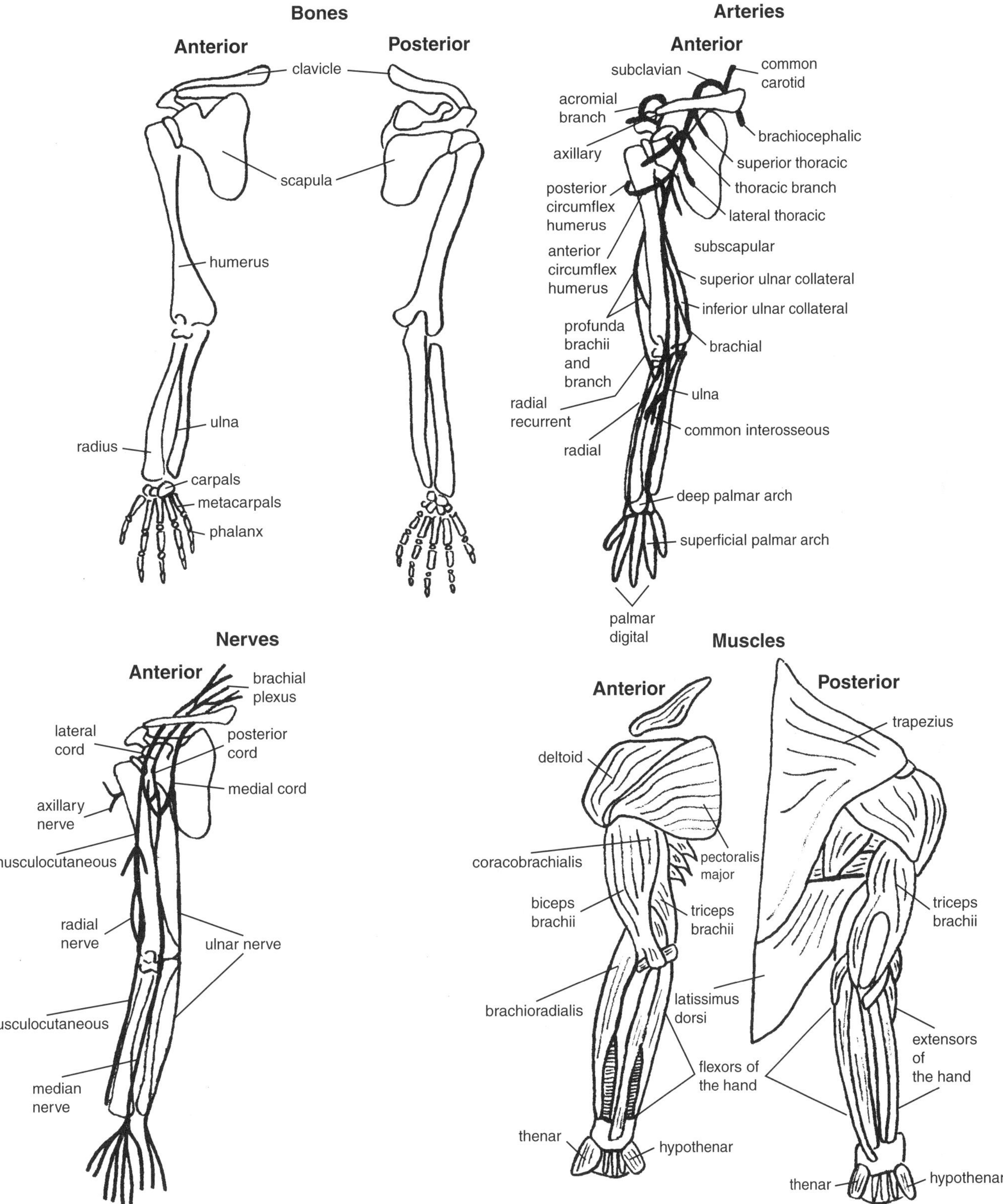
Bones
Anterior
Posterior
clavicle
scapula
humerus
ulna
radius
carpals
metacarpals
phalanx
Arteries
Anterior
subclavian
common carotid
acromial branch
brachiocephalic
axillary
superior thoracic
thoracic branch
posterior circumflex humerus
lateral thoracic
anterior circumflex humerus
subscapular
superior ulnar collateral
inferior ulnar collateral
profunda brachii and branch
brachial
radial recurrent
ulna
common interosseous
radial
deep palmar arch
superficial palmar arch
palmar digital
Nerves
Anterior
brachial plexus
lateral cord
posterior cord
medial cord
axillary nerve
musculocutaneous
radial nerve
ulnar nerve
musculocutaneous
median nerve
Muscles
Anterior
Posterior
trapezius
deltoid
coracobrachialis
pectoralis major
biceps brachii
triceps brachii
triceps brachii
brachioradialis
latissimus dorsi
extensors of the hand
flexors of the hand
thenar
hypothenar
thenar
hypothenar

NOTES

See Tables 14.1 and 14.2 in Appendix.

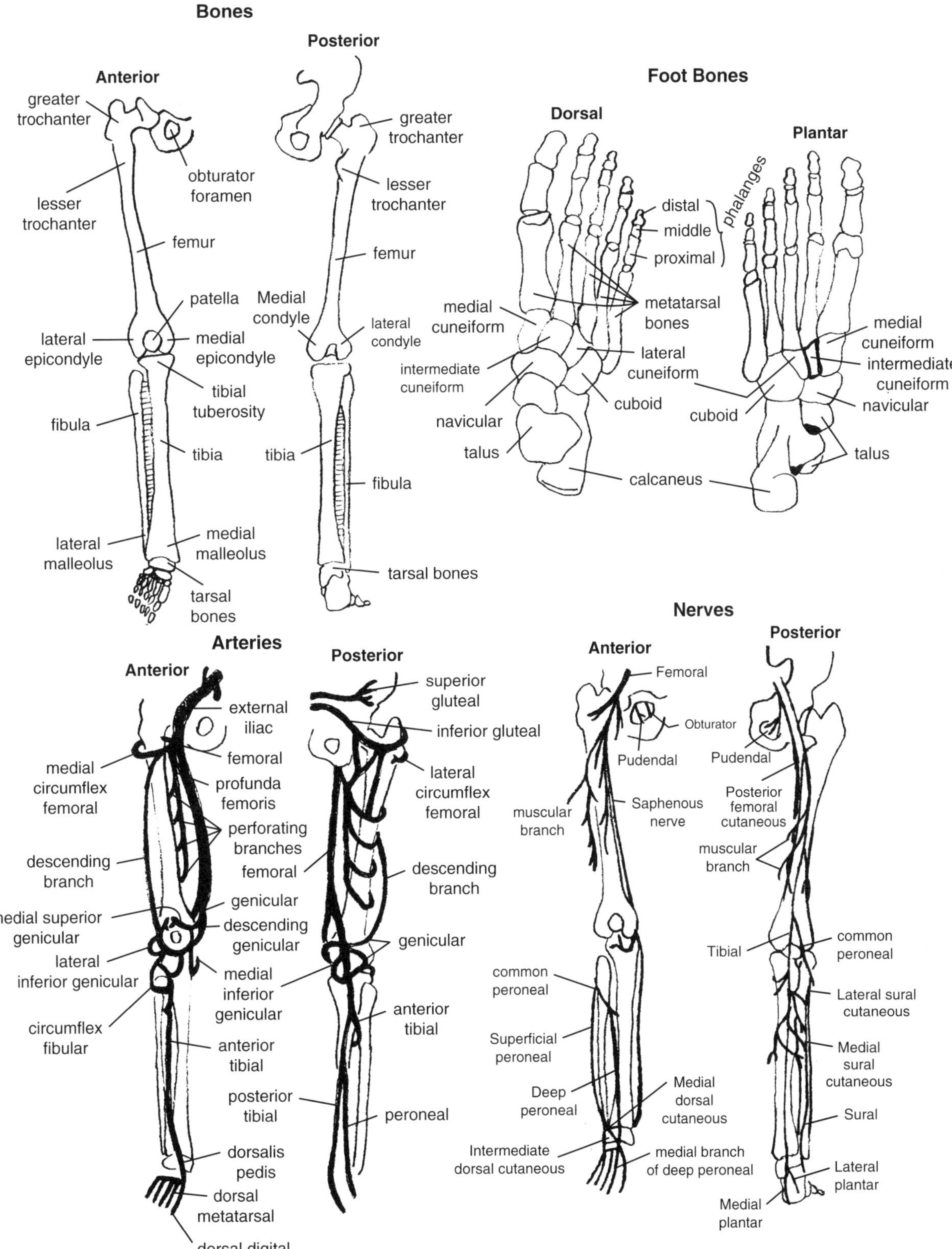
Bones
Anterior
greater trochanter
lesser trochanter
obturator foramen
femur
patella
lateral epicondyle
medial epicondyle
tibial tuberosity
fibula
tibia
lateral malleolus
medial malleolus
tarsal bones
Posterior
greater trochanter
lesser trochanter
femur
Medial condyle
lateral condyle
tibia
fibula
tarsal bones
Foot Bones
Dorsal
distal
middle
proximal
phalanges
metatarsal bones
medial cuneiform
intermediate cuneiform
lateral cuneiform
navicular
cuboid
talus
calcaneus
Plantar
medial cuneiform
intermediate cuneiform
navicular
cuboid
talus
Arteries
Anterior
external iliac
medial circumflex femoral
femoral
profunda femoris
perforating branches
descending branch
medial superior genicular
descending genicular
lateral inferior genicular
medial inferior genicular
circumflex fibular
anterior tibial
posterior tibial
dorsalis pedis
dorsal metatarsal
dorsal digital
Posterior
superior gluteal
inferior gluteal
lateral circumflex femoral
femoral
genicular
descending branch
genicular
anterior tibial
peroneal
Nerves
Anterior
Femoral
Obturator
Pudendal
muscular branch
Saphenous nerve
common peroneal
Superficial peroneal
Deep peroneal
Medial dorsal cutaneous
Intermediate dorsal cutaneous
medial branch of deep peroneal
Posterior
Pudendal
Posterior femoral cutaneous
muscular branch
Tibial
common peroneal
Lateral sural cutaneous
Medial sural cutaneous
Sural
Lateral plantar
Medial plantar

NOTES

See Tables 14.1 and 14.2 in Appendix.

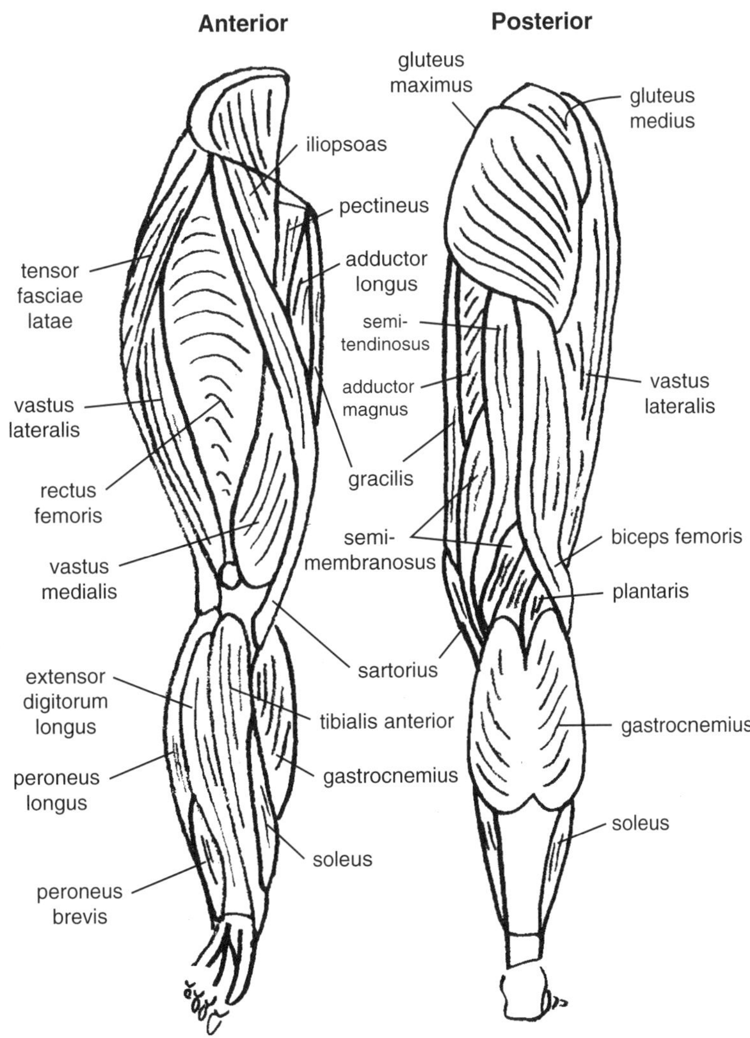
Muscles
Anterior
Posterior
gluteus maximus
gluteus medius
iliopsoas
pectineus
adductor longus
tensor fasciae latae
semi-tendinosus
adductor magnus
vastus lateralis
vastus lateralis
rectus femoris
gracilis
semi-membranosus
biceps femoris
vastus medialis
plantaris
sartorius
extensor digitorum longus
tibialis anterior
gastrocnemius
gastrocnemius
peroneus longus
soleus
soleus
peroneus brevis

NOTES

SACRAL PLEXUS

DALLEY/VOSS RULE OF 3'S OF 2'S*

- Instructions: The rules of 3's and 2's is as follows and will give 3 sets of nerves.
- The first set of 3 nerves will all have 3 spinal contributions.
- The second set will have 2 nerves with 3 spinal contributions and 1 nerve with 2 spinal contributions.
- The third set will only have 1 nerve with 3 spinal contributions and 2 nerves with 2 spinal contributions.
- The pattern to keep in mind is the following:
    - 3,3,3; 3,3,2; and 3,2,2
- Beginning with L4, take the first 3 nerves. This is the superior gluteal.
- Skip to L5 and take 3 nerves. This is the inferior gluteal.
- Skip to S1 and take 3 nerves. This is the posterior femoral cutaneous.
- Begin once again at L4 and do the same as above to get the spinal contributions for the next three nerves (quadratus femoris, obturator internus, and piriformis), the only difference being that the piriformis will only have 2 spinal contributions.
- On the last set of nerves, begin at S2 (where you left off with the piriformis), and take 3 nerves. This is the pudendal (remember, it gives 4 branches).
- Next, skip to S3 and take 2 nerves (levator ani).
- Finally, skip to S4 and take 2 nerves (coccygeus).

*Reprinted with permission from Dr. Bernell Dalley, Texas Tech University Health Sciences Center School of Medicine, Lubbock, TX.

See Tables 14.1 and 14.2 in Appendix.

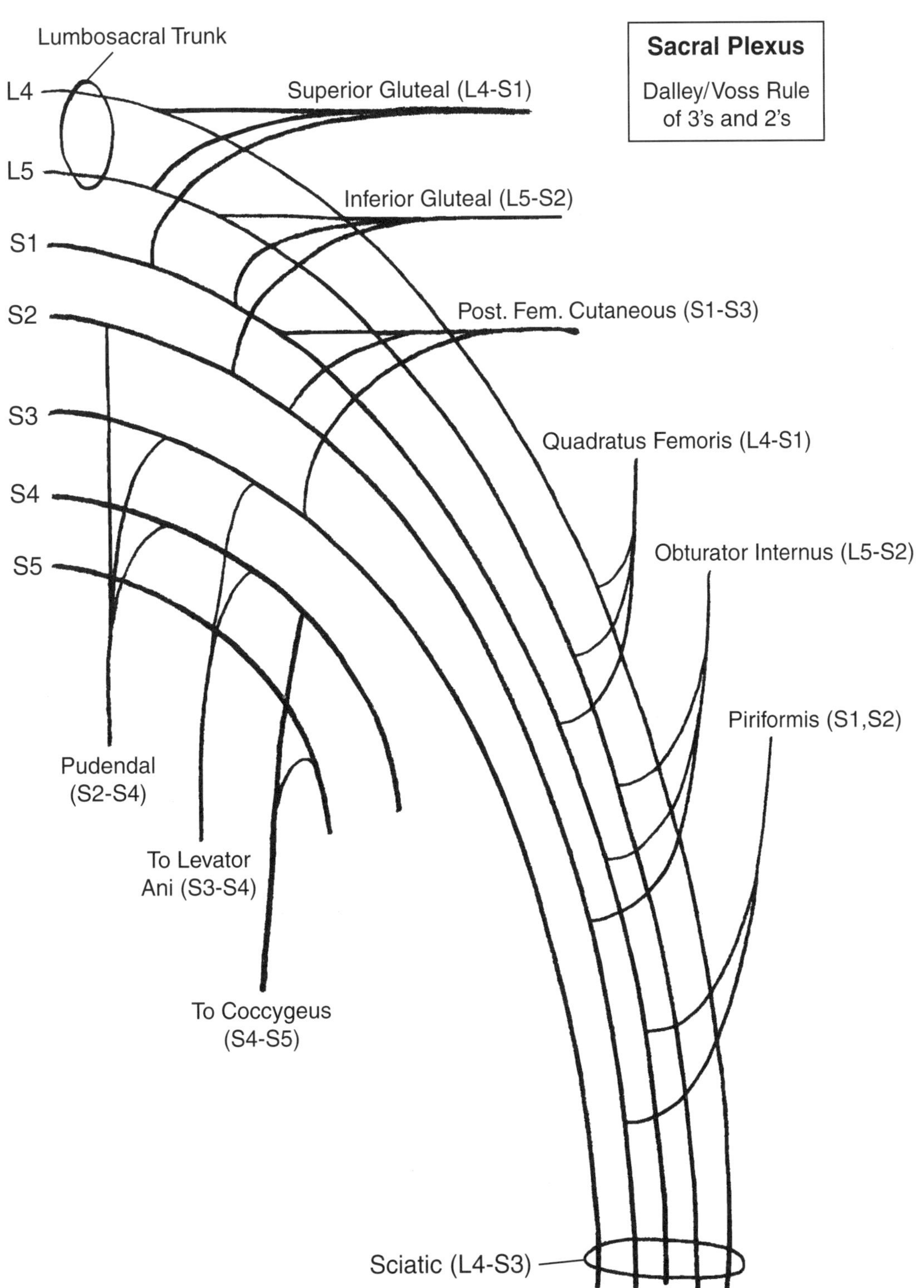
Sacral Plexus
Dalley/Voss Rule of 3's and 2's
Lumbosacral Trunk
L4
L5
S1
S2
S3
S4
S5
Superior Gluteal (L4-S1)
Inferior Gluteal (L5-S2)
Post. Fem. Cutaneous (S1-S3)
Quadratus Femoris (L4-S1)
Obturator Internus (L5-S2)
Piriformis (S1,S2)
Pudendal (S2-S4)
To Levator Ani (S3-S4)
To Coccygeus (S4-S5)
Sciatic (L4-S3)

NOTES

See Tables 15.1 and 15.2 in Appendix.

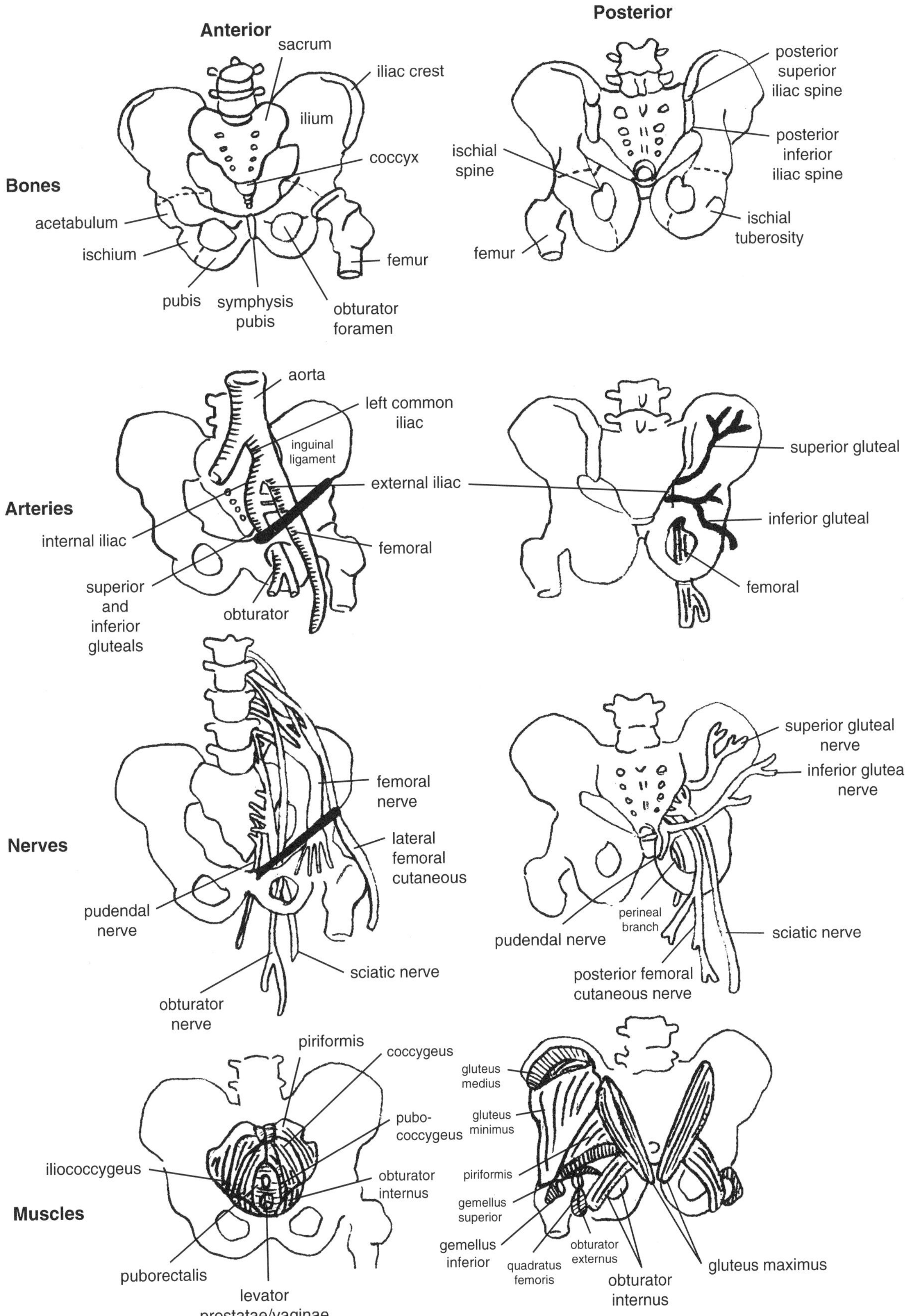
Anterior
Posterior
Bones
sacrum
iliac crest
ilium
coccyx
acetabulum
ischium
pubis
symphysis pubis
obturator foramen
femur
posterior superior iliac spine
ischial spine
posterior inferior iliac spine
ischial tuberosity
femur
Arteries
aorta
left common iliac
inguinal ligament
external iliac
internal iliac
femoral
superior and inferior gluteals
obturator
superior gluteal
inferior gluteal
femoral
Nerves
femoral nerve
lateral femoral cutaneous
pudendal nerve
sciatic nerve
obturator nerve
superior gluteal nerve
inferior gluteal nerve
perineal branch
pudendal nerve
sciatic nerve
posterior femoral cutaneous nerve
Muscles
piriformis
coccygeus
pubo-coccygeus
iliococcygeus
obturator internus
puborectalis
levator prostatae/vaginae
gluteus medius
gluteus minimus
piriformis
gemellus superior
gemellus inferior
quadratus femoris
obturator externus
obturator internus
gluteus maximus

NOTES

Steroid Hormone Synthesis

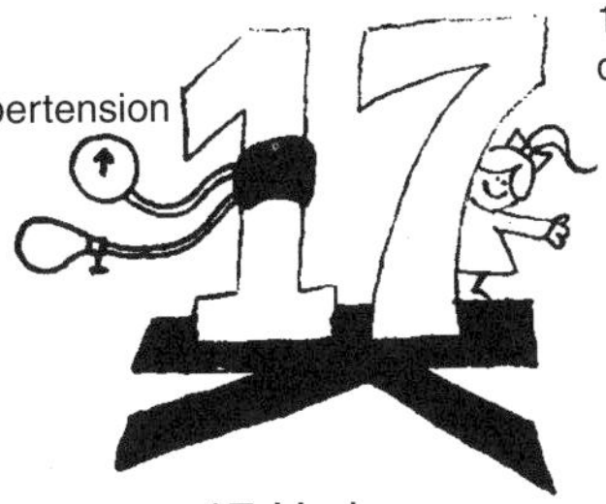

17-α-hydroxylase deficiency
hypertension
phenotypic female (no maturation)
hypokalemia

Cholesterol → (desmolase) → Pregnenolone

Pregnenolone → 17-Hydroxypregnenolone → (17,20-lyase) → Dehydroepiandrosterone

Pregnenolone → (3-β-dehydrogenase isomerase) → Progesterone

17-Hydroxypregnenolone → (3-β-dehydrogenase isomerase) → 17-α-Hydroxyprogesterone

Dehydroepiandrosterone → (3-β-dehydrogenase isomerase) → Androstenedione

Progesterone → 17-α-Hydroxyprogesterone → (17,20-lyase) → Androstenedione → Estrogen

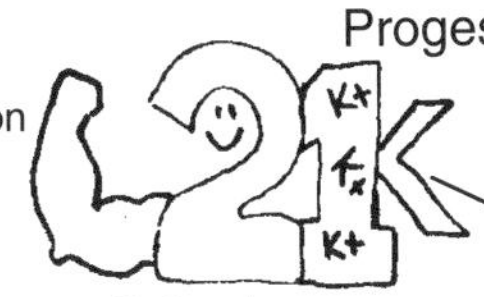

Hypotension
masculinization

Progesterone → (21-β-hydroxylase) → 11-Deoxycorticosterone
21-β-hydroxylase Deficiency → hyperkalemia, hypotension, masculinization

17-α-Hydroxyprogesterone → (21-β-hydroxylase) → 11-Deoxycortisol

Androstenedione → Testosterone (androgens) → (aromatase) → Estradiol (estrogens)

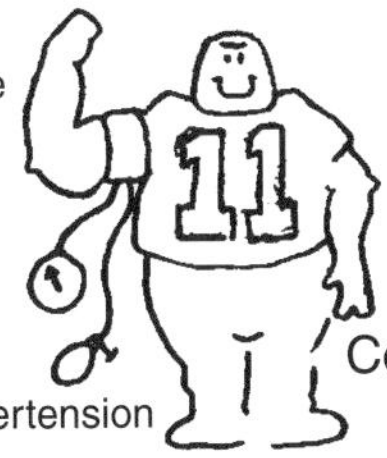

11-β-hydroxylase deficiency
hypertension

11-Deoxycorticosterone → (11-β-hydroxylase) → Corticosterone
(acts as weak mineralocorticoid which results in hypertension during 11-β-hydroxylase deficiency)

Corticosterone → (aldosterone synthase) → Aldosterone (mineralocorticoids)

11-Deoxycortisol → (11-β-hydroxylase) → Cortisol (glucocorticoids)

Testosterone → (5-α-reductase) → DHT

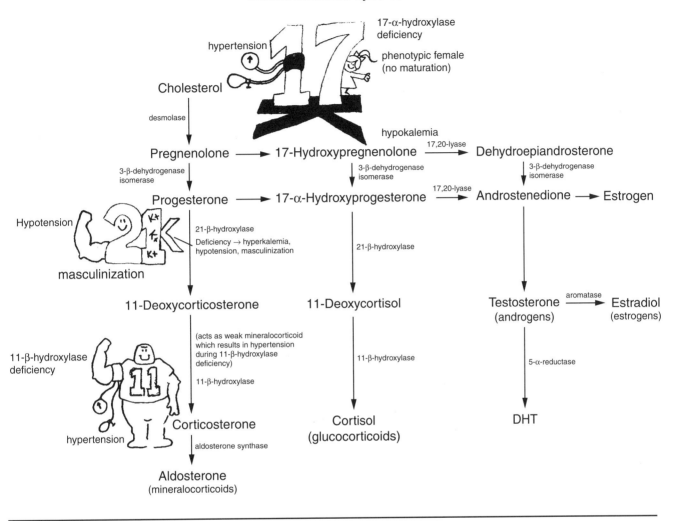

Protein Hormone Synthesis

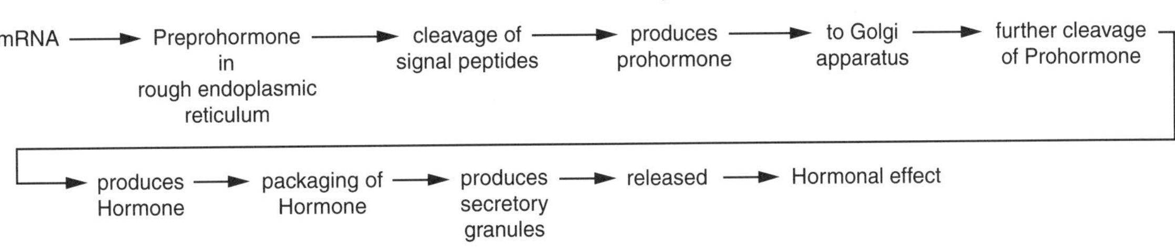

Amine Hormone Synthesis

(occurs in adrenal medulla and neural tissue)

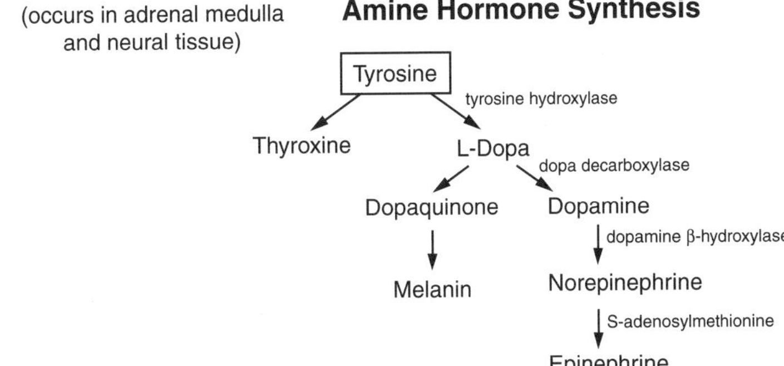

NOTES

cAMP (CYCLIC ADENOSINE MONOPHOSPHATE)

- Hormones that use the cAMP mechanism of action
    - "**A**denosine **C**yclase **L**oves **T**eaming with **H**er **G**TP-**B**inding protein to **F**orm **cAMP**"
        - A → ACTH (adrenocorticotropic hormone)
        - C → CRH (corticotropin-releasing hormone)
        - L → LH (luteinizing hormone)
        - T → TSH (thyroid-stimulating hormone)
        - H → HCG (human chorionic gonadotropin)
        - G → glucagon
        - B → β1 and β2 receptors
        - F → FSH (follicle-stimulating hormone)
        - c → calcitonin
        - A → ADH (V2 receptor) (antidiuretic hormone or vasopressin)
        - M → MSH (melanocyte-stimulating hormone)
        - P → PTH (parathyroid hormone)
- Steps of mechanism
    1. Hormone binds to receptor
    2. GDP replaced by GTP on G protein
    3. Stimulatory G protein activated (or inhibitory G protein)
    4. Stimulatory G protein activates adenylate cyclase (inhibitory G protein inhibits adenylate cyclase)
    5. Adenylate cyclase converts ATP → ADP
    6. cAMP activates protein kinase A
    7. Activated protein kinase A phosphorylates proteins
    8. Initiates physiological effects

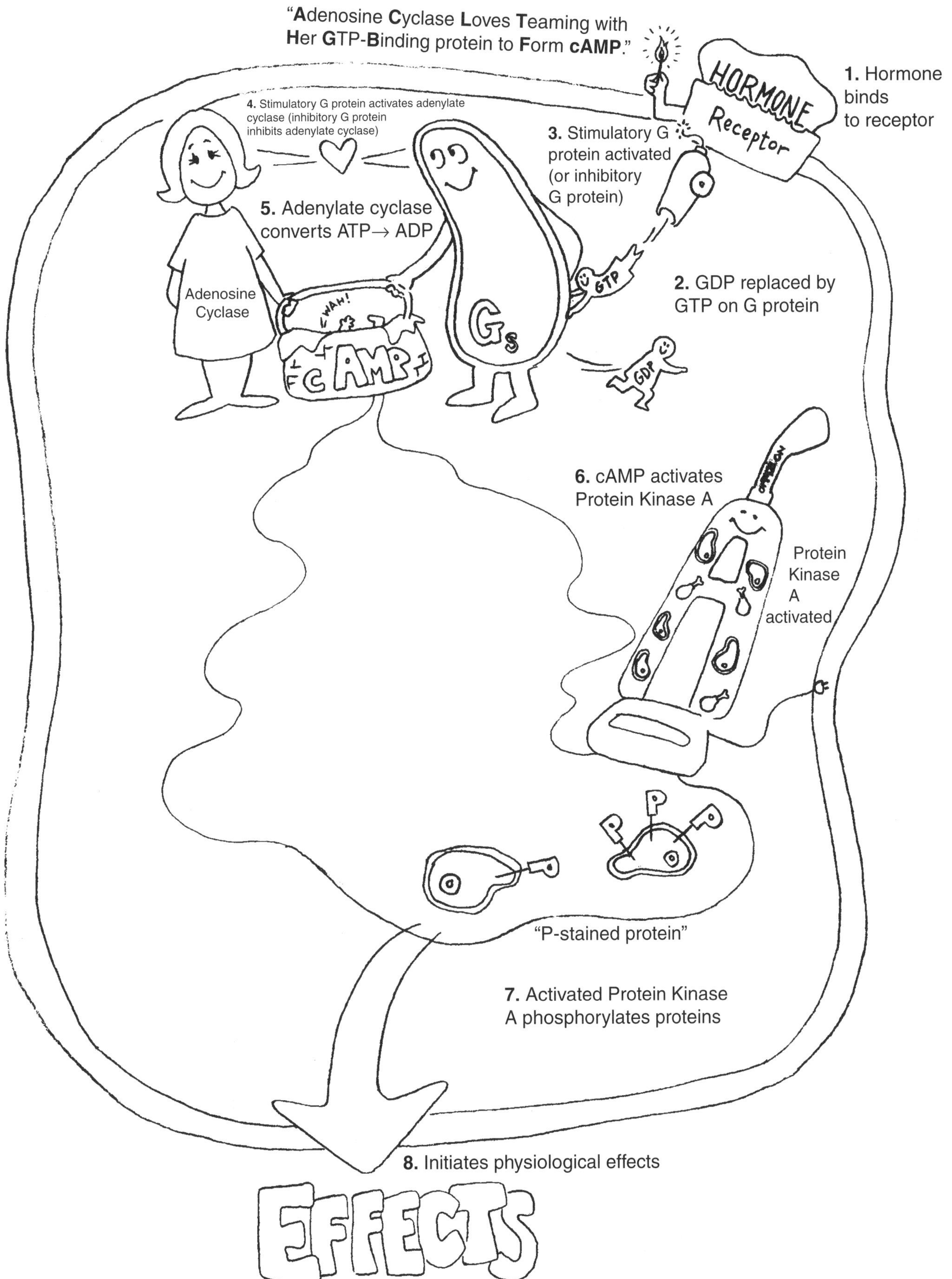
"Adenosine Cyclase Loves Teaming with Her GTP-Binding protein to Form cAMP."
HORMONE
Receptor
1. Hormone binds to receptor
4. Stimulatory G protein activates adenylate cyclase (inhibitory G protein inhibits adenylate cyclase)
3. Stimulatory G protein activated (or inhibitory G protein)
5. Adenylate cyclase converts ATP→ ADP
GTP
2. GDP replaced by GTP on G protein
Adenosine Cyclase
WAH!
cAMP
Gs
GDP
6. cAMP activates Protein Kinase A
Protein Kinase A activated
P
"P-stained protein"
7. Activated Protein Kinase A phosphorylates proteins
8. Initiates physiological effects
EFFECTS

NOTES

IP_3 (INOSITOL 1,4,5-TRIPHOSPHATE) MECHANISM

- Hormones that activate the IP_3 mechanism
  - ADH (V1 receptor) (antidiuretic hormone or vasopressin)
  - $\alpha 1$ receptors
  - TRH (thyrotropin-releasing hormone)
  - angiotensin II
  - GHRH (growth-releasing hormone)
  - GnRH (gonadotropin-releasing hormone)
  - oxytocin
- Steps in mechanism
  1. Hormone bound to receptor
  2. G-protein activated
  3. G-protein activates phospholipase C
  4. Phospholipase C breaks down phospholipids
  5. Destruction of phospholipids produces IP_3 and diacylglycerol
  6. Endoplasmic reticulum (ER) releases calcium
  7. Diacylglycerol + calcium activates protein kinase C
  8. Protein kinase C phosphorylates proteins
  9. Initiates physiological effects
- Diacylglycerol $\rightarrow$ arachidonic acid $\rightarrow$ prostaglandins

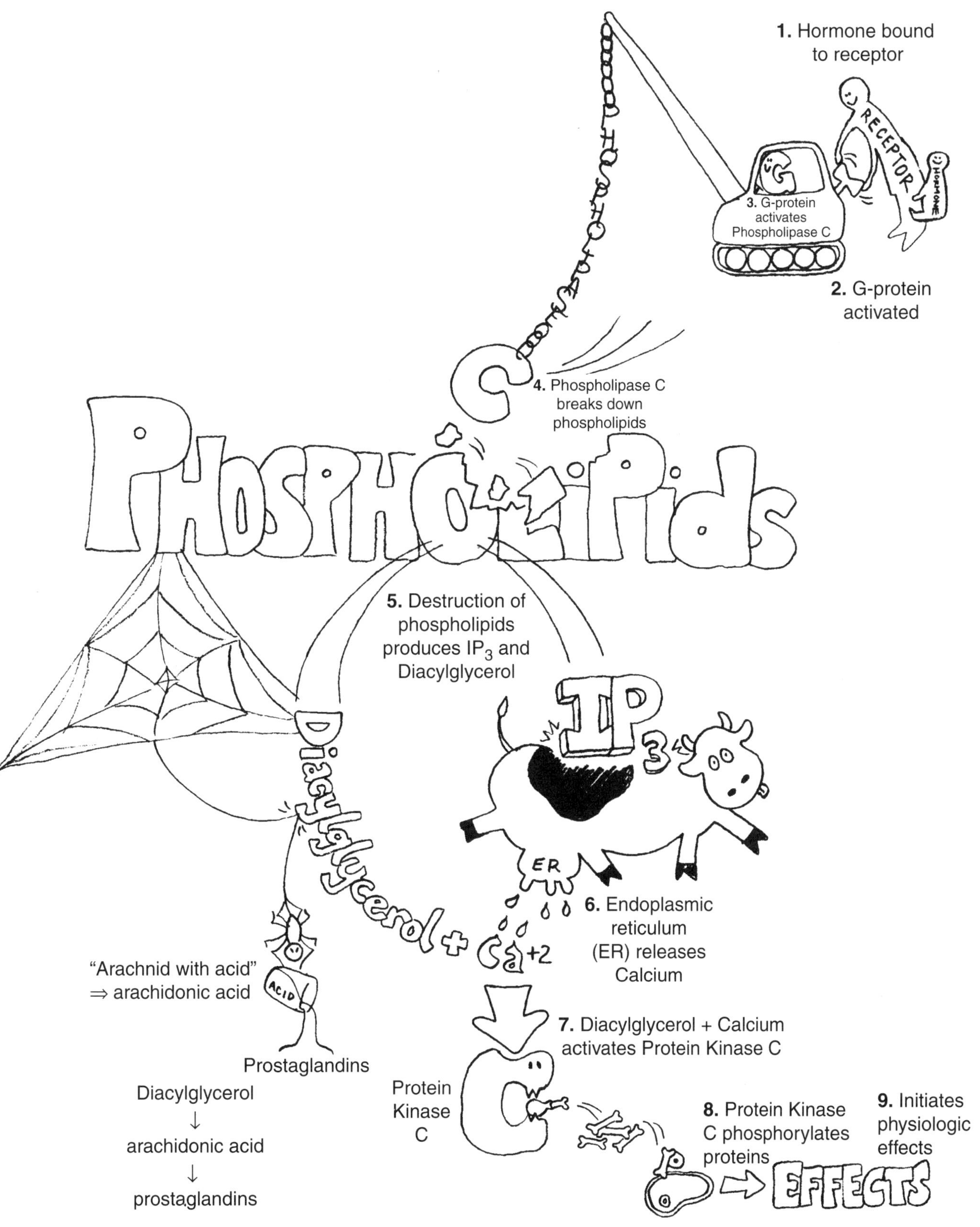
1. Hormone bound to receptor
RECEPTOR
HORMONE
3. G-protein activates Phospholipase C
2. G-protein activated
4. Phospholipase C breaks down phospholipids
PHOSPHOLIPIDS
5. Destruction of phospholipids produces IP3 and Diacylglycerol
IP3
Diacylglycerol + Ca+2
ER
6. Endoplasmic reticulum (ER) releases Calcium
"Arachnid with acid" ⇒ arachidonic acid
ACID
Prostaglandins
Diacylglycerol
↓
arachidonic acid
↓
prostaglandins
7. Diacylglycerol + Calcium activates Protein Kinase C
Protein Kinase C
8. Protein Kinase C phosphorylates proteins
9. Initiates physiologic effects
EFFECTS

NOTES

STEROID AND THYROID HORMONE MECHANISM

- Hormones that utilize mechanism
  - aldosterone
  - progesterone
  - testosterone
  - estrogen
  - glucocorticoids
  - vitamin D
  - thyroid hormone
- Steps in mechanism
  1. Steroid diffuses across cell membrane
  2. Steroid binds cytoplasmic receptor
  3. Steroid binds to nuclear receptor
  4. Conformational change of receptor → DNA-binding domain revealed
  5. DNA reacts with DNA-binding domain
  6. Transcription of mRNA
  7. mRNA translation
  8. Protein production responsible for initiating physiological effects

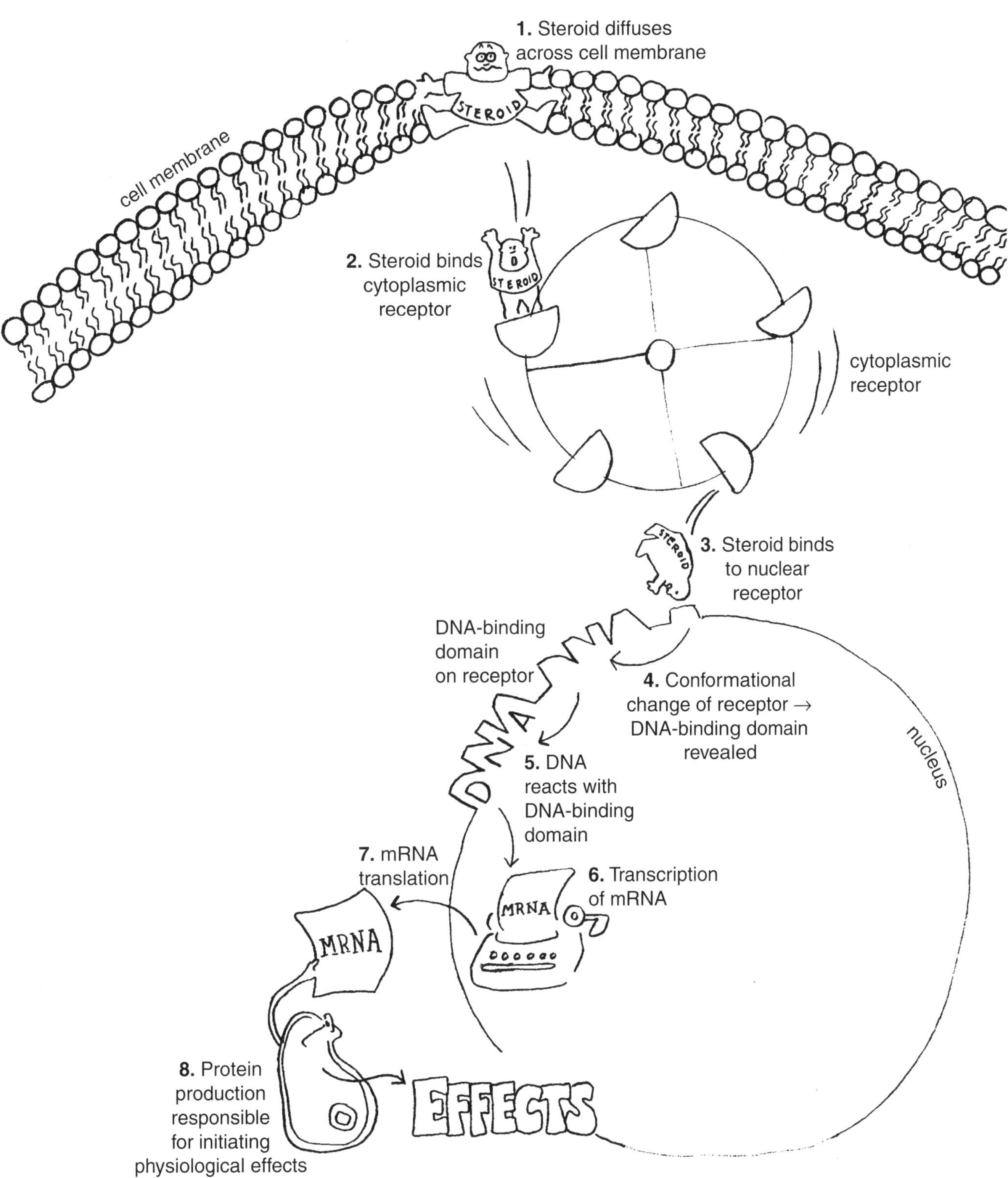
1. Steroid diffuses across cell membrane
STEROID
cell membrane
2. Steroid binds cytoplasmic receptor
STEROID
cytoplasmic receptor
STEROID
3. Steroid binds to nuclear receptor
DNA-binding domain on receptor
4. Conformational change of receptor → DNA-binding domain revealed
nucleus
DNA
5. DNA reacts with DNA-binding domain
7. mRNA translation
6. Transcription of mRNA
MRNA
MRNA
8. Protein production responsible for initiating physiological effects
EFFECTS

NOTES

CALCIUM-CALMODULIN MECHANISM

- Steps in mechanism
  1. Hormone bound to receptor
  2. G-protein activates cell membrane calcium channel
  3. G-protein activates release of calcium from endoplasmic reticulum (ER)
  4. Increase in intracellular calcium concentration
  5. Calcium binds to calmodulin
  6. Calmodulin initiates physiological effects

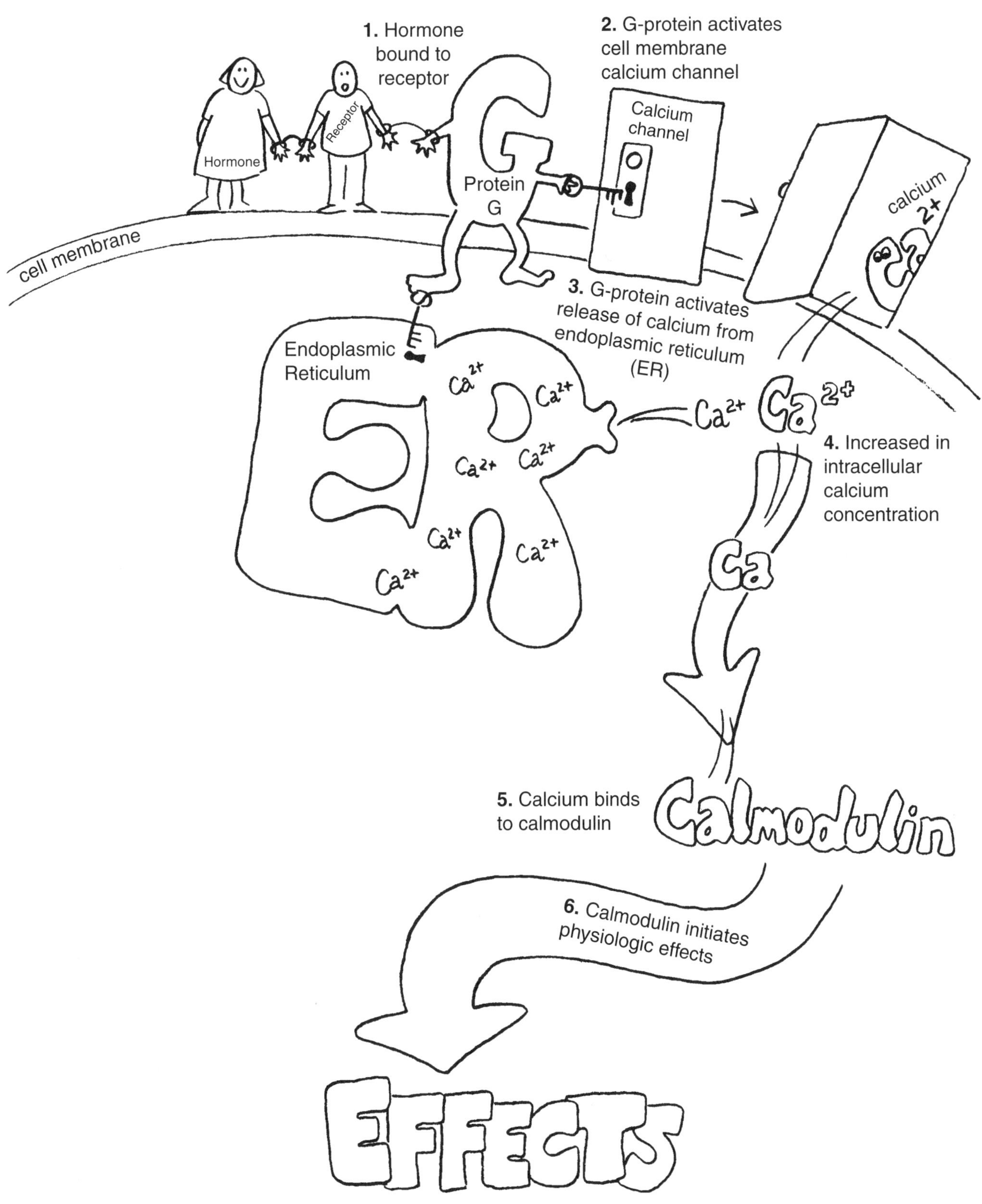
1. Hormone bound to receptor
2. G-protein activates cell membrane calcium channel
Hormone
Receptor
Protein G
Calcium channel
calcium 2+
cell membrane
3. G-protein activates release of calcium from endoplasmic reticulum (ER)
Endoplasmic Reticulum
ER
Ca2+
Ca2+
4. Increased in intracellular calcium concentration
Ca
5. Calcium binds to calmodulin
Calmodulin
6. Calmodulin initiates physiologic effects
EFFECTS

PITUITARY GLAND

- Composed of two lobes: anterior (adenohypophysis) and posterior (neurohypophysis)
- Anterior pituitary derived from Rathke pouch (extension of oral cavity); produces following hormones: somatotrophs (growth hormone), lactotrophs (produce prolactin), corticotrophs (adrenocorticotropic hormone → ACTH, pro-opiomelanocortin, melanocyte-stimulating hormone → MSH, endorphins, and lipotropin), thyrotrophs (thyroid-stimulating hormone → TSH), and gonadotrophs (follicle-stimulating hormone → FSH, luteinizing hormone → LSH)
- Posterior pituitary consists of modified glial cells (pituicytes) and axonal processes from hypothalamic nuclei (supraoptic and paraventricular); produces oxytocin and vasopressin; hormones released directly into systemic circulation

HYPERPITUITARISM AND PITUITARY ADENOMAS

- Anterior pituitary hormone production most often caused by anterior lobe adenoma; other causes → primary hypothalamic disorders and anterior pituitary carcinomas
- Adenomas may be functional (produce hormone or hormones) or nonfunctional and cause hypopituitarism by encroaching on surrounding pituitary tissue
- Adenomas usually monoclonal in origin
- Morphology: adenomas divided into macroadenomas (>1 cm diameter) and microadenomas (<1 cm diameter)
- Pituitary apoplexy → acute hemorrhage into adenoma with symptoms of rapidly enlarging intracranial lesion
- Present as endocrine abnormalities and mass effects; radiographic abnormalities of sella turcica; visual field abnormalities (due to close proximity of optic nerve fibers) classically present as bitemporal hemianopsia; increased intracranial pressure symptoms; or compression of adjacent nonneoplastic tissue may result in hypopituitarism

PROLACTINOMA

- Most frequent hyperfunctioning pituitary adenoma (30% of pituitary adenomas)
- Symptoms: amenorrhea, galactorrhea, libido loss, and infertility
- Other causes of hyperprolactinemia → lactotroph hyperplasia (occurs when there is interference with dopamine inhibition of prolactin secretion) that may be due to head trauma (causing pituitary stalk section) or antidopaminergic drugs; stalk effect → mass in adjacent area interferes with hypothalamic inhibition of prolactin by protruding into stalk
- Prolactinomas are treated with bromocriptine

GROWTH HORMONE ADENOMA

- GH hypersecretion causes hepatic secretion of insulin-like growth factor–I (IGF-I) that causes many symptoms; in children before the epiphyses have closed, increased GH levels result in gigantism (increase in body size especially in arm and legs); in adults after epiphyses have closed, increased GH results in acromegaly (growth in soft tissues, skin, viscera → thyroid, heart, liver, and adrenals), bones of face, hands, and feet; bone density increased in spine and hips; enlarged and protruding jaw (prognathism); hands and feet are enlarged with broad, sausage-like fingers

CORTICOTROPH CELL ADENOMA

- Corticotroph adenoma production of excess ACTH results in adrenal hypersecretion of cortisol known as Cushing syndrome (hypercortisolism)
- Cushing disease → hypercortisolism caused by excess excretion of ACTH by pituitary

HYPOPITUITARISM

- Decreased secretion of pituitary hormones most often from destructive processes (tumors of anterior pituitary, ischemia, empty sella syndrome)
- Other causes include pituitary surgery or radiation; genetic defects; Rathke cleft cyst; pituitary apoplexy (with sudden onset of extremely painful headache, diplopia, and hypopituitarism); Sheehan syndrome (postpartum necrosis of anterior pituitary)
- Empty sella syndrome → any condition that destroys part or all of pituitary gland
- Present with hypothyroidism, hypoadrenalism, pallor, amenorrhea, impotence, loss of libido, loss of pubic and axillary hair

POSTERIOR PITUITARY SYNDROMES

- Posterior pituitary secretes oxytocin and vasopressin (ADH)
- Oxytocin stimulates uterine smooth muscle and cells surrounding lactiferous ducts of mammary glands; excess oxytocin release has no clinical significance
- ADH excess production causes clinical syndromes including diabetes insipidus and secretion of inappropriately high levels of ADH (SIADH)
- Diabetes insipidus: ADH deficiency causes excessive urination due to kidney's inability to reabsorb water from urine, which leads to large amounts of dilute urine, increased serum sodium and osmolality, resulting in thirst and polydipsia
- Syndrome of inappropriate ADH (SIADH): ADH excess causes resorption of excessive amounts of free water, resulting in hyponatremia; most frequent causes include the secretion of ectopic ADH by malignant neoplasms (especially small cell carcinoma of lung); clinical manifestations → hyponatremia, cerebral edema, and neurological dysfunction; total body water increased, blood volume remains normal → peripheral edema does not develop

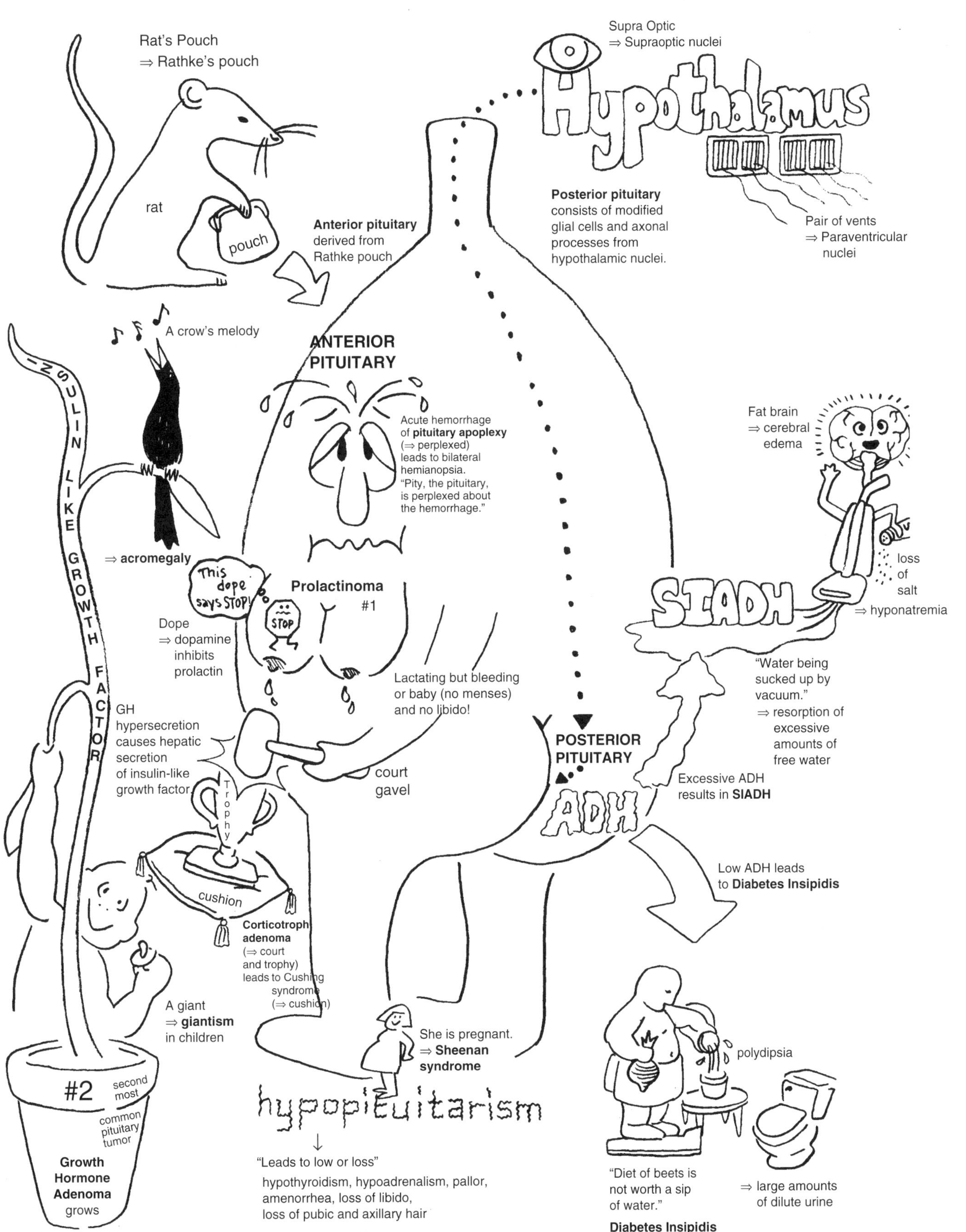
Rat's Pouch
⇒ Rathke's pouch
rat
pouch
Anterior pituitary
derived from
Rathke pouch
Supra Optic
⇒ Supraoptic nuclei
Hypothalamus
Posterior pituitary
consists of modified
glial cells and axonal
processes from
hypothalamic nuclei.
Pair of vents
⇒ Paraventricular
nuclei
A crow's melody
ANTERIOR
PITUITARY
INSULIN LIKE GROWTH FACTOR
Acute hemorrhage
of pituitary apoplexy
(⇒ perplexed)
leads to bilateral
hemianopsia.
"Pity, the pituitary,
is perplexed about
the hemorrhage."
Fat brain
⇒ cerebral
edema
⇒ acromegaly
This dope says STOP!
STOP
Prolactinoma
#1
Dope
⇒ dopamine
inhibits
prolactin
loss
of
salt
SIADH
⇒ hyponatremia
"Water being
sucked up by
vacuum."
⇒ resorption of
excessive
amounts of
free water
Lactating but bleeding
or baby (no menses)
and no libido!
GH
hypersecretion
causes hepatic
secretion
of insulin-like
growth factor
court
gavel
POSTERIOR
PITUITARY
Excessive ADH
results in SIADH
Trophy
ADH
cushion
Low ADH leads
to Diabetes Insipidis
Corticotroph
adenoma
(⇒ court
and trophy)
leads to Cushing
syndrome
(⇒ cushion)
A giant
⇒ giantism
in children
She is pregnant.
⇒ Sheenan
syndrome
polydipsia
#2
second
most
common
pituitary
tumor
hypopituitarism
↓
"Leads to low or loss"
hypothyroidism, hypoadrenalism, pallor,
amenorrhea, loss of libido,
loss of pubic and axillary hair
Growth
Hormone
Adenoma
grows
"Diet of beets is
not worth a sip
of water."
Diabetes Insipidis
⇒ large amounts
of dilute urine

NOTES

THYROID HORMONE SYNTHESIS

- Steps in thyroid hormone synthesis
  1. Iodide pump transports I- into thyroid follicular cells
  2. Peroxidase enzyme catalyzes I- + I- → I_2 and tyrosine + I_2 on thyroglobulin (=> glob) in follicular cell forming MIT (monoiodotyrosine) and DIT (diiodotyrosine)
  3. Coupling reactions form T_3 and T_4
  4. T_3 and T_4 on iodinated thyroglobulin in lumen
  5. TSH stimulates thyroid to secrete T_3 and T_4
  6. Deionization occurs as lysosomes digest thyroglobulin; then T_3 and T_4 released into circulation
  7. T_3 and T_4 bound to thyroid-binding globulin (TBG) in circulation
  8. T_4 heads to target tissues
  9. T_4 converted to T_3—the active form of thyroid hormone, or rT_3—the inactive form of thyroid hormone
- rT_3 is an inactive form of thyroid hormone

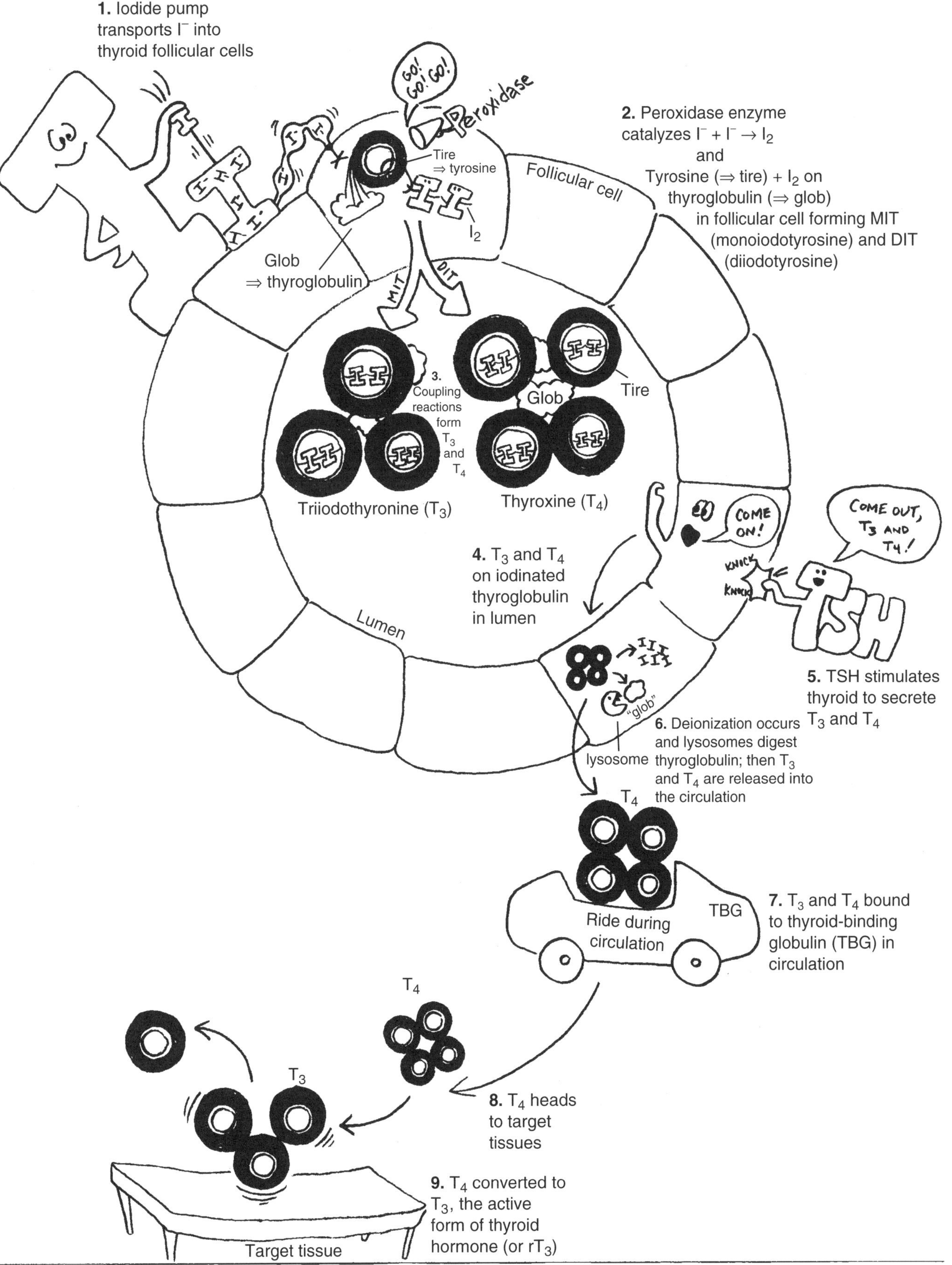
1. Iodide pump transports I^- into thyroid follicular cells
GO! GO! GO!
Peroxidase
Tire ⇒ tyrosine
Follicular cell
I_2
Glob ⇒ thyroglobulin
MIT
DIT
2. Peroxidase enzyme catalyzes $I^- + I^- \rightarrow I_2$ and Tyrosine (⇒ tire) + I_2 on thyroglobulin (⇒ glob) in follicular cell forming MIT (monoiodotyrosine) and DIT (diiodotyrosine)
3. Coupling reactions form T_3 and T_4
Glob
Tire
Triiodothyronine (T_3)
Thyroxine (T_4)
COME ON!
COME OUT, T_3 AND T_4!
KNOCK
KNOCK
TSH
4. T_3 and T_4 on iodinated thyroglobulin in lumen
Lumen
5. TSH stimulates thyroid to secrete T_3 and T_4
"glob"
lysosome
6. Deionization occurs and lysosomes digest thyroglobulin; then T_3 and T_4 are released into the circulation
T_4
TBG
Ride during circulation
7. T_3 and T_4 bound to thyroid-binding globulin (TBG) in circulation
T_4
T_3
8. T_4 heads to target tissues
9. T_4 converted to T_3, the active form of thyroid hormone (or rT_3)
Target tissue

NOTES

THYROID

- Develops from evagination of developing pharyngeal epithelium, then descends to anterior neck position
- TSH causes follicular epithelial cells to pinocytize colloid and convert thyroglobulin into thyroxine (T_4) and triiodothyronine (T_3)
- T_3 and T_4 are released into the systemic circulation and transported by plasma proteins to peripheral tissues where the net effect is increased basal metabolic rate
- Goitrogens → inhibit thyroid function by suppressing T_3 and T_4 synthesis; this in turn causes an increase in TSH (thyroid stimulating hormone) → the increased amounts of TSH cause hyperplastic gland enlargement or goiter
  - large amounts of iodide inhibit thyroid hormone release when patient has a hyperactive thyroid
- Parafollicular cells (C cells) → synthesize and secrete calcitonin, which increases bone absorption of calcium and decreases osteoclast bone reabsorption

HYPERTHYROIDISM

- Elevated T_3 and T_4 levels (thyrotoxicosis when due to excessive leakage of hormone from a nonhyperfunctioning gland; known as hyperthyroidism when due to hyperfunctioning thyroid)
- Physical manifestations → nervousness; palpitations; heat intolerance; weight loss (even with good appetite); excessive perspiration; osteoporosis; warm, moist, flushed skin; overactivity of sympathetic nervous system; diarrhea; and ocular changes
- Causes → diffuse hyperplasia, exogenous thyroid hormone, thyroiditis, hyperfunctioning multinodular goiter or adenoma
- Diagnosis → TSH and unbound T_4 measurement—a low TSH and high T_4 indicate primary hyperthyroidism due to intrinsic thyroid disease not thyrotoxicosis, which is caused by hypothalamic or pituitary disease (a.k.a. secondary hyperthyroidism)
- TRH stimulation test—determination of primary vs. secondary → a rise in TSH after a TRH injection excludes secondary hyperthyroidism
- T_3 hyperthryroidism → high serum T_3, low TSH, and normal T_4 → due to increased T_3 secretion and peripheral conversion of T_4 to T_3
- Treatment → β-blockers, thionamide, iodine, inhibitors of T_4 to T_3 conversion, and radioiodine

HYPOTHYROIDISM

- Low levels of thyroid hormone
- Primary hypothyroidism → most common cause in iodine-sufficient areas is chronic autoimmune thyroiditis or Hashimoto thyroiditis; other causes → radiation, drugs, surgery
- Secondary hypothyroidism → TSH deficiency and tertiary hypothyroidism are caused by TRH deficiency
- Clinical → cretinism and myxedema
- Cretinism—hypothyroidism in childhood or infancy; clinical manifestations: severe mental retardation, short stature, coarse facial features, protruding tongue, and umbilical hernia
- Myxedema—hypothyroidism in child or adult; slowing of physical and mental activity including fatigue, apathy, cold intolerance, overweight, reduced cardiac output, shortness of breath, decreased exercise capacity, constipation, decreased sweating; skin is cool and pale
- TSH increases in patients with intrinsic thyroid disease because of T_4 loss and T_3 feedback inhibition on pituitary TSH production
- TSH is NOT increased in patients with hypothalamic or pituitary disease
- In all cases T_4 is decreased

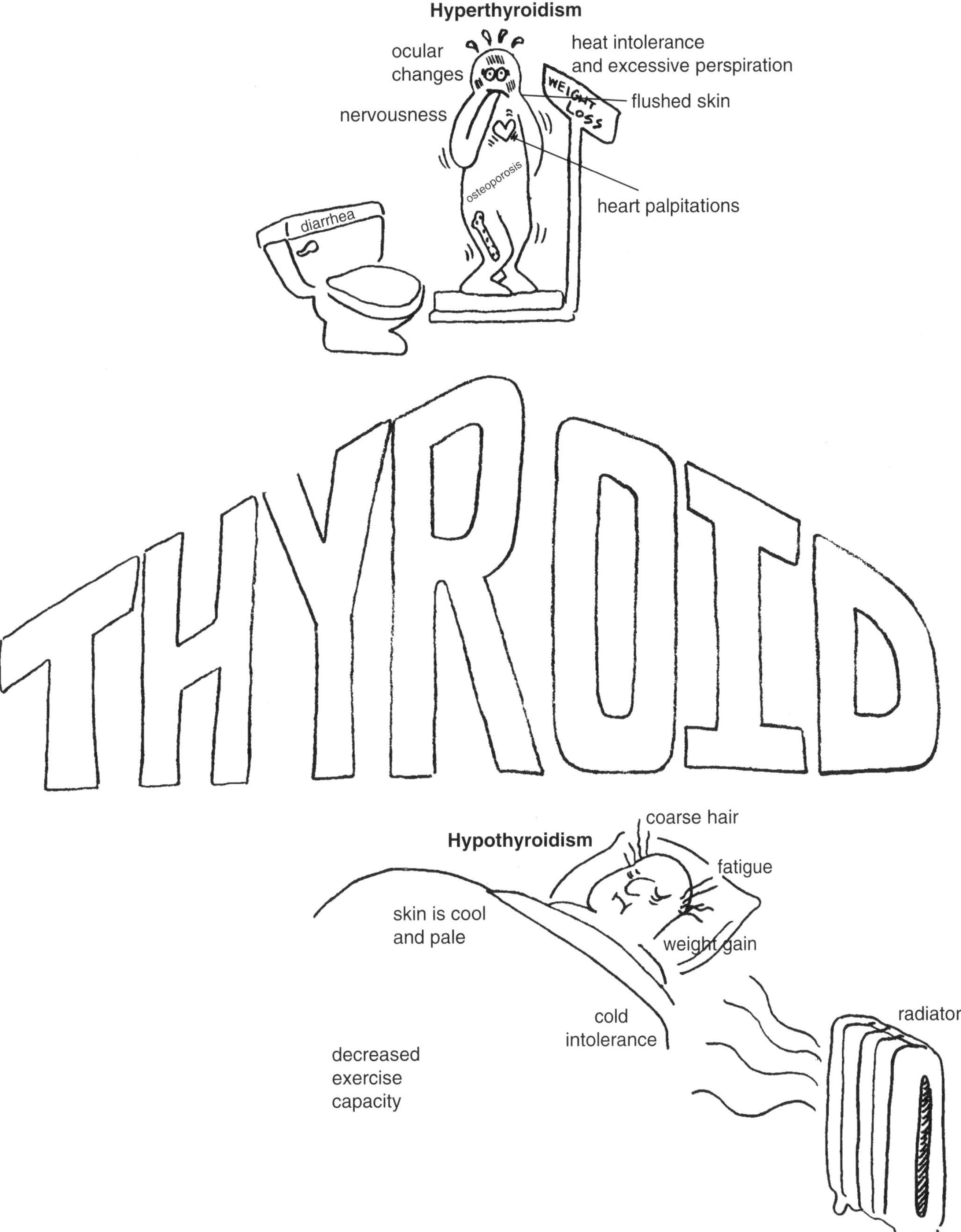
Hyperthyroidism
ocular changes
heat intolerance and excessive perspiration
WEIGHT LOSS
flushed skin
nervousness
osteoporosis
heart palpitations
diarrhea
THYROID
Hypothyroidism
coarse hair
fatigue
skin is cool and pale
weight gain
cold intolerance
radiator
decreased exercise capacity

NOTES

GRAVES' DISEASE

- Most common cause of endogenous hyperthyroidism
- Triad of findings: hyperthyroidism, infiltrative ophthalmopathy (exophthalmos), localized infiltrative dermopathy (pretibial myxedema)
- Common in women between age 20–40; associated with HLA-B8 and DR3
- Autoimmune disorder with autoantibodies to TSH receptor, which is specific for Graves' disease
- Ophthalmopathy → retro-orbital connective tissue and extraocular muscles' volume increased due to inflammation
- Morphology: symmetrically enlarged; diffuse hypertrophy and hyperplasia; histologically, there are too many cells; follicular epithelial cells tall and crowded; crowding results in papillae that project into lumen and encroach on the colloid; colloid is pale with scalloped margins
- Clinical: diffuse thyroid enlargement; audible bruit due to increased flow of blood through hyperactive gland; ophthalmopathy; wide staring gaze and lid lag; exophthalmos; pretibial myxedema (scaly thickening and induration of skin over shins)
- Radioactive iodine uptake is increased

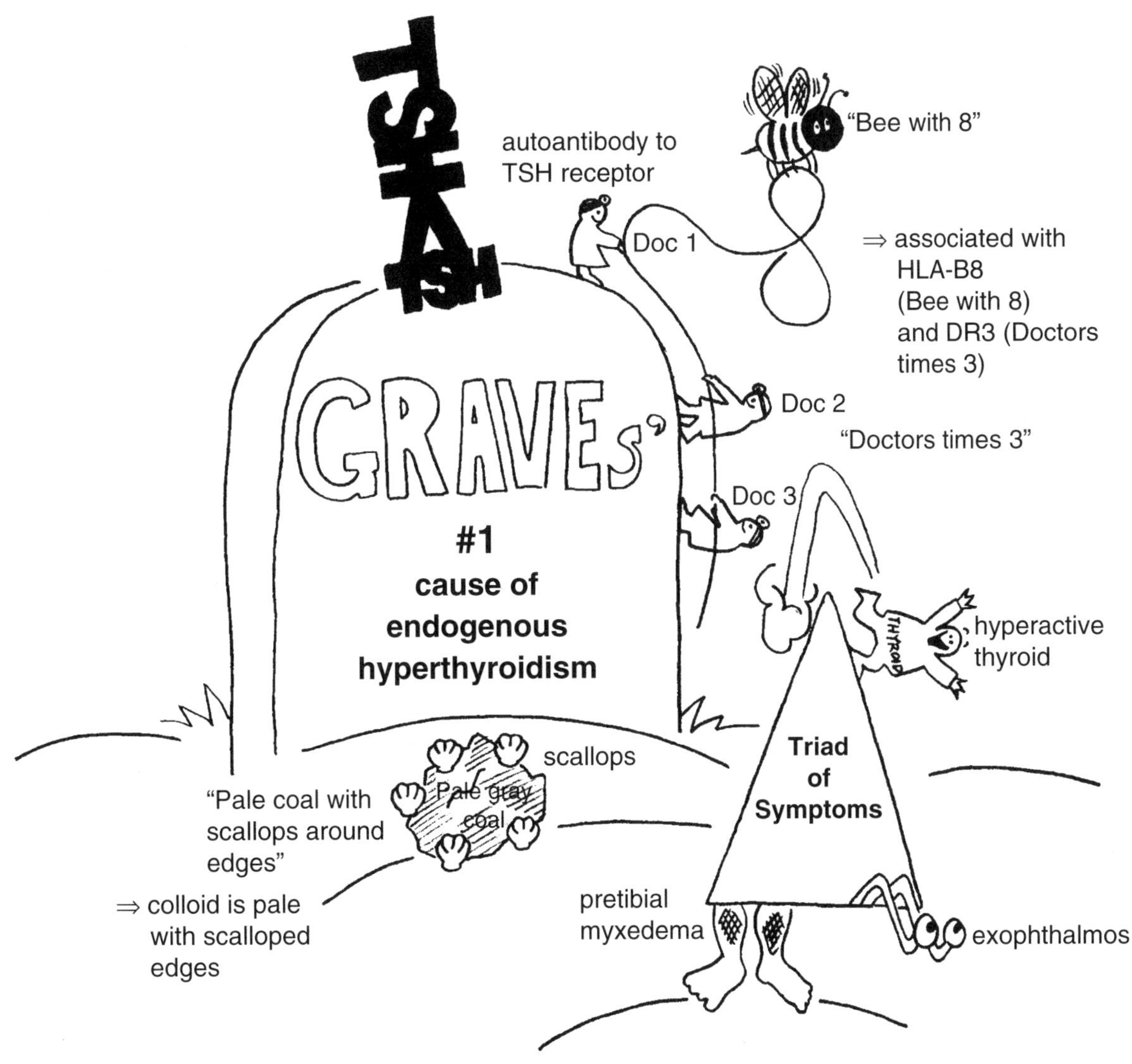
TSH
TSH
GRAVEs'
#1
cause of
endogenous
hyperthyroidism
autoantibody to
TSH receptor
"Bee with 8"
Doc 1
⇒ associated with
HLA-B8
(Bee with 8)
and DR3 (Doctors
times 3)
Doc 2
"Doctors times 3"
Doc 3
THYROID
hyperactive
thyroid
scallops
Pale gray
coal
"Pale coal with
scallops around
edges"
⇒ colloid is pale
with scalloped
edges
Triad
of
Symptoms
pretibial
myxedema
exophthalmos

NOTES

ADRENAL CORTEX

Layers

- Capsule
- Zona glomerulosa → produces mineralocorticoids (aldosterone)
- Zona fasciculata → produces glucocorticoids (cortisol)
- Zona reticularis → produces androgens and glucocorticoids
- Medulla → chromaffin cells produce catecholamines (epinephrine)

HYPERADRENALISM

- Three types: Cushing syndrome (excess cortisol); hyperaldosteronism; adrenogenital or virilizing syndromes (excess androgens)

ADRENAL INSUFFICIENCY

- Types: primary acute adrenocortical insufficiency (adrenal crisis); primary chronic adrenocortical insufficiency (Addison's disease); secondary adrenocortical insufficiency

⇒ a drain and a core + Tex

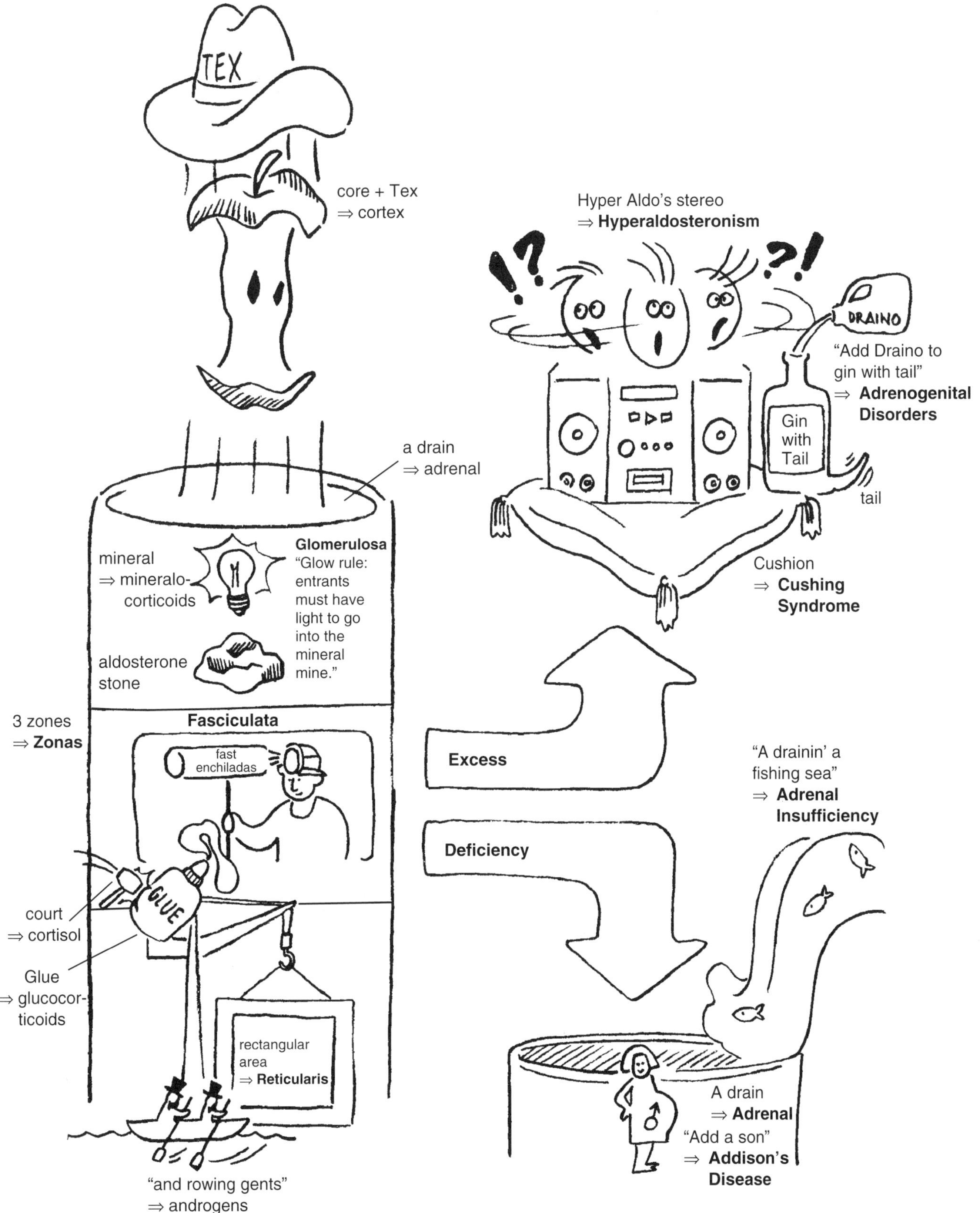
TEX
core + Tex
⇒ cortex
a drain
⇒ adrenal
mineral
⇒ mineralo-corticoids
Glomerulosa
"Glow rule: entrants must have light to go into the mineral mine."
aldosterone stone
3 zones
⇒ **Zonas**
Fasciculata
fast enchiladas
GLUE
court
⇒ cortisol
Glue
⇒ glucocor-ticoids
rectangular area
⇒ **Reticularis**
"and rowing gents"
⇒ androgens
Hyper Aldo's stereo
⇒ **Hyperaldosteronism**
DRAINO
"Add Draino to gin with tail"
⇒ **Adrenogenital Disorders**
Gin with Tail
tail
Cushion
⇒ **Cushing Syndrome**
Excess
Deficiency
"A drainin' a fishing sea"
⇒ **Adrenal Insufficiency**
A drain
⇒ **Adrenal**
"Add a son"
⇒ **Addison's Disease**

NOTES

HYPERALDOSTERONISM

- Chronic excess aldosterone secretion causes sodium retention (results in hypertension) and potassium excretion (results in hypokalemia)
- Primary hyperaldosteronism: autonomous overproduction of aldosterone → results in suppression of renin-angiotensin system; caused by aldosterone-producing adrenocortical neoplasm or adrenocortical hyperplasia; Conn's syndrome → aldosterone-secreting adenoma in one adrenal gland (more common in middle-aged women)
- Secondary hyperaldosteronism: aldosterone release occurs in response to renin-angiotensin system activation, which occurs in congestive heart failure, decreased renal perfusion, hypoalbuminemia, and pregnancy
- Clinical: primary → hypertension, hypokalemia, low serum renin, muscle weakness, paresthesias, visual disturbances, tetany, sodium retention

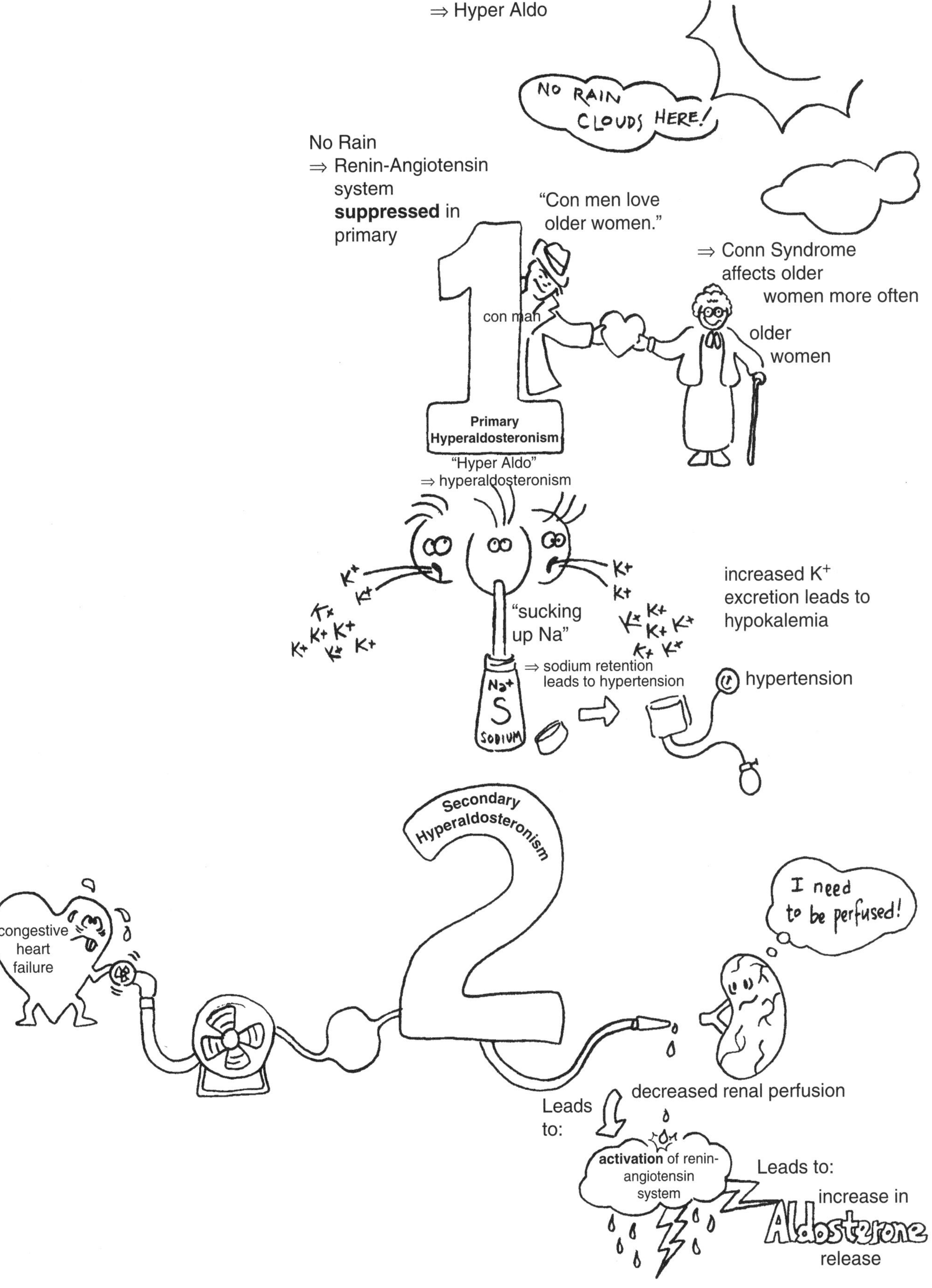
⇒ Hyper Aldo
NO RAIN CLOUDS HERE!
No Rain
⇒ Renin-Angiotensin system **suppressed** in primary
"Con men love older women."
⇒ Conn Syndrome affects older women more often
con man
older women
Primary Hyperaldosteronism
"Hyper Aldo"
⇒ hyperaldosteronism
K+
increased K+ excretion leads to hypokalemia
"sucking up Na"
⇒ sodium retention leads to hypertension
Na+
S
SODIUM
hypertension
Secondary Hyperaldosteronism
congestive heart failure
I need to be perfused!
decreased renal perfusion
Leads to:
activation of renin-angiotensin system
Leads to:
increase in
Aldosterone
release

NOTES

CUSHING'S SYNDROME (HYPERCORTISOLISM)

- Four sources of excess cortisol: primarily caused by intake of exogenous glucocorticoids and others associated with endogenous cortisol production from → primary hypothalamic-pituitary diseases associated with hypersecretion of ACTH; hypersecretion of cortisol by adrenal adenoma, carcinoma, or nodular hyperplasia; secretion of ectopic ACTH by nonendocrine neoplasm
- Primary hypersecretion of ACTH: most common in women in 20s to 30s; most patients have small ACTH-producing adenoma in pituitary
- Primary adrenal neoplasms: ACTH-independent Cushing syndrome or adrenal Cushing syndrome because adrenals function autonomously; with unilateral neoplasm → uninvolved adrenal cortex and opposite adrenal gland cortex undergoes atrophy because ACTH secretion suppressed; patient will therefore have elevated cortisol levels but low levels of ACTH
- Secretion of ectopic ACTH by nonpituitary tumors → most often small cell carcinoma of lung; adrenal glands undergo bilateral cortical hyperplasia
- Morphology: pituitary → most common change is due to high levels of glucocorticoids and results in accumulation of keratin in cytoplasm called Crooke's hyaline change
- Clinical: early symptoms include hypertension and weight gain; later central pattern of adipose tissue deposition (truncal obesity, moon facies, accumulation of fat in posterior neck and back) → buffalo hump; proximal muscle weakness; induction of gluconeogenesis and inhibition of glucose uptake by cells → results in hyperglycemia, glucosuria, and polydipsia; loss of collagen and bone resorption → resulting in thin skin and easy bruising; poor wound healing; abdominal cutaneous striae; suppression of immune response; mental disturbances; hirsutism; menstrual abnormalities
- Diagnosis: 24-hour urine where free cortisol level is increased and loss of normal diurnal pattern of cortisol secretion (normally cortisol released in the morning and gradually reduces throughout the day; in Cushing syndrome no reduction occurs)
- Determining cause: by administration of dexamethasone, then measure resulting ACTH and urinary excretion of steroid → in pituitary, Cushing syndrome ACTH levels are elevated but can be reduced with HIGH doses of dexamethasone with resultant suppression of urinary steroid secretion; other causes are not at all affected by dexamethasone

⇒ cushion

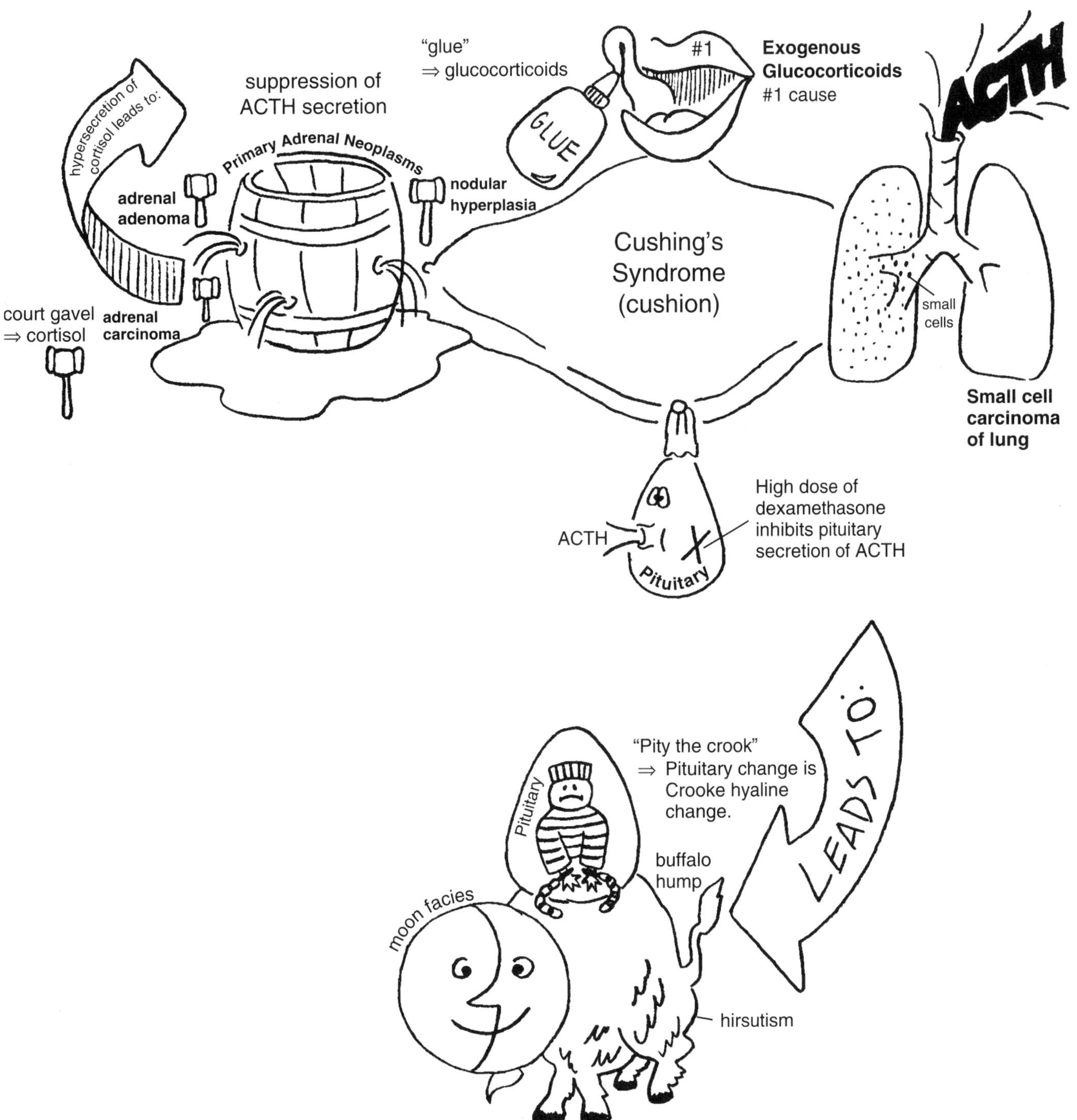
"glue"
⇒ glucocorticoids
#1
Exogenous Glucocorticoids
#1 cause
GLUE
ACTH
suppression of ACTH secretion
hypersecretion of cortisol leads to:
Primary Adrenal Neoplasms
adrenal adenoma
nodular hyperplasia
court gavel
⇒ cortisol
adrenal carcinoma
Cushing's Syndrome (cushion)
small cells
Small cell carcinoma of lung
ACTH
Pituitary
High dose of dexamethasone inhibits pituitary secretion of ACTH
"Pity the crook"
⇒ Pituitary change is Crooke hyaline change.
LEADS TO:
Pituitary
buffalo hump
moon facies
hirsutism

NOTES

ADRENOGENITAL SYNDROMES

- Disorders of sexual differentiation (e.g., virilization); caused by gonadal disorders, adrenocortical neoplasms, and congenital adrenal hyperplasia
- Adrenal neoplasms more likely to be carcinomas
- Congenital adrenal hyperplasia → autosomal recessive; inherited metabolic errors; deficiency of particular enzyme involved in biosynthesis of cortical steroids (especially cortisol); when deficiency occurs steroidogenesis is channeled to other pathways resulting in increased androgen production, which results in virilization; there is also simultaneous deficiency of cortisol leading to increased ACTH secretion and adrenal hyperplasia

21-hydroxylase deficiency

- Adrenal steroid synthesis: cholesterol → pregnenolone → progesterone and 17α-hydroxyprogesterone (21-hydroxylase is needed to convert progesterone to deoxycorticosterone and to convert 17α-hydroxyprogesterone to deoxycortisol)
- Deficiency of 21-hydroxylase therefore inhibits aldosterone and cortisol synthesis, which in turn causes steroid synthesis to be shifted to androgen production, resulting in three syndromes (depending on the severity of mutation):
  - salt-wasting adrenogenitalism
  - simple virilizing adrenogenitalism
  - nonclassic adrenogenitalism
- Salt-wasting syndrome results from total lack of hydroxylase; deficient mineralo-corticoid and glucocorticoid synthesis; clinical → salt wasting, hyponatremia, hyperkalemia, which causes acidosis, hypotension, cardiovascular collapse, and possible death; excess production of androgens leads to virilization; because there is no cortisol negative feedback to the pituitary, ACTH production is increased, causing bilateral adrenal hyperplasia
- Simple virilizing adrenogenital syndrome without salt wasting; less than total hydroxylase defect → enough enzyme to allow salt reabsorption but low gluco-corticoid levels are not sufficient for negative feedback and ACTH is elevated, resulting in adrenal hyperplasia
- Nonclassic or late-onset adrenal virilism: usually asymptomatic with only mild manifestations such as hirsutism
- Treatment of congenital adrenal hyperplasia → exogenous glucocorticoids

21- hydroxylase deficiency

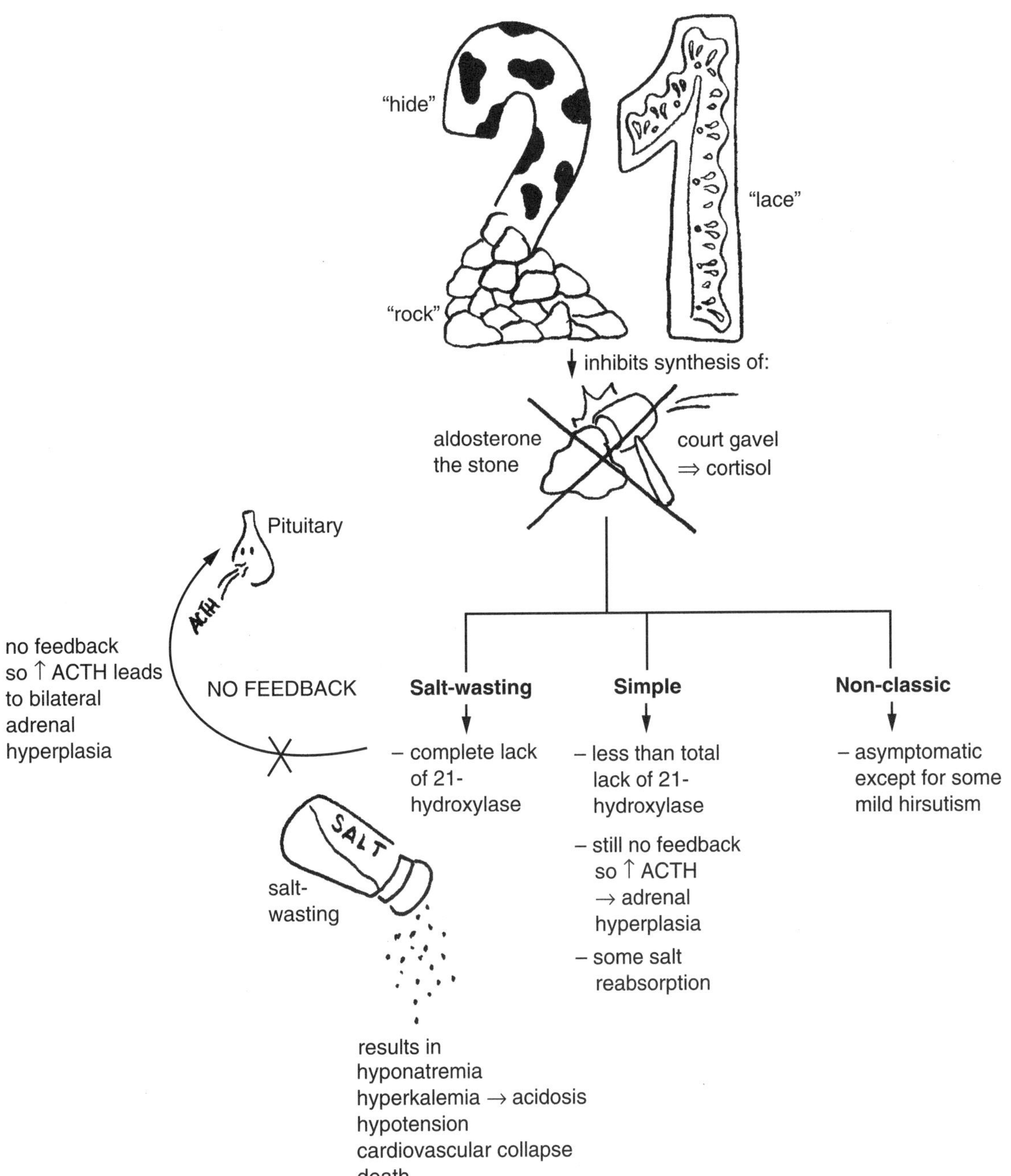
"21 + hide + rock + lace"
⇒ **21-hydroxylase deficiency**
"hide"
"lace"
"rock"
inhibits synthesis of:
aldosterone the stone
court gavel ⇒ cortisol
Pituitary
ACTH
no feedback so ↑ ACTH leads to bilateral adrenal hyperplasia
NO FEEDBACK
Salt-wasting
– complete lack of 21-hydroxylase
Simple
– less than total lack of 21-hydroxylase
– still no feedback so ↑ ACTH → adrenal hyperplasia
– some salt reabsorption
Non-classic
– asymptomatic except for some mild hirsutism
SALT
salt-wasting
results in hyponatremia hyperkalemia → acidosis hypotension cardiovascular collapse death

NOTES

ADRENAL INSUFFICIENCY

- Types: primary acute adrenocortical insufficiency (adrenal crisis); primary chronic adrenocortical insufficiency (Addison's disease); secondary adrenocortical insufficiency
- Primary acute adrenocortical insufficiency: adrenal crisis occurs when → a patient already suffering from chronic adrenocortical insufficiency cannot adequately react to stress because his or her adrenal glands are incapable of responding with immediate steroid output; when patients taking exogenous corticosteroids either withdraw from steroid use rapidly or do not increase steroid dose in response to acute stress; when there is massive adrenal hemorrhage (e.g., newborns following traumatic birth); patients on anticoagulant therapy; patients who suffer from disseminated intravascular coagulation with resultant infarction of adrenals; and when massive adrenal hemorrhage complicates bacteremic infection (Waterhouse-Friderichsen syndrome)
- Waterhouse-Friderichsen syndrome: associated with overwhelming bacterial infection, usually *Neisseria meningitidis* septicemia; rapidly progressive hypotension leading to shock; disseminated intravascular coagulation with extensive purpura, especially of skin

PRIMARY CHRONIC ADRENOCORTICAL INSUFFICIENCY (ADDISON'S DISEASE)

- Results from progressive destruction of the adrenal cortex; more common in white women
- 90% associated with autoimmune adrenalitis, tuberculosis, or metastatic cancers
- Clinical: Addison's disease is not symptomatic until 90% of cortex is destroyed or nonfunctional; initially → weakness and fatigue; GI disturbances (anorexia, nausea, vomiting, weight loss, and diarrhea); hyperpigmentation of skin (from ACTH precursor hormones that stimulate melanocytes)

SECONDARY ADRENOCORTICAL INSUFFICIENCY

- Disorder of hypothalamus and pituitary that reduce ACTH output or prolonged administration of exogenous glucocorticoids that suppress ACTH release
- No hyperpigmentation
- Characterized by deficient cortisol and androgen output but normal aldosterone synthesis (because aldosterone is influenced by the renin system)

ADRENOCORTICAL NEOPLASMS

- Most adenomas are nonfunctional
- Carcinomas: occur at any age; functional; associated with symptoms of hyperadrenalism; highly malignant; strong propensity to invade adrenal vein, vena cava, and lymphatics

⇒ a drainin' a fishing sea
Addison's Disease ⇒ add a son
and
Waterhouse-Friderichsen Syndrome
⇒ water house

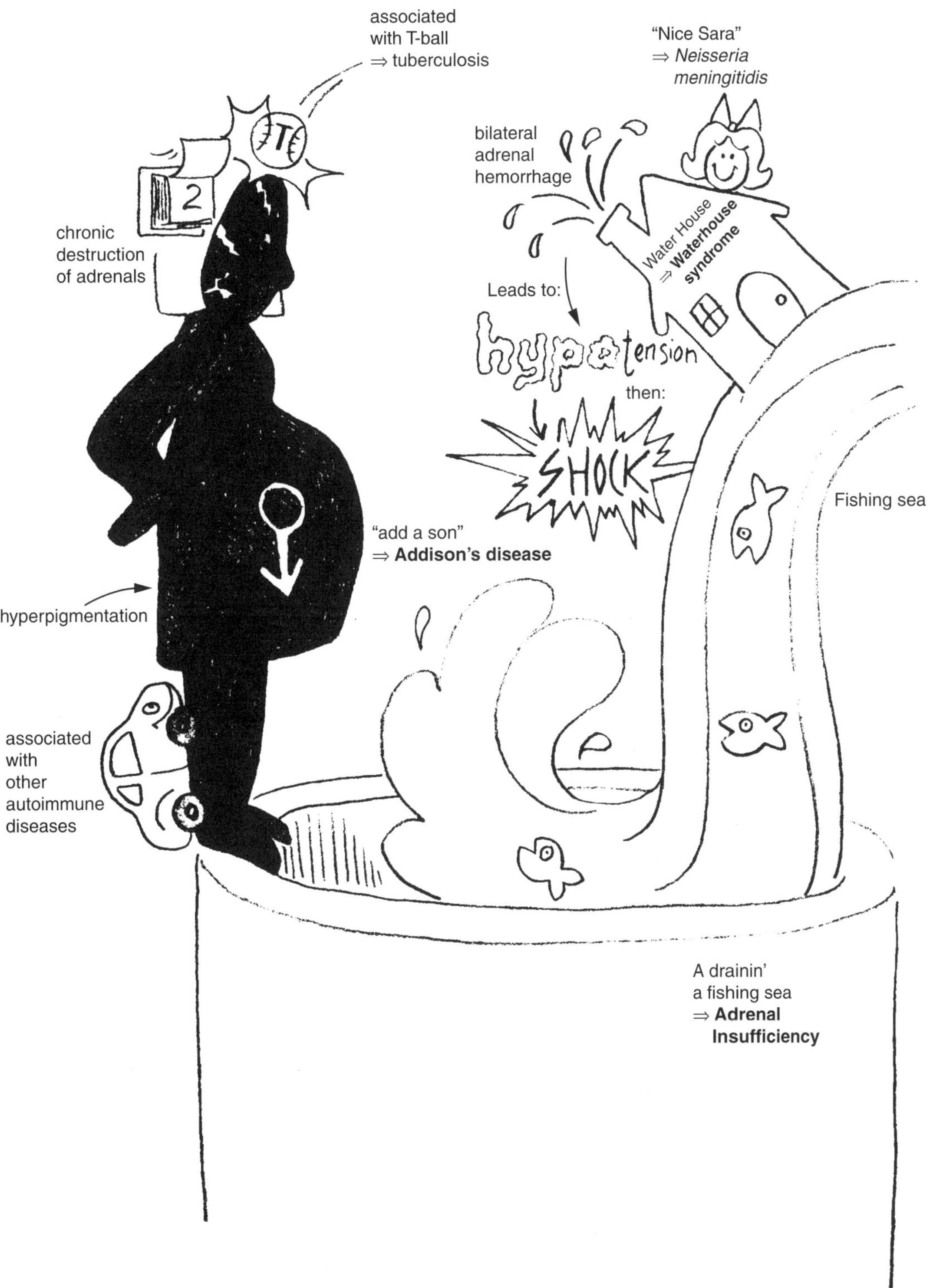

NOTES

ADRENAL MEDULLA

- Composed of specialized neural crest (neuroendocrine) cells → chromaffin cells
- Synthesize and secrete catecholamines (epinephrine and norepinephrine) in response to preganglionic sympathetic nervous system
- Neuroendocrine cells also produce other substances such as histamine, serotonin, renin, chromegranin A, and neuropeptide hormones
- Paraganglion system: neuroendocrine cells dispersed in an extra-adrenal system of clusters and nodules; closely associated with autonomic nervous system; divided according to anatomic position → branchiomeric, intravagal, aorticosympathetic; examples include carotid bodies

PHEOCHROMOCYTOMA

- Neoplasms composed of chromaffin cells
- Synthesize and release catecholamines and sometimes peptide hormones
- Most arise in adrenal medulla, but can also arise in extra-adrenal paraganglia known as paragangliomas (more often below diaphragm)
- Occur sporadically or as familial syndrome (autosomal dominant and include MEN syndromes, type I neurofibromatosis, von Hippel-Lindau disease, and Sturge-Weber syndrome)
- Histology: composed of polygonal to spindle-shaped chromaffin cells, clustered with their supporting cells into small nests or alveoli (zellballen)
- Diagnosis: based exclusively on the presence of metastases
- Clinical: dominant symptom is abrupt hypertension associated with tachycardia, palpitations, headache, sweating, tremor, and sense of apprehension; catecholamine cardiomyopathy (catecholamine-induced myocardial instability and ventricular arrhythmias)
- Lab diagnosis: increased urinary excretion of free catecholamines and their metabolites (vanillylmandelic acid [VMA]) and metanephrines

NEUROBLASTOMA

- Most common extracranial solid tumor of childhood; originates in adrenal medulla or anywhere in sympathetic nervous system; sporadic or familial

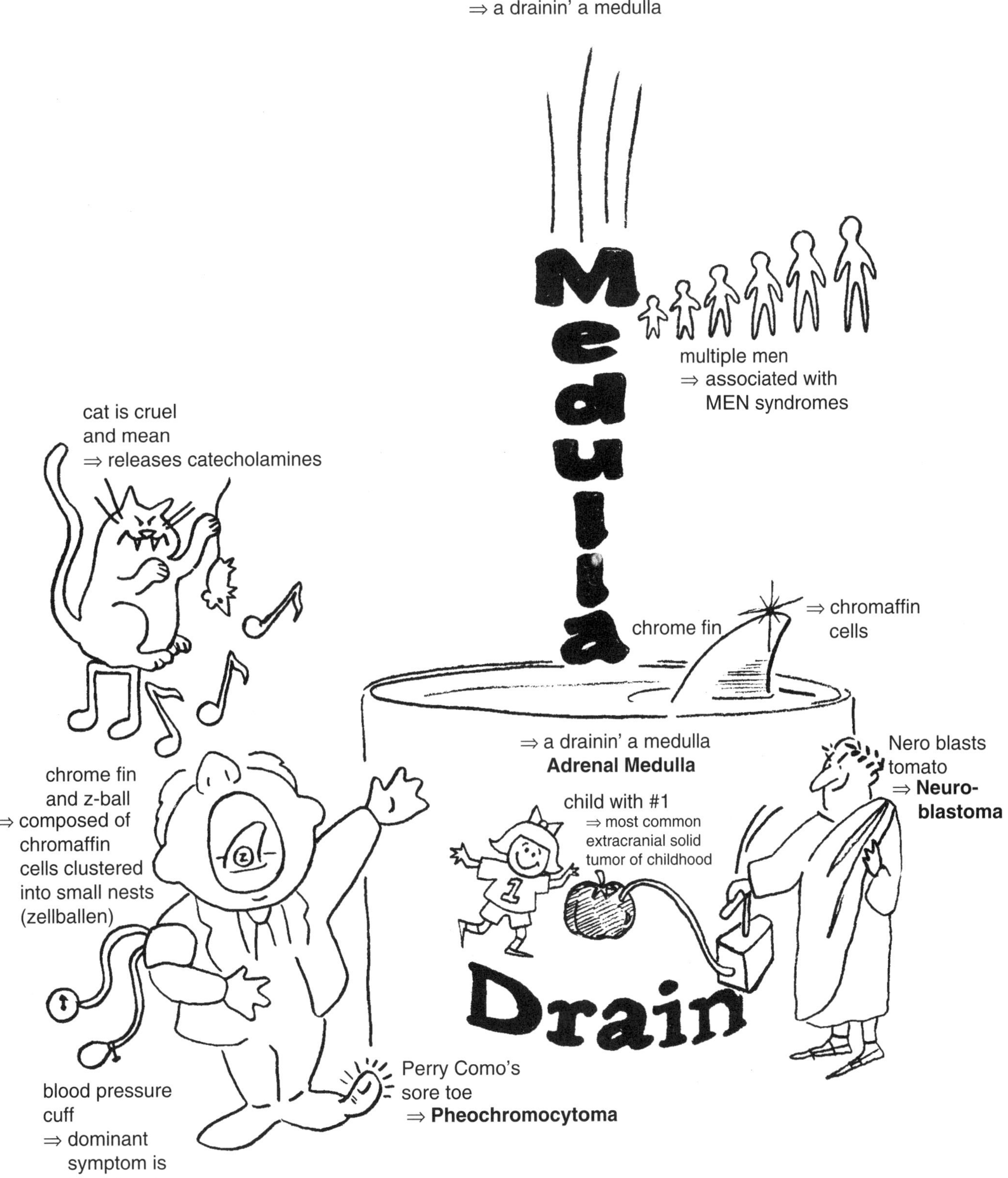
⇒ a drainin' a medulla
Medulla
multiple men
⇒ associated with MEN syndromes
cat is cruel and mean
⇒ releases catecholamines
chrome fin
⇒ chromaffin cells
⇒ a drainin' a medulla
Adrenal Medulla
Nero blasts tomato
⇒ **Neuro-blastoma**
child with #1
⇒ most common extracranial solid tumor of childhood
chrome fin and z-ball
⇒ composed of chromaffin cells clustered into small nests (zellballen)
Drain
blood pressure cuff
⇒ dominant symptom is hypertension
Perry Como's sore toe
⇒ **Pheochromocytoma**

NOTES

PARATHYROID

- Derived from developing pharyngeal pouches that also give rise to thymus
- Lie in close proximity to the upper and lower poles of each thyroid lobe
- Mostly composed of chief cells that contain secretory granules of parathyroid hormone (PTH); also contain oxyphil cells
- Activity controlled by level of free (ionized) calcium in blood; decreased calcium stimulates synthesis and secretion of PTH
- Metabolic functions of PTH: activates osteoclasts; increases the renal tubular reabsorption of calcium; increases the conversion of vitamin D to its active dihydroxy form in kidneys (this form of vitamin D is important for calcium transport across the GI tract); increases urinary phosphate excretion; augments gastrointestinal calcium absorption
- Hypercalcemia → result of elevated levels of PTH and malignancy
- Hypercalcemia due to malignancy occurs because of osteolytic metastases and local release of cytokines (which induce local osteolysis) and release of PTH-related protein (binds to PTH receptors and causes same reactions as PTH)

HYPERPARATHYROIDISM

- Primary (due to autonomous PTH overproduction); secondary and tertiary (due to chronic renal insufficiency)
- **Primary** → caused by adenoma; primary hyperplasia; and parathyroid carcinoma
- More common in women in their 50s; patients have a history of irradiation 30–40 years before onset
- Clinically may be asymptomatic (only manifestation is increased serum ionized calcium level) or symptomatic (painful bones, renal stones, abdominal groans, and psychic moans)
- Patients with primary hyperparathyroidism have an increased serum PTH level, whereas PTH levels are low in hypercalcemia caused by nonparathyroid disease
- **Secondary** → renal failure most common cause; other causes include inadequate intake of calcium, steatorrhea, and vitamin D deficiency
- Renal insufficiency also decreases phosphate excretion resulting in hyperphosphatemia, which further depresses serum calcium levels (formation of calcium phosphate) and by so doing stimulates parathyroid activity

HYPOPARATHYROIDISM

- Deficient PTH
- Causes: surgical removal; congenital absence of all glands; idiopathic atrophy; familial (associated with candidiasis and adrenal insufficiency)
- Clinically present with tetany; neuromuscular irritability (with positive Chvostek sign → tapping of facial nerve induces facial contractions of eye, nose, and mouth; and positive Trousseau sign → occluding forearm circulation induces carpal spasm that disappears when occlusion taken away)
- Mental status changes; ocular disease (calcification of lens); cardiovascular (prolonged QT interval)

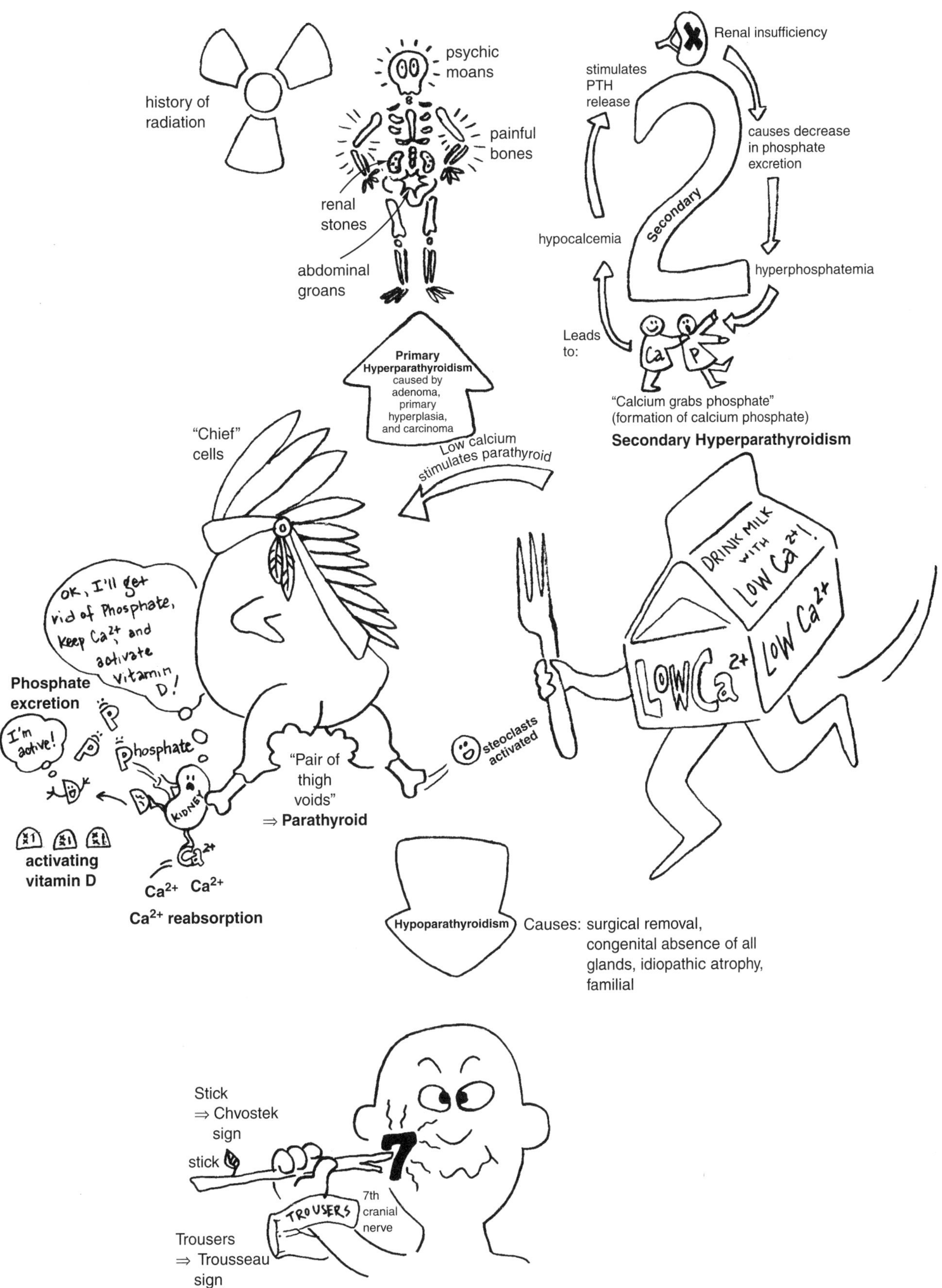
history of radiation
psychic moans
painful bones
renal stones
abdominal groans
Renal insufficiency
stimulates PTH release
causes decrease in phosphate excretion
Secondary
hypocalcemia
hyperphosphatemia
Leads to:
Ca
P
"Calcium grabs phosphate" (formation of calcium phosphate)
Secondary Hyperparathyroidism
Primary Hyperparathyroidism caused by adenoma, primary hyperplasia, and carcinoma
"Chief" cells
Low calcium stimulates parathyroid
DRINK MILK WITH LOW Ca2+!
LOW Ca2+
LOW Ca2+
OK, I'll get rid of Phosphate, keep Ca2+ and activate vitamin D!
Phosphate excretion
I'm active!
Phosphate
KIDNEY
activating vitamin D
Ca2+ Ca2+
Ca2+ reabsorption
"Pair of thigh voids" ⇒ Parathyroid
steoclasts activated
Hypoparathyroidism
Causes: surgical removal, congenital absence of all glands, idiopathic atrophy, familial
Stick ⇒ Chvostek sign
stick
7
7th cranial nerve
TROUSERS
Trousers ⇒ Trousseau sign

NOTES

ENDOCRINE PANCREAS

- Three types of cells:
  - α-cells secrete glucagon
  - β-cells secrete insulin
  - Δ-cells secrete somatostatin
- Glucagon
  - increases the amount of glucose in circulation
  - increases gluconeogenesis, glycogenolysis, lipolysis, insulin secretion, ketogenesis, and catecholamine secretion
  - decreases lipogenesis and inhibits glycogen synthetase
  - secretion stimulated by hypoglycemia and inhibited by hyperglycemia
  - diabetic malfunction leads to increased glucose level → insulin is required by α-cells to transport glucose into the cell; when insulin is not available (as with diabetics) glucose will not enter the cell and hence will not inhibit production of glucagons; glucagons therefore continue to produce, resulting in a further increase in serum glucose concentrations
  - diabetic ketoacidosis (DKA) → hyperglycemia (decreased insulin); protein destruction and lipolysis, which leads to ketosis and metabolic acidosis; sodium and potassium electrolyte imbalances; dehydration
    - treatment of **DKA**: for **D** (dehydration) → normal saline; for **K+** (potassium deficiency) → administer potassium phosphate; for **A** (acidosis) administer insulin and glucose
- Insulin
  - increases glycogenesis, protein synthesis, lipogenesis; and glucose uptake by muscle and fat cells
  - decreases glycogenolysis, proteolysis, lipolysis, and ketogenesis and gluconeogenesis of liver (inhibits glucagon secretion)
  - stimulated by increased serum glucose, free fatty acids, gastric inhibitory peptide, or increase in arginine or leucine
  - inhibited by exercise (or decreases need for insulin)
  - β-cell's insulin production dependent upon amount of glucose taken up by β-cell; glucose uptake in β-cell is insulin-independent
  - production of insulin
    - preproinsulin → proinsulin → insulin + C-peptide
      - C-peptide marker for β-cell function
- Somatostatin
  - inhibits insulin, glucagon, and gastrin secretion

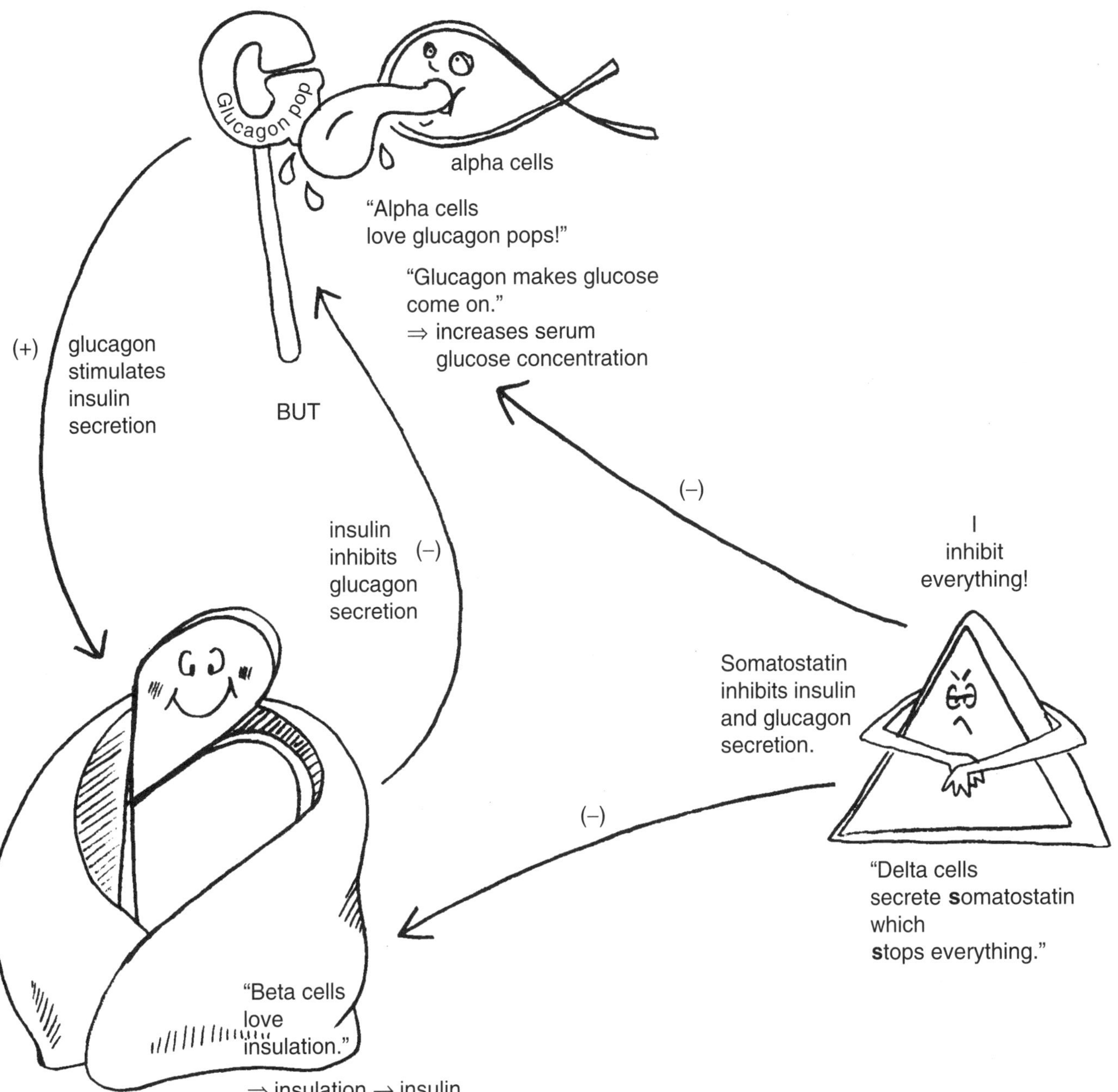
Glucagon pop
alpha cells
"Alpha cells
love glucagon pops!"
"Glucagon makes glucose
come on."
⇒ increases serum
glucose concentration
(+) glucagon
stimulates
insulin
secretion
BUT
(–)
insulin
inhibits
glucagon
secretion
(–)
I
inhibit
everything!
Somatostatin
inhibits insulin
and glucagon
secretion.
(–)
"Delta cells
secrete **s**omatostatin
which
stops everything."
"Beta cells
love
insulation."
⇒ insulation → insulin

NOTES

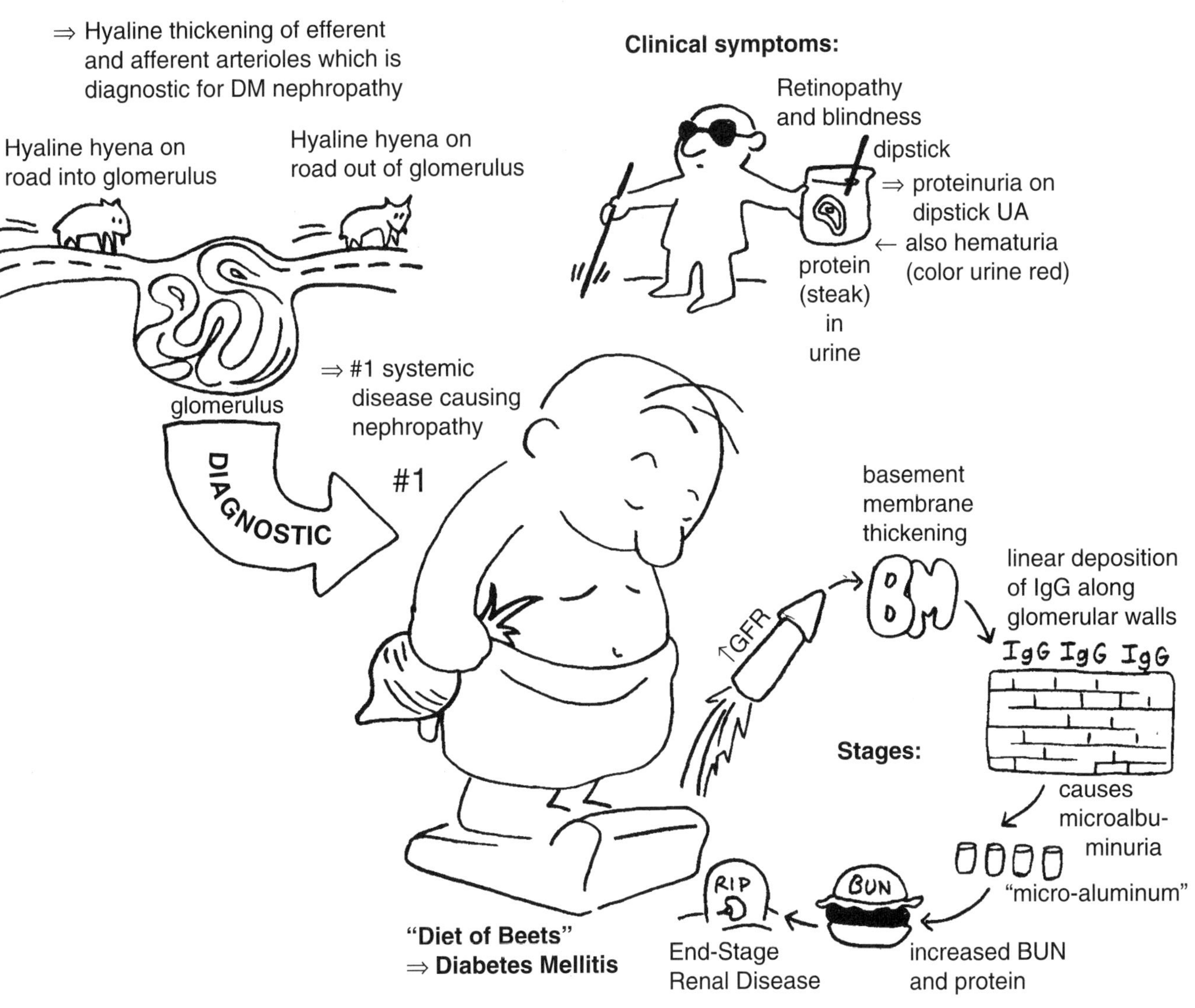
⇒ Diet of Beets
⇒ Hyaline thickening of efferent and afferent arterioles which is diagnostic for DM nephropathy
Hyaline hyena on road into glomerulus
Hyaline hyena on road out of glomerulus
glomerulus
DIAGNOSTIC
⇒ #1 systemic disease causing nephropathy
#1
Clinical symptoms:
Retinopathy and blindness
dipstick
⇒ proteinuria on dipstick UA
← also hematuria (color urine red)
protein (steak) in urine
basement membrane thickening
BM
linear deposition of IgG along glomerular walls
IgG IgG IgG
↑GFR
Stages:
causes microalbu-minuria
"micro-aluminum"
BUN
increased BUN and protein
RIP
End-Stage Renal Disease
"Diet of Beets"
⇒ Diabetes Mellitis

NOTES

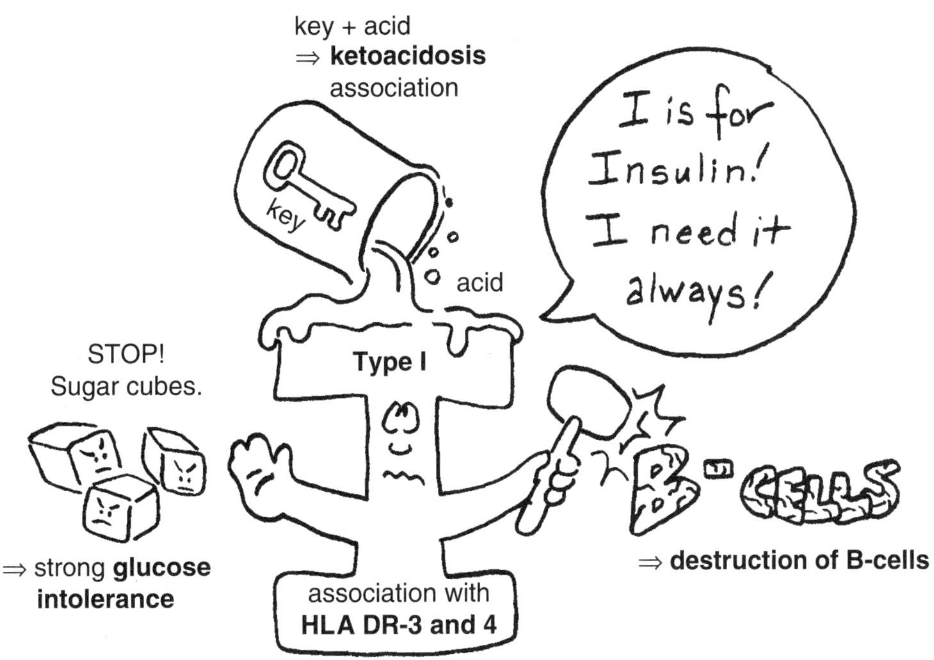
key + acid
⇒ **ketoacidosis** association
key
acid
I is for Insulin! I need it always!
Type I
STOP! Sugar cubes.
⇒ strong **glucose intolerance**
association with **HLA DR-3 and 4**
B-CELLS
⇒ **destruction of B-cells**

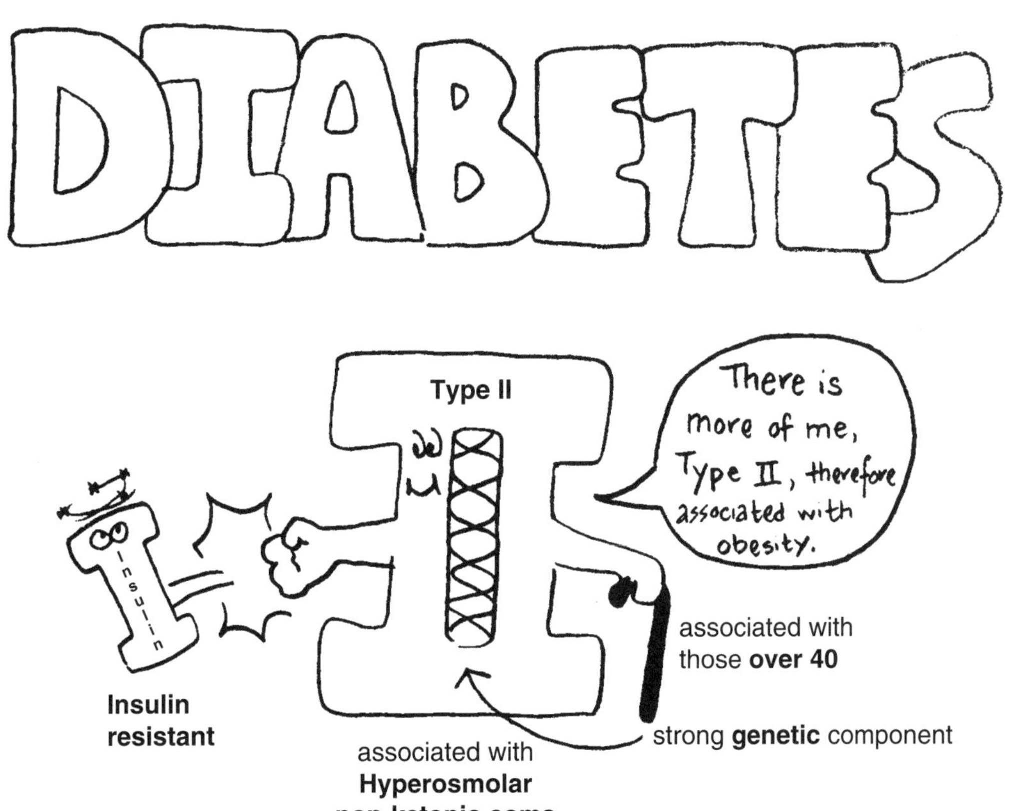
DIABETES
Type II
There is more of me, Type II, therefore associated with obesity.
Insulin
Insulin resistant
associated with those **over 40**
strong **genetic** component
associated with **Hyperosmolar non-ketonic coma**

NOTES

SKIN LAYERS

- Superficial to deep
  - stratum corneum → most superficial layer; many flat layers of keratinized dead cells
  - stratum lucidum → clear layer only in palms of hands and soles of feet
  - stratum granulosum → layer of granular cells
  - stratum spinosum → layer of cells with spinelike processes
  - stratum germinativum → basal cell layer; deepest layer; single layer of columnar cells; contains melanocytes

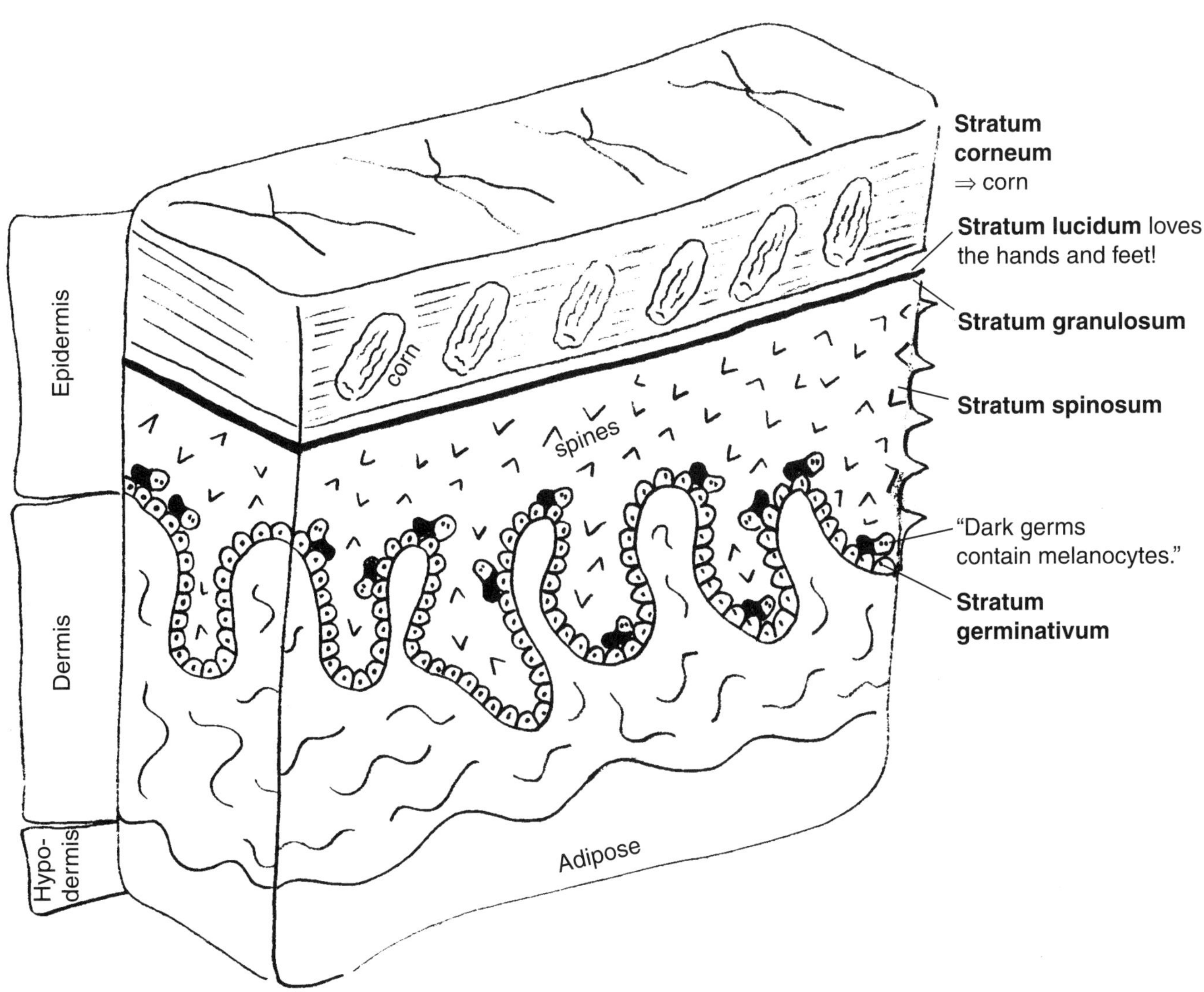
Stratum corneum
⇒ corn
Stratum lucidum loves the hands and feet!
Stratum granulosum
Stratum spinosum
"Dark germs contain melanocytes."
Stratum germinativum
corn
spines
Epidermis
Dermis
Hypo-dermis
Adipose

NOTES

SKIN GLANDS

- Sebaceous glands → secrete sebum into hair shaft
- Sudoriferous (sweat) glands
  - eccrine → distributed over entire body; formed before birth; evaporative cooling function
  - apocrine → larger glands found in axillary and pubic areas; associated with hair follicles; not functional until puberty

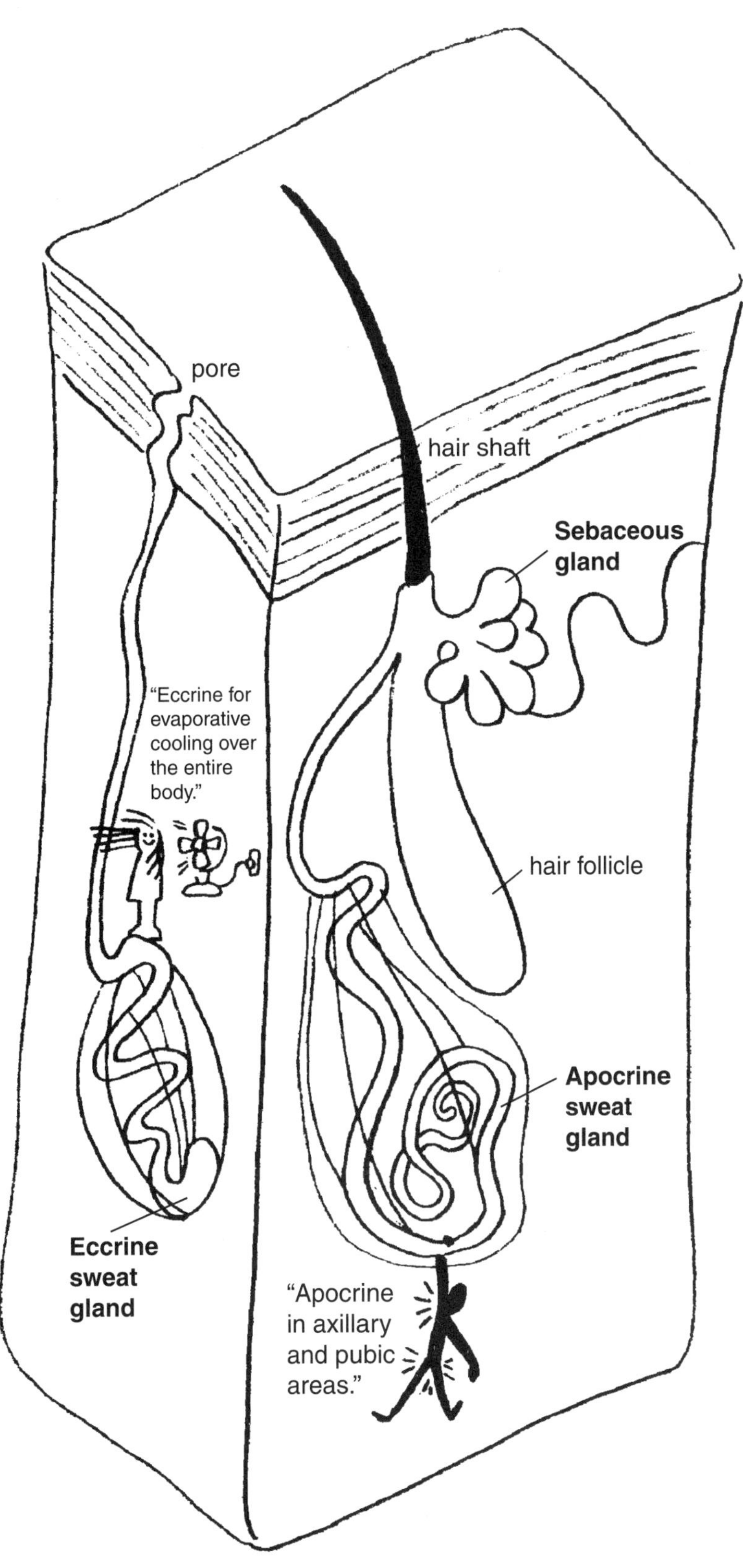
pore
hair shaft
Sebaceous gland
"Eccrine for evaporative cooling over the entire body."
hair follicle
Apocrine sweat gland
Eccrine sweat gland
"Apocrine in axillary and pubic areas."

NOTES

MELANOMA ABCDs

- **A**symmetry
- **B**order irregularity → notched border
- **C**olor variation → red, white, and blue
- **D**iameter > 6 mm

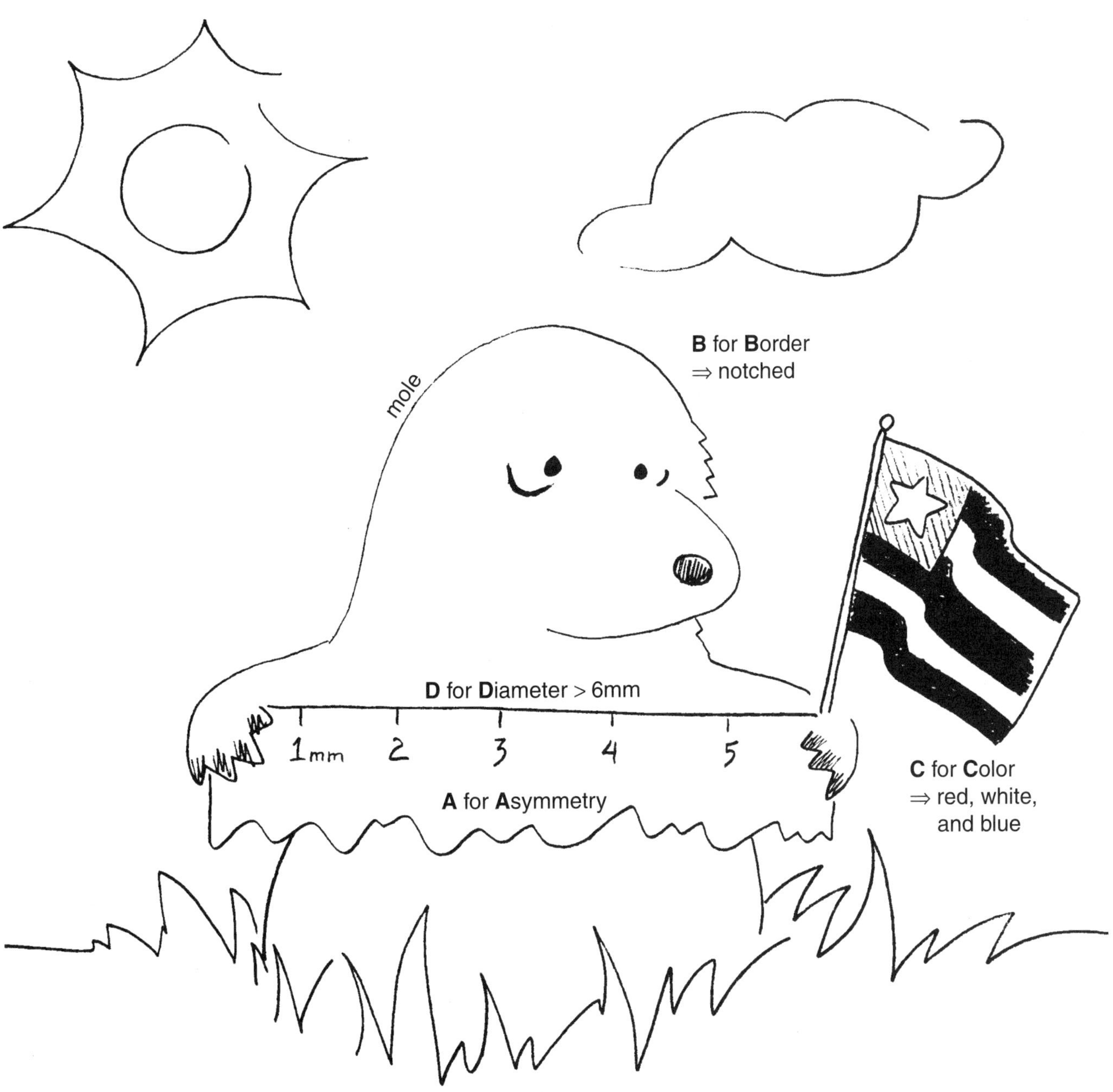
B for Border
⇒ notched
mole
D for Diameter > 6mm
1mm 2 3 4 5
A for Asymmetry
C for Color
⇒ red, white,
and blue

TABLE 1.1 BONES OF THE HEAD AND NECK

BONE/CARTILAGE	STRUCTURE	DESCRIPTION
arytenoid cartilage		pyramid shaped; located on superior margin of cricoid lamina
corniculate cartilage		located at arytenoid cartilage apex
cricoid cartilage		inferior and posterior cartilage of the larynx; complete cartilaginous ring
cuneiform cartilage		located in aryepiglottic fold
epiglottis		superior aspect of larynx
ethmoid		located between the two orbits
	cribriform plate	perforated portion of ethmoid bone
	superior nasal concha	
	middle nasal concha	
	ethmoidal air cells	pneumatized spaces within the ethmoid bone
frontal		anterior skull bone
hyoid		consists of body, 2 greater horns, 2 lesser horns
inferior nasal concha		on the lateral wall of the nasal cavity
lacrimal		part of orbital medial wall
mandible		lower jaw
	mental foramen	opening on anterior body of the mandible
	ramus	the angled portion of the mandible
	mandibular foramen	the opening on the medial surface of the ramus
maxilla		bone forming the midface
	orbital process	forms the floor of orbit
	zygomatic process	lateral projection
	infraorbital groove	groove in orbital process of the maxilla located in the posterior part of the orbit
	maxillary sinus	pneumatized center of maxilla
nasal		bone that forms part of the nasal bridge
occipital		bone of posterior skull
	foramen magnum	opening in inferior occipital bone
ossicles		series of three bones in middle ear connecting the tympanic membrane to the oval window; malleus, incus, stapes
	incus	middle ossicle
	malleus	lateral ossicle
	stapes	medial ossicle
palatine		posterior part of the hard palate
parietal		lateral bone of skull
thyroid cartilage		the large anterior cartilage of the larynx that consists of laminae (2), superior horns (2), inferior horns (2)
sphenoid		irregular bone forming of central skull
	chiasmatic sulcus	the groove for the optic chiasm
temporal		bone of lateral skull
vomer		posteroinferior part of the nasal septum
zygomatic		cheek bone

TABLE 1.2 MUSCLES, ARTERIES, AND NERVES OF THE HEAD AND NECK

MUSCLE	ORIGIN	INSERTION	ACTION	INNERVATION	ARTERY
aryepiglottic	apex of the arytenoid cartilage	epiglottis	draws the epiglottis posteriorly and downward during swallowing	inferior laryngeal nerve, from recurrent laryngeal nerve, a branch of the vagus (X)	laryngeal br. of the superior thyroid a.
auricular	anterior: galea aponeurotica anterior to ear; superior: galea aponeurotica superior to ear; posterior: mastoid process	auricle anteriorly, superiorly and posteriorly	wiggle the ears	anterior and superior: temporal branches of facial nerve (VII); posterior: posterior auricular branch of facial nerve (VII)	superficial temporal a., posterior auricular a.
buccinator	pterygomandibular raphe, mandible, and maxilla	angle of mouth and the lateral portion of the upper and lower lips	pulls the corner of mouth laterally; presses the cheek against the teeth	buccal branches of the facial nerve (VII)	facial a.
cricothyroid	cricoid cartilage	thyroid cartilage	draws the thyroid cartilage forward, lengthening the vocal ligaments	external branch of superior laryngeal nerve, a branch of the vagus nerve (X)	cricothyroid branch of the superior thyroid a.
depressor anguli oris	mandible	angle of the mouth	pulls corner of the mouth downward	marginal mandibular and buccal branches of the facial nerve (VII)	inferior labial branch of the facial a., mental a.
depressor labii inferioris	mandible	skin of the lower lip	depresses the lower lip	marginal mandibular branch of the facial nerve (VII)	inferior labial branch of the facial a., mental a.
depressor septi	maxilla	nasal septum	depresses the nasal septum	buccal branch of facial nerve (VII)	superior labial branch of the facial a.
digastric	anterior belly: digastric fossa of the mandible; posterior belly: mastoid notch of the temporal bone	body of the hyoid	elevates the hyoid bone; depresses the mandible	anterior belly: mylohyoid nerve, from the mandibular division of the trigeminal nerve (V); posterior belly: facial nerve (VII)	anterior belly: submental a.; posterior belly: occipital a.
frontalis	galea aponeurotica	skin of the eyebrow	elevates the eyebrows and wrinkles the forehead	temporal branches of the facial nerve (VII)	supraorbital and supratrochlear aa.
genioglossus	inner aspect of the mental symphysis	inserts into the tongue from the tip to the base	protrudes and depresses tongue	hypoglossal nerve (XII)	lingual a.
geniohyoid	mandible	hyoid bone	elevates the hyoid bone; depresses the mandible	ventral primary ramus of spinal nerve C1 via fibers carried by the hypoglossal nerve	lingual a., submental a.

TABLE 1.2 MUSCLES, ARTERIES, AND NERVES OF THE HEAD AND NECK (CONT.)

MUSCLE	ORIGIN	INSERTION	ACTION	INNERVATION	ARTERY
hyoglossus	hyoid bone	spreads out into the intrinsic muscles of the tongue	depresses the sides of the tongue; retracts the tongue	hypoglossal nerve (XII)	lingual a.
inferior oblique	floor of the orbit	inferior eyeball	elevates and abducts eye	oculomotor nerve (III), inferior division	ophthalmic a.
inferior pharyngeal constrictor	oblique line of the thyroid cartilage, lateral surface of cricoid cartilage	midline pharyngeal raphe	constricts pharyngeal cavity	vagus (X), via the pharyngeal plexus, with aid from the superior laryngeal and recurrent laryngeal nerves	ascending pharyngeal a., superior thyroid a., inferior thyroid a.
lateral cricoary-tenoid	cricoid cartilage	arytenoid cartilage	draws arytenoid cartilage anteriorly	inferior laryngeal nerve, from the recurrent laryngeal nerve, a branch of the vagus nerve (X)	superior laryngeal a., cricothyroid branch of the superior thyroid a.
lateral pterygoid	superior head: greater wing of the sphenoid bone; inferior head: lateral pterygoid plate	superior head: capsule and articular disk of the temporo-mandibular joint; inferior head: neck of the mandible	protracts the mandible; opens the mouth; aids in chewing	mandibular division of the trigeminal nerve (V)	pterygoid branch of the maxillary a.
levator anguli oris	maxilla	angle of the mouth	elevates the angle of the mouth	buccal branch of the facial nerve (VII)	infraorbital a., superior labial branch of the facial a.
levator labii superioris	inferior orbit	skin of the upper lip	elevates the upper lip	buccal branch of the facial nerve (VII)	infraorbital a., superior labial branch of the facial a.
levator labii superioris alaque nasi	frontal process of maxilla	ala of the nose and skin of the upper lip	elevates the upper lip and flares the nostril	buccal branch of the facial nerve (VII)	infraorbital a., superior labial branch of the facial a.
levator palpebrae superioris	orbital apex	skin and fascia of upper eyelid and the superior tarsal plate	elevates the upper eyelid	oculomotor nerve (III) and sympathetics (to the superior tarsal portion)	ophthalmic a.
levator scapulae	transverse processes of C1-4 vertebrae	medial border of the scapula from the superior angle to the spine	elevates scapula	dorsal scapular nerve (C5); the upper part of the muscle receives branches of C3 and C4 spinal nerves	dorsal scapular a.
levator veli palatini	petrous part of the temporal bone and the medial auditory tube cartilage	muscles and fascia of the soft palate; palatine aponeurosis	elevates the soft palate	vagus nerve (X) via the pharyngeal plexus	ascending pharyngeal a.

TABLE 1.2 MUSCLES, ARTERIES, AND NERVES OF THE HEAD AND NECK (CONT.)

MUSCLE	ORIGIN	INSERTION	ACTION	INNERVATION	ARTERY
longus capitis	anterior tubercles of vertebrae C3-6	basilar portion of the occipital bone	flex the head and neck	cervical plexus, ventral primary rami of spinal nerves C1-4	deep cervical a.
longus colli	anterior tubercles and anterior surfaces of the bodies of vertebrae C3-T3	anterior arch of atlas, anterior tubercles of C5-6, anterior surfaces of bodies of vertebrae C2-4	flex neck, rotate and laterally bend neck	cervical and brachial plexus, C2-7	deep cervical a.
masseter	zygomatic arch and zygomatic bone	lateral surface of the ramus and angle of the mandible	elevates the mandible	nerve to the masseter, from the mandibular division of the trigeminal nerve (V)	masseteric branch of the maxillary a.
medial pterygoid	medial surface of lateral pterygoid plate, pyramidal process of the palatine bone, tuberosity of the maxilla	medial surface of the ramus and angle of the mandible	elevates and protracts the mandible	medial pterygoid branch of the mandibular division of the trigeminal nerve (V)	pterygoid branch of the maxillary a.
mentalis	anterior mandible	skin of the chin	elevates the skin of chin	marginal mandibular branch of the facial nerve (VII)	mental a., inferior labial branch of the facial a.
middle pharyngeal constrictor	lesser and greater horns of the hyoid bone	midline pharyngeal raphe	constricts the pharyngeal cavity	vagus (X)	ascending pharyngeal a.
mylohyoid	mylohyoid line of mandible	hyoid bone	elevates the hyoid bone and the tongue; depresses the mandible	branch of the mandibular division of the trigeminal nerve (V)	mylohyoid branch of the inferior alveolar a.
nasalis pars alaris	maxilla	ala of the nose	flares the nostrils	buccal branch of facial nerve (VII)	superior labial branch of the facial a.
nasalis pars transversa	maxilla	midline aponeurosis	flattens the nose	buccal branch of facial nerve (VII)	superior labial branch of the facial a.
occipitalis	superior nuchal line	galea aponeurotica	pulls the scalp posteriorly; elevates the eyebrows	posterior auricular branch of the facial nerve (VII)	occipital a.
occipito-frontalis	frontalis: galea aponeurotica; occipitalis: superior nuchal line	frontalis: skin of the eyebrows; occipitalis: galea aponeurotica	elevates eyebrows and wrinkles the forehead	frontalis: temporal branches of the facial nerve (VII); occipitalis: posterior auricular branch of the facial nerve (VII)	frontalis: supraorbital and supratrochlear aa.; occipitalis: occipital a.

TABLE 1.2 MUSCLES, ARTERIES, AND NERVES OF THE HEAD AND NECK (CONT.)

MUSCLE	ORIGIN	INSERTION	ACTION	INNERVATION	ARTERY
omohyoid	inferior belly: upper border of the scapula; superior belly: intermediate tendon	inferior belly: intermediate tendon; superior belly: lower border of the hyoid bone	depresses the hyoid bone	ansa cervicalis	transverse cervical a.
orbicularis oculi	orbital part: medial orbital margin and the medial palpebral ligament; palpebral part: medial palpebral ligament	orbital part: skin of the lateral cheek; palpebral part: lateral palpebral raphe	closes the eyelids	temporal and zygomatic branches of the facial nerve (VII)	supraorbital a., supratrochlear a., infraorbital a., angular branch of the facial a.
orbicularis oris	skin and fascia of lips	skin and fascia of the lips	purses the lips	buccal branch of the facial nerve (VII)	superior and inferior labial branches of the facial a., mental a., infraorbital a.
palato-glossus	palatine aponeurosis	side of the tongue	elevates and retracts the tongue	vagus nerve (X) via the pharyngeal plexus	tonsilar branch of the facial a., ascending pharyngeal a.
palatopha-ryngeus	posterior bony palate and palatine aponeurosis	posterior pharynx and posterior thyroid cartilage	elevates the larynx	vagus nerve (X) via pharyngeal plexus	ascending pharyngeal a.
platysma	fascia overlying the pectoralis major and deltoid muscles	inferior mandible	draws the mouth down	cervical branch of the facial nerve (VII)	facial a.
procerus	nasal bone	skin between the eyebrows	depresses the medial eyebrows	temporal branch of the facial nerve (VII)	supratrochlear a.
rectus capitis anterior	atlas	basilar portion of occipital bone	flexes the head	ventral primary ramus of spinal nerve C1	deep cervical a.
rectus capitis lateralis	transverse process of atlas	occipital bone	laterally bends the head	ventral primary ramus of spinal nerve C1	deep cervical a.
rectus, inferior	common tendinous ring at orbital apex	inferior eyeball	depresses and adducts the eyeball	oculomotor nerve (III), inferior division	ophthalmic a.
rectus, lateral	common tendinous ring at orbital apex	lateral eyeball	abducts the eyeball	abducens nerve (VI)	ophthalmic a.
rectus, medial	common tendinous ring at orbital apex	medial eyeball	adducts the eyeball	oculomotor nerve (III)	ophthalmic a.
rectus, superior	common tendinous ring at orbital apex	superior eyeball	elevates and adducts the eyeball	oculomotor nerve (III)	ophthalmic a.

TABLE 1.2 MUSCLES, ARTERIES, AND NERVES OF THE HEAD AND NECK (CONT.)

MUSCLE	ORIGIN	INSERTION	ACTION	INNERVATION	ARTERY
risorius	fascia of the lateral cheek	skin of the angle of mouth	draws corner of mouth laterally	buccal branches of the facial nerve (VII)	transverse facial a., facial a.
scalene, anterior	transverse processes of vertebrae C3-C6	scalene tubercle of the first rib	elevates the first rib; flexes and laterally bends the neck	brachial plexus, C5-C7	ascending cervical a., a branch of the thyrocervical trunk
scalene, middle	transverse processes of vertebrae C2-C7	upper surface of the first rib	elevates the first rib; flexes and laterally bends the neck	brachial plexus, C3-C8	ascending cervical a.
scalene, posterior	transverse processes of vertebrae C5-C7	lateral portion of second rib	elevates the second rib; flexes and laterally bends the neck	brachial plexus, C7-C8	ascending cervical a.
splenius	ligamentum nuchae and spines C7-T6	capitis: mastoid process and superior nuchal line laterally; cervicis: posterior tubercles of C1-3	extends and laterally bends neck and head; rotates head to same side	dorsal primary rami of spinal nerves C2-6	supplied segmentally by: deep cervical a., posterior intercostal aa.
stapedius	walls of the pyramidal eminence	neck of the stapes	dampens vibration of the stapes	facial nerve (VII)	anterior tympanic a.
sternocleido-mastoid	sternal head: anterior manubrium; clavicular head: medial 1/3 of the clavicle	mastoid process and lateral 1/2 of the superior nuchal line	draws the mastoid process down toward the same side which causes the chin to turn up toward the opposite side; together flex the neck	spinal accessory nerve (XI), with sensory supply from C2 and C3 (for proprioception)	sternocleido-mastoid branch of the occipital a.
sternohyoid	posterior manubrium and clavicle	lower border of the hyoid bone	depresses the hyoid bone	ansa cervicalis	superior thyroid a.
sternothyroid	posterior manubrium	thyroid cartilage oblique line	depresses the hyoid bone	ansa cervicalis	superior thyroid a.
styloglossus	anterior styloid process	posterolateral tongue	retracts and elevates the tongue	hypoglossal nerve (XII)	ascending pharyngeal a., ascending palatine branch of the facial a.
stylohyoid	posterior styloid process	divides around the intermediate tendon of the digastric m. and inserts on hyoid bone body	elevates and retracts the hyoid bone	facial nerve (VII)	ascending pharyngeal a.

TABLE 1.2 MUSCLES, ARTERIES, AND NERVES OF THE HEAD AND NECK (CONT.)

MUSCLE	ORIGIN	INSERTION	ACTION	INNERVATION	ARTERY
stylopharyngeus	medial styloid process	superior border of the thyroid cartilage	elevates the larynx	glossopharyngeal nerve (IX)	ascending pharyngeal a.
superior oblique	orbital apex	posterior superior surface of eyeball	depresses and abducts the eyeball	trochlear nerve (IV)	ophthalmic a.
superior pharyngeal constrictor	medial pterygoid plate, pterygoid hamulus, pterygomandibular raphe, mylohyoid line of mandible	pharyngeal tubercle and midline pharyngeal raphe	constricts the pharyngeal cavity	vagus (X), via the pharyngeal plexus	ascending pharyngeal a.
temporalis	temporal fossa and the temporal fascia	mandibular coronoid process and anterior mandible	elevates the mandible	mandibular division of the trigeminal nerve (V)	anterior and posterior deep temporal aa.
tensor tympani	cartilagenous auditory tube and the greater wing of the sphenoid bone	manubrium of the malleus	dampens vibrations of the tympanic membrane	medial pterygoid branch of the mandibular division of the trigeminal nerve (V)	superior tympanic branch of the middle meningeal a.
tensor veli palatini	scaphoid fossa, lateral wall of the auditory tube cartilage	palatine aponeurosis	opens the auditory tube; tenses the soft palate	mandibular division of the trigeminal nerve (V)	ascending pharyngeal a.
zygomaticus major	upper lateral zygomatic bone	skin of the angle of the mouth	elevates corner of the mouth laterally	zygomatic and buccal branches of the facial nerve (VII)	transverse facial a., facial a.
zygomaticus minor	lower zygomatic bone	lateral upper lip	elevates upper lip	buccal branch of the facial nerve (VII)	transverse facial a., facial a.

TABLE 6.1 GASTROINTESTINAL SECRETIONS

	SOURCE OF SECRETION	MAJOR EFFECT	STIMULATES SECRETION	INHIBITS SECRETION
Pepsin	Chief cells of stomach	Starts protein digestion	Acid and vagal stimulus	
Gastric Acid	Parietal cells of stomach	Lowers pH for function of pepsin	ACh, gastrin, histamine	Somatostatin and gastric inhibitory peptide
Intrinsic Factor	Parietal cells of stomach	Required for vit. B12 uptake in terminal ileum		
Gastrin	G cells of stomach and duodenum	Increases secretion of HCl, intrinsic factor, pepsinogen Stimulates motility and mucosal growth	Amino acids and peptides Stomach distention Vagal stimulus	Secretin Gastric Acid
Cholecystokinin	I cells of duodenum and jejunum	Stimulates gallbladder contraction Increases pancreatic enzyme and HCO_3^- secretion Inhibits gastric emptying	Amino acids, small peptides, and fatty acids	
Secretin	S cells of duodenum	Increases pancreatic HCO_3^- secretion Decreases gastric acid secretion	Acid and fatty acids in duodenum	
Somatostatin	D cells in pancreas GI mucosa	Inhibits gastric acid and pepsinogen secretion Inhibits release of insulin and glucagon Inhibits gallbladder contraction Inhibits digestion and absorption	Acid	Vagus

TABLE 7.1 ENDOCRINE PANCREAS

	GENERAL	STIMULATES SECRETION	MAJOR EFFECTS	EFFECTS ON BLOOD LEVELS	INHIBITS SECRETION
Insulin	Beta cells secrete A chain and B chain Tyrosine kinase receptor Acts on muscle, liver, and adipose	Increased blood glucose Increased amino acids Increased fatty acids Glucagon, Acetylcholine, Cortisol, Growth Hormone, Gastric Inhibitory Peptide	Increases glucose uptake into cells Decreases glycogenolysis and gluconeogenesis Increases protein synthesis Increases fat synthesis Decreases lipolysis Increases in K^+ uptake	Decreases blood glucose Decreases amino acids Decreases fatty acids Hypokalemia	Decreased blood glucose Norepi, Epinephrine Somatostatin
Glucagon	Alpha cells secrete 2nd messenger is cAMP Acts on liver and adipose	Decreased blood glucose Increased amino acids Acetylcholine Norepi, epinephrine Cholecystokinin	Increases gluconeogenesis and glycogenolysis Increases lipolysis	Increased blood glucose Increased fatty acids	Increased blood glucose Increased fatty acids Insulin Somatostatin

TABLE 11.1 BONES OF THE BACK

BONE	STRUCTURE	DESCRIPTION
vertebra		series of irregular bones that form the spine
cervical vertebrae		seven vertebrae of the neck
	atlas (C1)	first cervical vertebra
	axis (C2)	second cervical vertebra
thoracic vertebrae		12 vertebrae of thoracic region
lumbar vertebrae		5 vertebrae of lumbar region
sacrum		triangular bone of posterior pelvis
	promontory	anterior projection of superior sacrum
coccyx		most inferior portion of vertebral column

TABLE 11.2 MUSCLES, ARTERIES, AND NERVES OF THE BACK

MUSCLE	ORIGIN	INSERTION	ACTION	INNERVATION	ARTERY
latissimus dorsi	vertebral spines from T7 to the sacrum, posterior third of the iliac crest, lower 3 or 4 ribs	intertubercular groove	extends the arm and medial rotation of the arm	thoracodorsal nerve (C7,8) of brachial plexus	thoracodorsal a.
levator scapulae	C1-C4 vertebrae transverse processes	medial border of the scapula from the superior angle to the spine	elevates the scapula	dorsal scapular nerve (C5); the upper part of the muscle receives branches of C3 and C4	dorsal scapular a.
rhomboideus major	spines of vertebrae T2-T5	medial border of the scapula inferior to the spine of the scapula	retracts, elevates and rotates the scapula inferiorly	dorsal scapular nerve (C5)	dorsal scapular a.
rhomboideus minor	inferior ligamentum nuchae, spines of vertebrae C7 and T1	medial border of the scapula at the root of the spine of the scapula	retracts, elevates, and rotates the scapula inferiorly	dorsal scapular nerve (C5)	dorsal scapular a
serratus anterior	ribs 1-8	scapula's deep medical border	moves scapula forward; rotates scapula superiorly	long thoracic nerve (from ventral rami C5-C7)	lateral thoracic a.

TABLE 11.2 MUSCLES, ARTERIES, AND NERVES OF THE BACK (CONT.)

MUSCLE	ORIGIN	INSERTION	ACTION	INNERVATION	ARTERY
trapezius	medial third of the superior nuchal line, external occipital protuberance, ligamentum nuchae, spinous processes of vertebrae C7-T12	lateral third of the clavicle, medial side of the acromion and the upper crest of the scapular spine, tubercle of the scapular spine	elevates and depresses the scapula; rotates the scapula superiorly; retracts scapula	spinal accessory (XI)	transverse cervical a.
erector spinae	iliac crest, sacrum, transverse and spinous processes of vertebrae and supraspinal ligament	angles of the ribs, transverse and spinous processes of vertebrae, posterior aspect of the skull	extends and laterally bends the trunk, neck, and head	segmentally innervated by dorsal primary rami of spinal nerves C1-S5	supplied segmentally by: deep cervical a., posterior intercostal aa., subcostal aa., lumbar aa.
iliocostalis	iliac crest and sacrum	angles of the ribs	extends and laterally bends the trunk and neck	dorsal primary rami of spinal nerves C4-S5	supplied segmentally by: deep cervical a., posterior intercostal aa., subcostal aa., lumbar aa.
interspinales	upper border of spinous process	lower border of spinous process	extend trunk and neck	dorsal primary rami of spinal nerves C1-L5	supplied segmentally by: deep cervical a., posterior intercostal aa., subcostal aa., lumbar aa.
intertransversarii	upper border of transverse process	lower border of transverse process	laterally bend trunk and neck	dorsal primary rami of spinal nerves C1-L5	supplied segmentally by: deep cervical a., posterior intercostal aa., subcostal aa., lumbar aa.
longissimus	transverse process at inferior vertebral levels	transverse process at superior vertebral levels and mastoid process	extends and laterally bends the trunk, neck, and head	dorsal primary rami of spinal nerves C1-S1	supplied segmentally by: deep cervical a., posterior intercostal aa., subcostal aa., lumbar aa.
multifidus	sacrum, transverse processes of C3-L5	spinous processes 2-4 vertebral levels superior to their origin	extend and laterally bend trunk and neck, rotate to opposite side	dorsal primary rami of spinal nerves C1-L5	supplied segmentally by: deep cervical a., posterior intercostal aa., subcostal aa., lumbar aa.
obliquus capitis inferior	spinous process of the axis	transverse process of atlas	rotates the head to the same side	suboccipital nerve	occipital a.
obliquus capitis superior	transverse process of atlas	occipital bone above inferior nuchal line	extends the head, rotates the head to the same side	suboccipital nerve	occipital a.
rectus capitis posterior major	spinous process of axis	inferior nuchal line	extends the head, rotates it to same side	suboccipital nerve	occipital a.
rectus capitis posterior minor	posterior tubercle of atlas	inferior nuchal line medially	extends the head	suboccipital nerve	occipital a.

TABLE 11.2 MUSCLES, ARTERIES, AND NERVES OF THE BACK (CONT.)

MUSCLE	ORIGIN	INSERTION	ACTION	INNERVATION	ARTERY
rotatores	transverse processes	long rotatores: spines 2 vertebrae above origin; short rotatores: spines 1 vertebra above origin	rotates the vertebral column to the opposite side	dorsal primary rami of spinal nerves C1-L5	supplied segmentally by: deep cervical a., posterior intercostal aa., subcostal aa., lumbar aa.
semispinalis	transverse processes of C7-T12	capitis: back of skull between nuchal lines; cervicis and thoracis: spines 4-6 vertebra above origin	extends the trunk and laterally bends the trunk, rotates the trunk to the opposite side	dorsal primary rami of spinal nerves C1-T12	supplied segmentally by: deep cervical a., posterior intercostal aa., subcostal aa., lumbar aa.
serratus posterior inferior	thoracolumbar fascia, spines of vertebrae T11-T12 and L1-L2	ribs 9-12, lateral to the angles	pulls lower ribs inferiorly	branches of the ventral primary rami of spinal nerves T9-T12	lowest posterior intercostal a., subcostal a., first two lumbar aa.
serratus posterior superior	ligamentum nuchae, spines of vertebrae C7 and T1-T3	ribs 1-4, lateral to the angles	elevates the upper ribs	branches of the ventral primary rami of spinal nerves T1-T4	posterior intercostal aa. 1-4
spinalis	spinous processes at inferior vertebral levels	spinous processes at superior vertebral levels and base of the skull	extends and laterally bends trunk and neck	dorsal primary rami of spinal nerves C2-L3	supplied segmentally by: deep cervical a., posterior intercostal aa., subcostal aa., lumbar aa.
splenius capitis	ligamentum nuchae and spines of C7-T6 vertebrae	mastoid process and superior lateral nuchal line	extends and laterally bends the neck and head, rotates head to the same side	dorsal primary rami of spinal nerves C2-C6	supplied segmentally by: deep cervical a., posterior intercostal aa.
splenius cervicis	ligamentum nuchae and spines of C7-T6 vertebrae	posterior tubercles of the transverse processes of C1-C3 vertebrae	extends and laterally bends neck and head, rotates head to the same side	dorsal primary rami of spinal nerves C2-C6	supplied segmentally by: deep cervical a., posterior intercostal aa.

TABLE 11.3 BONES OF THE THORAX

BONE	STRUCTURE	DESCRIPTION
rib		bone of lateral thoracic wall
ribs 1-7		"true" ribs attach directly to the sternum
rib 8-10		"false" ribs
rib 11-12		"floating" ribs
sternum		broad flat bone of anterior thoracic wall
	manubrium	superior portion of sternum
	jugular (suprasternal) notch	notch on superior border of manubrium
	body	middle portion of sternum
	xiphoid process	inferior portion of sternum

TABLE 11.4 MUSCLES, ARTERIES, AND NERVES OF THE THORAX

MUSCLE	ORIGIN	INSERTION	ACTION	INNERVATION	ARTERY
pectoralis major	medial 1/2 of the clavicle, manubrium, and body of sternum, costal cartilages of ribs 2-6	crest of the greater tubercle of the humerus	flexes and adducts the arm, medially rotates the arm	medial and lateral pectoral nerves (C5-T1)	pectoral branch of the thoracoacromial trunk
pectoralis minor	ribs 3-5	coracoid process of the scapula	moves scapula anteriorly, medially, and posteriorly	medial pectoral nerve (C8, T1)	pectoral branch of the thoracoacromial trunk
diaphragm	xiphoid process, costal margin, fascia over the quadratus lumborum and psoas major mm., vertebral bodies L1-L3	central tendon of the diaphragm	pushes the abdominal viscera inferiorly, increasing the volume of the thoracic cavity (inspiration)	phrenic nerve (C3-C5)	musculophrenic a., superior phrenic a., inferior phrenic a.
external intercostal	lower border of rib within an intercostal space	upper border of the rib below, coursing caudally and medially	elevates the rib during inspiration	intercostal nerves (T1-T11)	intercostal a.
innermost intercostal	upper borders of a rib	fibers course up and medially to insert on the inferior margin of the rib above	aids in compressing thorax during expiration	intercostal nerves (T1-T11)	intercostal a.
internal intercostal	upper border of a rib	lower border of rib above, coursing up and medially	aids in compressing thorax during expiration	intercostal nerves (T1-T11)	intercostal a.
levatores costarum	transverse processes C7-T11	rib below its origin, medial to the angle	elevates the rib	dorsal primary rami of spinal nerves C7-T11	deep cervical a., intercostal aa.
subcostalis	angle of ribs	angle of a rib 2-3 ribs above origin	compresses the intercostal spaces	intercostal nerves	intercostal a.
transversus thoracis	posterior surface of the sternum	inner surfaces of costal cartilages 2-6	compresses the thorax for forced expiration	intercostal nerves 2-6	internal thoracic a.

TABLE 12.1 BONES OF THE ABDOMEN

BONE	STRUCTURE	DESCRIPTION
os coxae		one of three bones that form the pelvis
	acetabulum	cup-shaped depression in the lateral surface of the os coxae bone
	obturator foramen	a large foramen formed by the pubic and ischial rami
pubis		forms the anterior portion of the pelvis
ischium		the V-shaped bone that forms the posteroinferior part of the pelvis
ilium		fan-shaped bone that forms the lateral prominence of the pelvis
sacrum		a triangular bone of posterior pelvis
	promontory	anterior projection of the superior part of the sacrum
coccyx		the most inferior portion of the vertebral column

TABLE 12.2 MUSCLES, ARTERIES, AND NERVES OF THE ABDOMEN

MUSCLE	ORIGIN	INSERTION	ACTION	INNERVATION	ARTERY
cremaster	inguinal ligament	forms thin network of muscle fascicles around the spermatic cord and testis	elevates testis	genital branch of the genitofemoral nerve	cremasteric a., a branch of the inferior epigastric a.
dartos	subcutaneous connective tissue of the scrotum and the penis	skin of the scrotum and penis	elevates testis	postganglionic sympathetic nerve fibers via the ilioinguinal nerve and the posterior scrotal nerve	cremasteric a., posterior scrotal a.
diaphragm	xiphoid process, costal margin, fascia over the quadratus lumborum and psoas major mm., vertebral bodies L1-L3	central tendon of the diaphragm	pushes the abdominal viscera inferiorly, increasing the volume of the thoracic cavity (inspiration)	phrenic nerve (C3-C5)	musculophrenic a., superior phrenic a., inferior phrenic a.
external abdominal oblique	lower 8 ribs	linea alba, pubic crest and tubercle, anterior superior iliac spine and anterior half of iliac crest	flexes and laterally bends the trunk	intercostal nerves 7-11, subcostal, iliohypogastric and ilioinguinal nerves	musculophrenic a., superior epigastric a., intercostal aa. 7-11, subcostal a., lumbar aa., superficial circumflex iliac a., deep circumflex iliac a., superficial epigastric a., inferior epigastric a., superficial external pudendal a.
iliacus	iliac fossa and iliac crest; ala of sacrum	lesser trochanter of the femur	flexes the thigh; if the thigh is fixed it flexes the pelvis on the thigh	femoral nerve	iliolumbar a.

TABLE 12.2 MUSCLES, ARTERIES, AND NERVES OF THE ABDOMEN (CONT.)

MUSCLE	ORIGIN	INSERTION	ACTION	INNERVATION	ARTERY
iliopsoas	iliac fossa; bodies and transverse processes of lumbar vertebrae	lesser trochanter of the femur	flexes the thigh; flexes and laterally bends the lumbar vertebral column	branches of the ventral primary rami of spinal nerves L2-L4; branches of the femoral nerve	iliolumbar a.
interfoveolar	transversus abdominis fibers that lie superficial to the inferior epigastric vessels	anterior lamina of femoral sheath, immediately distal to origin of inferior epigastric vessels	compresses abdominal contents	iliohypogastric and ilioinguinal nerves	inferior epigastric a.
oblique, external abdominal	lower 8 ribs	linea alba, pubic crest and tubercle, anterior superior iliac spine and anterior half of iliac crest	flexes and laterally bends the trunk	intercostal nerves 7-11, subcostal, iliohypogastric and ilioinguinal nerves	musculophrenic a., superior epigastric a., intercostal aa. 7-11, subcostal a., lumbar aa., superficial circumflex iliac a., deep circumflex iliac a., superficial epigastric a., inferior epigastric a., superficial external pudendal a.
oblique, internal abdominal	thoracolumbar fascia, anterior two-thirds of the iliac crest, lateral two-thirds of the inguinal ligament	lower 3 or 4 ribs, linea alba, pubic crest	flexes and laterally bends the trunk	intercostal nerves 7-11, subcostal, iliohypogastric and ilioinguinal nerves	musculophrenic a., superior epigastric a., intercostal aa. 7-11, subcostal a., lumbar aa., superficial circumflex iliac a., deep circumflex iliac a., superficial epigastric a., inferior epigastric a., superficial external pudendal a.
psoas major	bodies and transverse processes of lumbar vertebrae	lesser trochanter of femur (with iliacus) via iliopsoas tendon	flexes the thigh; flexes and laterally bends the lumbar vertebral column	branches of the ventral primary rami of spinal nerves L2-L4	subcostal a., lumbar aa.
psoas minor	bodies of the T12 and L1 vertebrae	iliopubic eminence at the line of junction of the ilium and the superior pubic ramus	flexes and laterally bends the lumbar vertebral column	branches of the ventral primary rami of spinal nerves L1-L2	lumbar aa.
pyramidalis	pubis, anterior to the rectus abdominis	linea alba	draws the linea alba inferiorly	subcostal nerve	subcostal a., inferior epigastric a.
quadratus lumborum	posterior part of the iliac crest and the iliolumbar ligament	transverse processes of lumbar vertebrae 1-4 and the 12th rib	laterally bends the trunk, fixes the 12th rib	subcostal nerve and ventral primary rami of spinal nerves L1-L4	subcostal a., lumbar aa.
rectus abdominis	pubis and the pubic symphysis	xiphoid process of the sternum and costal cartilages 5-7	flexes the trunk	intercostal nerves 7-11 and subcostal nerve	superior epigastric a. intercostal aa., subcostal a., inferior epigastric a.
transversus abdominis	lower 6 ribs, thoracolumbar fascia, anterior three-fourths of the iliac crest, lateral one-third of inguinal ligament	linea alba, pubic crest and pecten of the pubis	compresses the abdomen	intercostal nerves 7-11; subcostal, iliohypogastric, and ilioinguinal nerves	musculophrenic a., superior epigastric a., intercostal aa. 7-11, subcostal a., lumbar aa., superficial circumflex iliac a., deep circumflex iliac a., superficial epigastric a., inferior epigastric a., superficial external pudendal a.

TABLE 13.1 BONES OF THE UPPER LIMB

BONE	STRUCTURE	DESCRIPTION
clavicle		an "S" shaped bone located between the sternum and the scapula
scapula		the bone of the shoulder
	spine	a heavy ridge that runs from the medial border of the scapula to the acromion process
	scapular notch	a notch on the superior border of the scapula located medial to the attachment of the coracoid process
	coracoid process	a beak-like process that projects anteriorly from the lateral end of the superior border of the scapula
	acromion	a broad, flat process located at the lateral end of the scapular spine
	supraspinatous fossa	a broad depression located superior to the spine of the scapula
	infraspinatous fossa	a broad depression located inferior to the spine of the scapula
humerus		the bone of the arm
ulna		the bone on the medial side of the forearm
	olecranon	the proximal end of the ulna
	styloid process	projection from the distal surface of the head of the ulna
radius		the bone on the lateral side of the forearm
	ulnar notch	a shallow notch located on the medial surface of the distal end of the radius
	styloid process	the distal-most projection from the lateral side of the radius
carpal bones		the bones of the wrist
	proximal row	lateral to medial: scaphoid, lunate, triquetrum, pisiform
	distal row	lateral to medial: trapezium, trapezoid, capitate, hamate
metacarpal bones		the bones located between the carpal bones and the phalanges of the hand
phalanx (phalanges)		the distal two or three bones in the digits of the hand

TABLE 13.2 MUSCLES, ARTERIES, AND NERVES OF THE UPPER LIMB

MUSCLE	ORIGIN	INSERTION	ACTION	INNERVATION	ARTERY
abductor digiti minimi (hand)	pisiform	base of the proximal phalanx of the 5th digit on its ulnar side	abducts the 5th digit	deep branch of the ulnar nerve	ulnar a.
abductor pollicis brevis	flexor retinaculum, scaphoid, trapezium	base of the proximal phalanx of the first digit	abducts thumb	recurrent branch of median nerve	superficial palmar br. of the radial a.
abductor pollicis longus	middle one-third of the posterior surface of the radius, interosseous membrane, mid-portion of posterolateral ulna	radial side of the base of the first metacarpal	abducts the thumb at carpometacarpal joint	radial nerve, deep branch	posterior interosseous a.
adductor pollicis	oblique head: capitate and base of the 2nd and 3rd metacarpals; transverse head: shaft of the 3rd metacarpal	base of the proximal phalanx of the thumb	adducts the thumb	ulnar nerve, deep branch	deep palmar arterial arch
anconeus	lateral epicondyle of the humerus	lateral side of the olecranon and the upper one-fourth of the ulna	extends the forearm	nerve to anconeus from the radial nerve	interosseous recurrent a.
biceps brachii	short head: tip of the coracoid process of the scapula; long head: supraglenoid tubercle of the scapula	tuberosity of the radius	flexes the forearm, flexes arm, supinates	musculocutaneous nerve (C5,6)	brachial a.
brachialis	anterior surface of the lower one-half of the humerus	coronoid process of the ulna	flexes the forearm	musculocutaneous nerve (C5,6)	brachial a., radial recurrent a.
brachioradialis	upper two-thirds of the lateral supracondylar ridge of the humerus	lateral styloid process of the radius	flexes the elbow, assists in pronation and supination	radial nerve	radial recurrent a.
coracobrachialis	coracoid process of the scapula	medial side of the humerus at mid-shaft	flexes and adducts the arm	musculocutaneous nerve (C5,6)	brachial a.
deltoid	lateral one-third of the clavicle, acromion, spine of the scapula	deltoid tuberosity of the humerus	abducts arm; anterior fibers flex and medially rotate the arm; posterior fibers extend and laterally rotate the arm	axillary nerve (C5,6) from the posterior cord of the brachial plexus	posterior circumflex humeral a.
dorsal interosseous (hand)	four muscles, each arising from two adjacent metacarpal shafts	base of the proximal phalanx and the extensor expansion on lateral side of the 2nd digit, lateral and medial sides of the 3rd digit, and medial side of the 4th digit	flexes the metacarpophalangeal joint, extends the proximal and distal interphalangeal joints of digits 2-4, abducts digits 2-4	ulnar nerve, deep branch	dorsal and palmar metacarpal aa.

TABLE 13.2 MUSCLES, ARTERIES, AND NERVES OF THE UPPER LIMB (CONT.)

MUSCLE	ORIGIN	INSERTION	ACTION	INNERVATION	ARTERY
extensor carpi radialis brevis	lateral supracondylar ridge of the humerus (common extensor tendon)	dorsum of the third metacarpal bone (base)	extends the wrist; abducts the hand	radial nerve	radial a.
extensor carpi radialis longus	lower one-third of the lateral supracondylar ridge of the humerus	dorsum of the second metacarpal bone (base)	extends the wrist; abducts the hand	deep radial nerve	radial a.
extensor carpi ulnaris	common extensor tendon and the middle one-half of the posterior border of the ulna	medial side of the base of the 5th metacarpal	extends the wrist; adducts the hand	deep radial nerve	ulnar a.
extensor digiti minimi	lateral epicondyle of the humerus	joins the extensor digitorum tendon to the 5th digit and inserts into the extensor expansion	extends the metacarpopha-langeal, proximal interphalangeal, and distal interphalangeal joints of the 5th digit	deep radial nerve	interosseous recurrent a.
extensor digitorum	lateral epicondyle of the humerus	extensor expansion of digits 2-5	extends the metacarpopha-langeal, proximal interphalangeal, and distal inter-phalangeal joints of the 2nd-5th digits; extends wrist	deep radial nerve	interosseous recurrent a. and posterior interosseous a.
extensor indicis	interosseous membrane and the posterolateral surface of the distal ulna	its tendon joins the tendon of the extensor digitorum to the second digit; both tendons insert into the extensor expansion	extends the index finger at the metacarpopha-langeal, proximal interphalangeal, and distal interphalangeal joints	deep radial nerve	posterior interosseous a.
extensor pollicis brevis	interosseous membrane and the posterior surface of the distal radius	base of the proximal phalanx of the thumb	extends the thumb at the metacarpopha-langeal joint	deep radial nerve	posterior interosseous a.
extensor pollicis longus	interosseous membrane and middle part of the posterolateral surface of the ulna	base of the distal phalanx of the thumb	extends the thumb at the interphalangeal joint	deep radial nerve	posterior interosseous a.
flexor carpi radialis	common flexor tendon from the medial epicondyle of the humerus	base of the second and third metacarpals	flexes the wrist, abducts the hand	median nerve	ulnar a.
flexor carpi ulnaris	common flexor tendon and (ulnar head) from medial border of olecranon and upper two-thirds of the posterior border of the ulna	pisiform, hook of hamate, and base of 5th metacarpal	flexes wrist, adducts hand	ulnar nerve	ulnar a.

TABLE 13.2 MUSCLES, ARTERIES, AND NERVES OF THE UPPER LIMB (CONT.)

MUSCLE	ORIGIN	INSERTION	ACTION	INNERVATION	ARTERY
flexor digiti minimi brevis (hand)	hook of hamate and the flexor retinaculum	proximal phalanx of the 5th digit	flexes the carpometacarpal and metacarpophalangeal joints of the 5th digit	ulnar nerve, deep branch	ulnar a.
flexor digitorum profundus	posterior border of the ulna, proximal two-thirds of medial border of ulna, interosseous membrane	base of the distal phalanx of digits 2-5	flexes the metacarpophalangeal, proximal interphalangeal, and distal interphalangeal joints	median nerve (radial one-half); ulnar nerve (ulnar one-half)	ulnar a., anterior interosseous a.
flexor digitorum superficialis	humeroulnar head: common flexor tendon; radial head: middle one-third of radius	shafts of the middle phalanges of digits 2-5	flexes the metacarpophalangeal and proximal interphalangeal joints	median nerve	ulnar a.
flexor pollicis brevis	flexor retinaculum, trapezium	proximal phalanx of the 1st digit	flexes the carpometacarpal and metacarpophalangeal joints of the thumb	recurrent branch of the median nerve	superficial palmar br. of the radial a.
flexor pollicis longus	anterior surface of radius and interosseous membrane	base of the distal phalanx of the thumb	flexes the metacarpophalangeal and interphalangeal joints of the thumb	median nerve	anterior interosseous a.
infraspinatus	infraspinatous fossa	greater tubercle of the humerus	laterally rotates the arm	suprascapular nerve	suprascapular a.
interosseous, dorsal (hand)	four muscles, each arising from two adjacent metacarpal shafts	base of the proximal phalanx and the extensor expansion on lateral side of the 2nd digit, lateral & medial sides of the 3rd digit, and medial side of the 4th digit	flexes the metacarpophalangeal joint, extends the proximal and distal interphalangeal joints of digits 2-4, and abducts digits 2-4	ulnar nerve, deep branch	dorsal and palmar metacarpal aa.
levator scapulae	transverse processes of C1-C4 vertebrae	medial border of the scapula from the superior angle to the spine	elevates the scapula	dorsal scapular nerve (C5); the upper part of the muscle receives branches of C3 and C4	dorsal scapular a.
lumbrical (hand)	flexor digitorum profundus tendons of digits 2-5	extensor expansion on the radial side of the proximal phalanx of digits 2-5	flexes the metacarpophalangeal joints, extends the proximal and distal interphalangeal joints of digits 2-5	median nerve via palmar digital nerves & ulnar nerve via deep branch	superficial palmar arterial arch

TABLE 13.2 MUSCLES, ARTERIES, AND NERVES OF THE UPPER LIMB (CONT.)

MUSCLE	ORIGIN	INSERTION	ACTION	INNERVATION	ARTERY
opponens digiti minimi	hook of hamate and flexor retinaculum	shaft of 5th metacarpal	opposes the 5th digit	ulnar nerve, deep branch	ulnar a.
opponens pollicis	flexor retinaculum, trapezium	shaft of 1st metacarpal	opposes the thumb	recurrent branch of median nerve	superficial palmar branch of the radial a.
palmar interosseous	three muscles, arising from the palmar surface of the shafts of metacarpals 2, 4, and 5	base of the proximal phalanx and extensor expansion of the medial side of digit 2, and lateral side of digits 4 & 5	flexes the metacarpophalangeal, extends proximal and distal interphalangeal joints, and adducts digits 2, 4, & 5	ulnar nerve, deep branch	palmar metacarpal aa.
palmaris brevis	fascia overlying the hypothenar eminence	skin of the palm near the ulnar border of the hand	draws the skin of the ulnar side of the hand toward the center of the palm	superficial br. of the ulnar n.	ulnar a.
palmaris longus	common flexor tendon, from the medial epicondyle of the humerus	palmar aponeurosis	flexes the wrist	median nerve	ulnar a.
pectoralis major	medial one-half of the clavicle, manubrium and body of sternum, costal cartilages of ribs 2-6	crest of the greater tubercle of the humerus	flexes and adducts the arm, medially rotates the arm	medial and lateral pectoral nerves (C5-T1)	pectoral branch of the thoracoacromial trunk
pectoralis minor	ribs 3-5	coracoid process of the scapula	draws the scapula forward, medialward, and downward	medial pectoral nerve (C8, T1)	pectoral branch of the thoracoacromial trunk
pronator quadratus	medial side of the anterior surface of the distal one-fourth of the ulna	anterior surface of the distal one-fourth of the radius	pronates the forearm	median nerve via the anterior interosseous nerve	anterior interosseous a.
pronator teres	common flexor tendon and medial side of ulnar coronoid process	midpoint of the lateral side of the shaft of the radius	pronates the forearm	median nerve	ulnar a., anterior ulnar recurrent a.
rhomboideus major	spines of vertebrae T2-T5	medial border of the scapula inferior to the spine of the scapula	retracts, elevates, and rotates the scapula inferiorly	dorsal scapular nerve (C5)	dorsal scapular a.
rhomboideus minor	inferior end of the ligamentum nuchae, spines of vertebrae C7 and T1	medial border of the scapula at the root of the spine of the scapula	retracts, elevates, and rotates the scapula inferiorly	dorsal scapular nerve (C5)	dorsal scapular a.
serratus anterior	ribs 1-8 or 9	medial border of the scapula on its costal (deep) surface	it draws the scapula forward; the inferior fibers rotate the scapula superiorly	long thoracic nerve (from ventral rami C5-C7)	lateral thoracic a.

TABLE 13.2 MUSCLES, ARTERIES, AND NERVES OF THE UPPER LIMB (CONT.)

MUSCLE	ORIGIN	INSERTION	ACTION	INNERVATION	ARTERY
serratus posterior inferior	thoracolumbar fascia, spines of vertebrae T11-T12 and L1-L2	ribs 9-12, lateral to the angles	pulls down lower ribs	branches of the ventral primary rami of spinal nerves T9-T12	lowest posterior intercostal a., subcostal a., first two lumbar aa.
serratus posterior superior	ligamentum nuchae, spines of vertebrae C7 and T1-T3	ribs 1-4, lateral to the angles	elevates the upper ribs	branches of the ventral primary rami of spinal nerves T1-T4	posterior intercostal aa. 1-4
subclavius	first rib and its cartilage	inferior surface of the clavicle	moves clavicle anteriorly and posteriorly	nerve to subclavius (C5)	clavicular br. of the thoraco-acromial trunk
subscapularis	subscapular fossa	lesser tubercle of the humerus	medially rotates the arm; assists arm extension	upper and lower subscapular nerves (C5,6)	subscapular a.
supinator	lateral epicondyle of the humerus, supinator crest and fossa of the ulna, radial collateral ligament, annular ligament	lateral side of proximal one-third of the radius	supinates the forearm	deep radial nerve	recurrent interosseous a.
supraspinatus	supraspinatous fossa	greater tubercle of the humerus	abducts the arm (initiates abduction)	suprascapular nerve (C5,6) from the superior trunk of the brachial plexus	suprascapular a.
teres major	dorsal surface of the inferior angle of the scapula	crest of the lesser tubercle of the humerus	adducts the arm, medially rotates the arm, assists in arm extension	lower subscapular nerve (C5,6) from the posterior cord of the brachial plexus	circumflex scapular a.
teres minor	upper two-thirds of the lateral border of the scapula	greater tubercle of the humerus (lowest facet)	laterally rotates the arm	axillary nerve (C5,6) from the posterior cord of the brachial plexus	circumflex scapular a.
trapezius	medial third of the superior nuchal line, external occipital protuberance, ligamentum nuchae, spinous processes of vertebrae C7-T12	lateral third of the clavicle, medial side of the acromion and the upper crest of the scapular spine, tubercle of the scapular spine	elevates and depresses the scapula; rotates the scapula superiorly; retracts scapula	motor: spinal accessory (XI), proprioception: C3-C4	transverse cervical a.
triceps brachii	long head: infraglenoid tubercle of the scapula; lateral head: posterolateral humerus and lateral intermuscular septum; medial head: posteromedial surface of the inferior one-half of the humerus	olecranon process of the ulna	extends the forearm; the long head extends and adducts arm	radial nerve	deep brachial (profunda brachii) a.

TABLE 14.1 BONES OF THE LOWER LIMB

BONE	STRUCTURE	DESCRIPTION
pubis		anterior portion of pelvis
ischium		the "V"-shaped bone of posteroinferior pelvis
ilium		fan-shaped bone of lateral pelvis
sacrum		a triangular bone of posterior pelvis
	promontory	anterior projection of superior sacrum
coccyx		the most inferior portion of the vertebral column
femur		the bone of the thigh
patella		knee cap
tibia		medial bone of lower leg
fibula		lateral bone of lower leg
tarsal		bones of the ankle
talus		most proximal tarsal bones
calcaneus		tarsal bone which forms the heel
navicular		tarsal bone located distal to the talus and proximal to cuneiform bones
cuneiform, medial		the most medial bone in the distal row of tarsal bones
cuneiform, middle		the intermediate bone of the three cuneiform bones
cuneiform, lateral		the bone that is located between the middle cuneiform and the cuboid bone
cuboid		the most lateral bone in the distal row of tarsal bones
metatarsals		the bones located between the tarsal bones and the phalanges
phalanx (phalanges)		the distal two or three bones in the digits of the foot

TABLE 14.2 MUSCLES, ARTERIES, AND NERVES OF THE LOWER LIMB

MUSCLE	ORIGIN	INSERTION	ACTION	INNERVATION	ARTERY
abductor digiti minimi (foot)	medial and lateral sides of the tuberosity of the calcaneus	lateral side of the base of the proximal phalanx of the 5th digit	abducts the 5th toe; flexes the metatarsophalageal joint	lateral plantar nerve	lateral plantar a.
abductor hallucis	medial side of the tuberosity of calcaneus	medial side of the base of the proximal phalanx of the great toe (hallux)	abducts the great toe; flexes the metatarsophalageal joint	medial plantar nerve	medial plantar a.
adductor brevis	inferior pubic ramus	pectineal line and linea aspera (deep to the pectineus and adductor longus mm.)	adducts, flexes, and medially rotates the femur	anterior division of the obturator nerve	obturator a., deep femoral a.
adductor hallucis	oblique head: bases of metatarsals 2-4; transverse head: heads of metatarsals 3-5	lateral side of base of the proximal phalanx of the great toe	adducts the great toe (moves it toward midline of the foot; i.e., toward the 2nd digit)	deep branch of the lateral plantar nerve	plantar arterial arch
adductor longus	medial portion of the superior pubic ramus	linea aspera of the femur	adducts, flexes, and medially rotates the femur	anterior division of the obturator nerve	obturator a., deep femoral a.
adductor magnus	ischiopubic ramus and ischial tuberosity	linea aspera of the femur; the ischiocondylar part inserts on the adductor tubercle of the femur	adducts, flexes, and medially rotates the femur; extends the femur (ischiocondylar part)	posterior division of the obturator nerve; tibial nerve (ischiocondylar part)	obturator a., deep femoral a., medial femoral circumflex a.
adductor minimus	lower portion of the inferior pubic ramus	gluteal ridge and upper part of the linea aspera of the femur	adducts and laterally rotates the femur	posterior division of the obturator nerve	obturator a., medial femoral circumflex a., deep femoral a.
articularis genu	anterior surface of the femur above the patellar surface	articular capsule of the knee	elevates the articular capsule of the knee joint	femoral nerve	descending genicular a.
biceps femoris	long head: ischial tuberosity; short head: lateral lip of the linea aspera	head of fibula and lateral condyle of the tibia	extends the thigh, flexes the leg	long head: tibial nerve; short head: common fibular (peroneal) nerve	perforating branches of the deep femoral a.
dorsal interosseous (foot)	shafts of adjacent metatarsal bones	bases of the proximal phalanges for digit 2 (both sides) and digits 3,4 (lateral side)	abducts digits 2-4, flexes the metatarsophalangeal joints, and extends the interphalangeal joints of those digits	deep branch of the lateral plantar nerve	dorsal metatarsal aa.
extensor digitorum brevis	superolateral surface of the calcaneus	extensor expansion of toes 1-4	extends toes 1-4	deep fibular (peroneal) nerve	dorsalis pedis a.

TABLE 14.2 MUSCLES, ARTERIES, AND NERVES OF THE LOWER LIMB (CONT.)

MUSCLE	ORIGIN	INSERTION	ACTION	INNERVATION	ARTERY
extensor digitorum longus	lateral condyle of the tibia, anterior surface of the fibula, lateral portion of the interosseous membrane	dorsum of the lateral 4 toes via extensor expansions	extends the metatarsophalangeal, proximal interphalangeal, and distal interphalangeal joints of the lateral 4 toes	deep fibular (peroneal) nerve	anterior tibial a.
extensor hallucis brevis	superolateral surface of the calcaneus	dorsum of base of proximal phalanx of the great toe	extends the great toe	deep fibular (peroneal) nerve	dorsalis pedis a.
extensor hallucis longus	middle half of the anterior surface of the fibula and the interosseous membrane	base of the distal phalanx of the great toe	extends the metatarsophalangeal interphalangeal joints of the great toe	deep fibular (peroneal) nerve	anterior tibial a.
fibularis (peroneus) brevis	lower one-third of the lateral surface of the fibula	tuberosity of the base of the 5th metatarsal	extends and everts the foot	superficial fibular (peroneal) nerve	fibular (peroneal) a.
fibularis (peroneus) longus	upper two-thirds of the lateral surface of the fibula	after crossing the plantar surface of the foot deep to the intrinsic muscles, it inserts on the medial cuneiform and the base of the 1st metatarsal bone	extends and everts the foot	superficial fibular (peroneal) nerve	fibular (peroneal) a.
fibularis (peroneus) tertius	distal part of the anterior surface of the fibula	dorsum of the shaft of the 5th metatarsal bone	everts the foot	deep fibular (peroneal) nerve	anterior tibial a.
flexor digiti minimi brevis (foot)	base of 5th metatarsal bone	lateral side of base of proximal phalanx of 5th digit	flexes the metatarsophalangeal joint of the 5th digit	lateral plantar nerve	lateral plantar a.
flexor digitorum brevis	tuberosity of the calcaneus, plantar aponeurosis, intermuscular septae	base of the middle phalanx of digits 2-5 after splitting to allow passage of the flexor digitorum longus tendons	flexes the metatarsophalangeal and proximal interphalangeal joints of digits 2-5	medial plantar nerve	medial and lateral plantar aa.
flexor digitorum longus	middle half of the posterior surface of the tibia	bases of the distal phalanges of digits 2-5	flexes the metatarsophalangeal, proximal interphalangeal and distal interphalangeal, joints of digits 2-5; plantar flexes the foot	tibial nerve	tibial a.
flexor hallucis brevis	cuboid, lateral cuneiform, medial side of the first metatarsal	medial belly: medial side of proximal phalanx of the great toe; lateral belly: lateral side of the proximal phalanx of the great toe	flexes the metatarsophalangeal joint of the great toe	medial plantar nerve	medial plantar a.

TABLE 14.2 MUSCLES, ARTERIES, AND NERVES OF THE LOWER LIMB (CONT.)

MUSCLE	ORIGIN	INSERTION	ACTION	INNERVATION	ARTERY
flexor hallucis longus	lower two-thirds of the posterior surface of the fibula	base of the distal phalanx of the great toe	flexes the metatarsophalangeal and proximal interphalangeal joints of the great toe; plantar flexes the foot	tibial nerve	fibular (peroneal) a. and tibial a.
gastrocnemius	femur; medial head: above the medial femoral condyle; lateral head: above the lateral femoral condyle	dorsum of the calcaneus via the calcaneal (Achilles) tendon	flexes leg; plantar flexes foot	tibial nerve	sural aa. (from the popliteal a.), posterior tibial a.
gemellus, inferior	ischial tuberosity	obturator internus tendon	laterally rotates the femur	nerve to the quadratus femoris m.	inferior gluteal a.
gemellus, superior	ischial spine	obturator internus tendon	laterally rotates the femur	nerve to the obturator internus m.	inferior gluteal a.
gluteus maximus	posterior gluteal line, posterior surface of sacrum and coccyx, sacrotuberous ligament	upper fibers: iliotibial tract; lowermost fibers: gluteal tuberosity of the femur	extends the thigh; laterally rotates the femur	inferior gluteal nerve	superior and inferior gluteal aa.
gluteus medius	external surface of the ilium between the posterior and anterior gluteal lines	greater trochanter of the femur	abducts the femur; medially rotates the thigh	superior gluteal nerve	superior gluteal a.
gluteus minimus	external surface of the ilium between the anterior and inferior gluteal lines	greater trochanter of the femur	abducts the femur; medially rotates the thigh	superior gluteal nerve	superior gluteal a.
gracilis	pubic symphysis and the inferior pubic ramus	medial surface of the tibia	adducts the thigh, flexes and medially rotates the thigh, flexes the leg	anterior division of the obturator nerve	obturator a.
iliacus	iliac fossa and iliac crest; ala of sacrum	lesser trochanter of the femur	flexes the thigh	femoral nerve	iliolumbar a.
iliopsoas	iliac fossa; bodies and transverse processes of lumbar vertebrae	lesser trochanter of the femur	flexes the thigh; flexes and laterally bends the lumbar vertebral column	branches of the ventral primary rami of spinal nerves L2-L4; branches of the femoral nerve	iliolumbar a.
lumbricals (foot)	tendons of the flexor digitorum longus	medial side of the extensor expansion of digits 2-5	flexes the metatarsophalangeal joint, extends the proximal interphalangeal and distal interphalangeal joints of digits 2-5	medial lumbrical: medial plantar nerve; lateral three lumbricals: lateral plantar nerve	medial and lateral plantar aa.

TABLE 14.2 MUSCLES, ARTERIES, AND NERVES OF THE LOWER LIMB (CONT.)

MUSCLE	ORIGIN	INSERTION	ACTION	INNERVATION	ARTERY
obturator externus	the external surface of the obturator membrane and the superior and inferior pubic rami	trochanteric fossa of the femur	laterally rotates the thigh	obturator nerve	obturator a.
obturator internus	the internal surface of the obturator membrane and margin of the obturator foramen	greater trochanter on its medial surface above the trochanteric fossa	laterally rotates and abducts the thigh	nerve to the obturator internus m.	obturator a.
pectineus	pecten of the pubis	pectineal line of the femur	adducts, flexes, and medially rotates the thigh	femoral nerve and possibly the anterior division of the obturator nerve	medial femoral circumflex a.
piriformis	anterior surface of sacrum	upper border of greater trochanter of femur	laterally rotates and abducts thigh	ventral rami of S1-S2	inferior gluteal superior gluteal lateral sacral
plantar interosseous	base and medial side of metatarsals 3-5	bases of proximal phalanges and extensor expansions of digits 3-5	adducts digits 3-5; flexes the metacar-pophalangeal and extends interphalangeal joints of digits 3-5	deep branch of the lateral plantar nerve	plantar metatarsal aa.
plantaris	above the lateral femoral condyle	dorsum of the calcaneus medial to the calcaneal tendon	flexes the leg; plantar flexes the foot	tibial nerve	popliteal a.
popliteus	lateral condyle of the femur	posterior surface of the tibia above soleal line	flexes and rotates the leg medially (with the foot planted, it rotates the thigh laterally)	tibial nerve	popliteal a.
psoas major	bodies and transverse processes of lumbar vertebrae	lesser trochanter of femur (with iliacus) via iliopsoas tendon	flexes the thigh; flexes and laterally bends the lumbar vertebral column	branches of the ventral primary rami of spinal nerves L2-L4	subcostal a., lumbar aa.
psoas minor	bodies of the T12 and L1 vertebrae	iliopubic eminence at the line of junction of the ilium and the superior pubic ramus	flexes and laterally bends the lumbar vertebral column	branches of the ventral primary rams of spinal nerves L1-L2	lumbar aa.
quadratus femoris	lateral border of the ischial tuberosity	quadrate line of the femur below the intertrochanteric crest	laterally rotates the thigh	nerve to the quadratus femoris m.	inferior gluteal a.
quadratus plantae	anterior portion of the calcaneus and the long plantar ligament	tendons of the flexor digitorum longus m.	assists the flexor digitorum longus in flexing the toes	lateral plantar nerve	lateral plantar a.

TABLE 14.2 MUSCLES, ARTERIES, AND NERVES OF THE LOWER LIMB (CONT.)

MUSCLE	ORIGIN	INSERTION	ACTION	INNERVATION	ARTERY
quadriceps femoris	anterior surface of the femur and the anterior side of the medial and lateral intermuscular septa	tibial tuberosity via the patellar ligament	extends the knee; rectus femoris flexes the thigh	femoral nerve	lateral circumflex femoral a., deep femoral a.
rectus femoris	straight head: anterior inferior iliac spine; reflected head: above the superior rim of the acetabulum	patella and tibial tuberosity (via the patellar ligament)	extends the leg, flexes the thigh	femoral nerve	lateral circumflex femoral a.
sartorius	anterior superior iliac spine	medial surface of the tibia	flexes, abducts, and laterally rotates the thigh; flexes leg	femoral nerve	lateral femoral circumflex a., saphenous a.
semimembranosus	upper, outer surface of the ischial tuberosity	medial condyle of the tibia	extends the thigh, flexes the leg	tibial nerve	perforating branches of the deep femoral a.
semitendinosus	lower, medial surface of ischial tuberosity	medial surface of tibia	extends the thigh, flexes the leg	tibial nerve	perforating branches of the deep femoral a.
soleus	posterior surface of head and upper shaft of the fibula, soleal line of the tibia	dorsum of the calcaneus via the calcaneal (Achilles) tendon	plantar flexes the foot	tibial nerve	posterior tibial a.
tensor fasciae latae	anterior part of the iliac crest, anterior superior iliac spine	iliotibial tract	flexes, abducts, and medially rotates the thigh	superior gluteal nerve	superior gluteal a.
tibialis anterior	lateral tibial condyle and the upper lateral surface of the tibia	medial surface of the medial cuneiform and the 1st metatarsal	dorsiflexes and inverts the foot	deep fibular (peroneal) nerve	anterior tibial a.
tibialis posterior	interosseous membrane, posteromedial surface of the fibula, posterolateral surface of the tibia	tuberosity of the navicular and medial cuneiform, metatarsals 2-4	plantar flexes the foot; inverts the foot	tibial nerve	fibular (peroneal) a. and tibial a.
vastus intermedius	anterior and lateral surface of the femur	patella	extends the leg	femoral nerve	lateral femoral circumflex a.
vastus lateralis	lateral intermuscular septum, lateral lip of the linea aspera and the gluteal tuberosity	patella and medial patellar retinaculum	extends the leg	femoral nerve	lateral femoral circumflex a., perforating branches of the deep femoral a.
vastus medialis	medial intermuscular septum, medial lip of the linea aspera	patella and medial patellar retinaculum	extends the leg	femoral nerve	lateral femoral circumflex a.

TABLE 15.1 BONES OF THE PELVIS AND PERINEUM

BONE	STRUCTURE	DESCRIPTION
os coxae		one of three bones that form the pelvis
	acetabulum	a cup-shaped depression in the lateral surface of the os coxae bone
	obturator foramen	a large foramen formed by the pubic and ischial rami
pubis		an angulated bone that forms the anterior part of the pelvis
ischium		the "V"-shaped bone that forms the posteroinferior part of the pelvis
ilium		fan-shaped bone that forms the lateral prominence of the pelvis
	iliac crest	arching superior edge of the ilium that forms the rim of the "fan"
sacrum		a triangular bone of posterior pelvis
coccyx		the most inferior portion of the vertebral column

TABLE 15.2 MUSCLES, ARTERIES, AND NERVES OF THE PELVIS AND PERINEUM

MUSCLE	ORIGIN	INSERTION	ACTION	INNERVATION	ARTERY
anal sphincter, external	perineal body	encircles the anal canal	constricts the anal canal	inferior rectal nerves of pudendal nerve	inferior rectal a.
anal sphincter, internal	encircles the anal canal	encircles the anal canal	constricts the anal canal	parasympathetic fibers from S4	middle rectal a.
bulbospongiosus, in female	perineal body and fascia of the bulb of the vestibule	perineal membrane and corpus cavernosum of the clitoris	compresses the vestibular bulb and constricts the vaginal orifice	deep branch of the perineal nerve of pudendal nerve	perineal a.
bulbospongiosus, in male	central tendinous point and the midline raphe on the bulb of the penis	perineal membrane, dorsal surface of the corpus spongiosum, deep penile fascia	compresses the bulb of the penis, compresses the spongy urethra	deep branch of the perineal nerve of pudendal nerve	perineal a.
coccygeus	ischial spine	side of the coccyx and lower sacrum	elevates the pelvic floor	branches of the ventral primary rami of spinal nerves S3-S4	inferior gluteal a.
deep transverse perineus	medial surface of the ischial ramus	contralateral muscle and perineal body/central tendinous point	fixes and stabilizes the perineal body/central tendinous point	deep branch of perineal nerve of pudendal nerve	internal pudendal a.
detruser of bladder	smooth muscle in the wall of the urinary bladder	fascicles are arranged roughly in three layers	compresses the urinary bladder	parasympathetic nerve fibers from the pelvic splanchnic nerves (S2-S4 spinal cord levels)	superior and inferior vesical aa.
iliococcygeus	arcus tendineus levator ani and the ischial spine	anococcygeal raphe and the coccyx	elevates the pelvic floor	branches of the ventral primary rami of spinal nerves S3-S4	inferior gluteal a.

TABLE 15.2 MUSCLES, ARTERIES, AND NERVES OF THE PELVIS AND PERINEUM (CONT.)

MUSCLE	ORIGIN	INSERTION	ACTION	INNERVATION	ARTERY
ischiocavernosus	medial surface of the ischial tuberosity and the ischiopubic ramus	corpus cavernosum and crus of the penis/clitoris	compresses the corpus cavernosum	deep branch of the perineal nerve (from pudendal nerve)	perineal a.
levator ani	posterior surface of the body of the pubis, fascia of the obturator internus m. (arcus tendineus levator ani), ischial spine	anococcygeal raphe and coccyx	elevates the pelvic floor	branches of the ventral primary rami of spinal nerves S3-S4	inferior gluteal a.
levator prostatae	posterior aspect of the pubis	fascia of the prostate	elevates the prostate	branches of the ventral primary rami of spinal nerves S3-S4	inferior gluteal a.
obturator internus	the internal surface of the obturator membrane and margin of the obturator foramen	greater trochanter on its medial surface above the trochanteric fossa	laterally rotates and abducts the thigh	nerve of obturator internus m.	obturator a.
piriformis	anterior surface of sacrum	upper border of greater trochanter of femur	laterally rotates and abducts thigh	ventral rami of S1-S2	
pubococcygeus	posterior aspect of the superior pubic ramis	coccyx	elevates the pelvic floor	branches of the ventral primary rami of spinal nerves S3-S4	inferior gluteal a.
puborectalis	posterior aspect of the body of the pubis	unites with the puborectalis m. of other side posterior to the rectum	draws the distal rectum forward and superiorly; aids in voluntary retention of feces	branches of the ventral primary rami of spinal nerves S3-S4	inferior gluteal a.
pubovaginalis	posterior aspect of the body of the pubis	fascia of the vagina and perineal body	draws the vagina forward and superiorly	branches of the ventral primary rami of spinal nerves S3-S4	inferior gluteal a.
sphincter urethrae, in female	encircles the urethra	encircles urethra and vagina; extends superiorly along the urethra to inferior bladder	compresses urethra and vagina	deep branch of perineal nerve of pudendal nerve	internal pudendal a.
sphincter urethrae, in male	encircles the urethra	encircles urethra, reaches lateral surface of prostate and inferior bladder	compresses urethra	deep branch of perineal nerve of pudendal nerve	internal pudendal a.
superficial transverse perineus	medial surface of the ischial ramus	contralateral muscle and the perineal body	fixes and stabilizes perineal body	deep branch of perineal nerve of pudendal nerve	perineal a.

INDEX

D

E

F